ADVANCE PRAISE F

HEALING WITH INFORMATION

by Dr Mária Sági

with István Sági

A renaissance in science is shattering old myths and rewriting the story of life. Profound insights offered by research in the frontier sciences have completely revised our understanding of health and disease. A 'new' biology is launching a revolution in healthcare by providing a scientific foundation for the emerging field of *energy medicine.*

The powerful role of energy healing practices in healthcare is grounded in the science of *quantum biophysics.* This new field of research expands our awareness of the mechanics of life far beyond the conventional knowledge currently offered in higher education and medical schools.

In *Healing With Information,* Mária Sági, with her brother István, integrate quantum physics principles with leading edge discoveries in cellular and molecular biology. The Ságis' valuable compilation introduces the revolutionary research of Erich Körbler (1935–1994), founder of 'New Homeopathy.' This new science, which presents an empirical healing system based on the reception of information by the organism, provides insight into the communication channels that link mind, body and spirit.

Conventional allopathic medical scientists perceive of energy's biological influence only in terms of a 'force' that can physically alter molecules and cells (ionizing energy). Additionally, the biological role of energy healing has been actively suppressed by pharmaceutical financial interests, for this industry profits from the antiquated classical (Newtonian) mechanics belief that a physical body can only be influenced by physical chemistry (i.e., drugs).

In contrast, Körbler's 'New Homeopathy' paradigm emphasizes the role of energy as 'information' that influences biological organization and controls function. A highlight of *Healing With Information* is the excellent in depth scientific assessment of the nature by which energy vibrations and resonance influence biological systems by shaping cell, organ and organismal behavior and gene activity. The described mechanisms underscore a fundamental role for entanglement, complexity, coherence and emergence, quantum mechanical principles that collectively provide a foundation for a new vitalism.

In addition, *Healing With Information* offers readers a unique opportunity to construct and use Körbler's dowsing rod, a device that translates subconscious information via micro-muscle movements. The Ságis have included a large number of dowsing experiments that enable the reader to personally assess the role of energy information fields in their own health and life experiences.

I highly recommend the contents of *Healing With Information,* especially for practitioners of allopathic and complementary medicine modalities. The knowledge offered in this important work will expand their horizons and further empower their healing work. The new insights provide a master key that unlocks the science by which energetic patterns in the environment, and those created by thoughts, attitudes and beliefs, create the conditions of our body and our experiences in the external world.

Thinking required ... and well worth the effort!

Bruce H. Lipton, PhD

Stem cell biologist and bestselling author of *The Biology of Belief, Spontaneous Evolution and The Honeymoon Effect*

Information, as it has been proven, is the basis of all phenomena, even those concerning the inorganic world. The aggregation and disintegration of atoms and subatomic particles are governed by complex interactions of energy and electromagnetic fields, namely energy. The suitable combination of the elements that is at the origin of the organic molecules, and therefore of life, arises from the energetic interactions, i.e. from the information conveyed by these substrates which in turn generate other information that must be stored. In the case of biological organisms, such task is carried out by the memory of the genetic code, of the immune system, of the nervous system, of the endocrine system and so on. The entire system, to work at its best and reproduce itself, must be consistent. Numerous studies prove that any alteration of the consistency generate misinformation and, therefore, a pathology but also, restoring the correct information, therapy.

This valuable text by Dr Sági, which takes up and continues Erich Körbler's research – Körbler is the founder of the discipline called 'New Homeopathy' – thoroughly analyzes and explains these mechanisms with the aid of numerous experiments and practical examples. In the wake of the studies of Popp, Del Giudice, Laszlo and others, the author explains how to detect the interference of subtle, electrical and electromagnetic energies acting on the cell, and the systems to restore the impaired balance.

Doctors can find surprising explanations that will help diagnosing and solving, whenever possible, a range of disorders that are extremely recurring nowadays – including chronic fatigue, insomnia, allergies, intolerances, musculoskeletal pain, chronic mycosis and even cancer – disorders for which doctors often lack appropriate responses. What doctors can generally offer is a generic reference to stress, and accordingly they prescribe a therapy that is completely inadequate, and sometimes even harmful. Reading Sági's illuminating study will therefore help them understanding and prevent errors in therapy.

Claudio Mazza

Publisher, Nuova Ipsa Editore, Palermo

If you are now holding this book in your hands it is probably because you have been attracted by its title or cover, or because someone suggested reading it, or for some other personal reasons. Whatever the reason, you need to know that this book is not the kind of book everyone can read.

It is a fascinating book, full of information and data which are completely new and original, but are, to be sure, definitely beyond the understanding of science, especially of mainstream Medicine. The concept of cause and effect in healing still is fundamental, obviously, but it is beyond the generally recognized paradigms, which are linear and mechanical. If you have a free spirit, interested in looking at reality with new eyes, don't be discouraged by the effort needed to address these new scenarios. They are worth it!!!

Alessandro Pizzoccaro

President Guna Pharmaceutical S.p.a. Milan

Dr Mária Sági's book offers a complete synthesis of the role of information in determining the events that are at the origin of life, and of all things in the universe. In addition, her book tells us how to view the information present in the human organism and assess whether we are in a state of health or of disease and also informs us of the role of the various substances with which our organism comes in contact that can have affect on the state of our health.

The book of Mária Sági provides a complete synthesis that every person should know in order not to damage his or her own organic equilibrium and the equilibrium of the ecology. It is a book that should be read particularly by physicians and all people interested in questions of health and healing.

Dr Pier Mario Biava

Istituto di Ricovero e Cura a Carattere Scientifico

Multimedica, Milan

I commend the wealth of knowledge contained in this book to all my *medical doctor colleagues* who have the dynamism, courage, motivation and love of the medical profession to acquire ever new knowledge and familiarize themselves with even lesser-known methods of treatment. Taking possession of such knowledge and forms of treatment and integrating further tools in the repertoire of our already existing therapeutic toolkit, they will be able to ensure an even better and more extensive treatment for their patients. I can vouch for their experiencing much success and appreciation in their practice.

I recommend this work to all *healers and practitioners* who have the self-knowledge and the devotion and respect for their profession to keep expanding their understanding in order to provide even better and more efficient help to those who seek their assistance.

I recommend it to all my *fellow humans* who choose the path of self-healing. I encourage them to immerse themselves with all due attention in the study of this wonderful method; to use it with circumspection and with the wisdom to discern the ways they can heal themselves and their family up to the point where they truly need to consult a physician.

I recommend this work to all the *readers,* suggesting that they immerse themselves without hesitation in this marvellous fountainhead of knowledge where they will find themselves in the domain of new energies and information.

When all is said and done, *everything in the world is information and energy.*

I wish you all much success, joy, health, and peace of mind.

Dr Erzsébet Tusor MD

Specialist of Rheumatology and Physiotherapy, Hypnotist, Symbol-therapist, NLP Master, Erich Körbler-method Practitioner

Erich Körbler was one of the greatest figures of the late 20th century. His theoretical and practical work has laid new foundations for our understanding of disease, its aetiology, diagnostics and therapy, as well as for our entire thinking about medicine. It is not easy to provide a commendation of such a massive scholarly activity, even less to summarize it.

A scientific discovery which modifies the very basis of previous thinking is called a paradigm shift. All paradigm shifts are revolutionary in their impact. The previous approach and its representatives become surpassed and outdated – they become orthodox. The transition is never easy or smooth.

Erich Körbler and the scientific approach he termed New Homeopathy integrate the physical concepts of energetics, informatics and wave theory into the conceptual structures not only of medicine but also of our everyday thinking. The authors of the present book trace this fascinating intellectual process, creating something that is of lasting value not only from the 'popular' but also from the scientific point of view. This is a seminal work which responds to a felt need, as life did not grant Erich Körbler the chance to provide a heritage of a completed work. His heritage consists of short articles and lecture notes that his students and disciples could rely on, following his abrupt and untimely death.

Dr Mária Sági and István Sági take on a momentous task 20 years after Körbler's death to reconstruct his teaching that lays the foundations for medical science in the 21st century. Regrettably, the dowsing rod ('bio-indicator') invented by Erich Körbler has not yet become a diagnostic tool in medicine, but hopefully in a short time it will become a common instrument in the hand of every healer.

Dr Róbert Csiszár MD
honoris causa Biological Dentistry Secretary General,
Acupuncture Hungarian Medical Association
Erich Körbler-method instructor

Healing with Information

Healing with Information

The New Homeopathy

by Dr Mária Sági

with István Sági

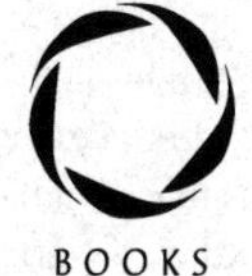

BOOKS

Winchester, UK
Washington, USA

First published by O-Books, 2018
O-Books is an imprint of John Hunt Publishing Ltd., Laurel House, Station Approach,
Alresford, Hants, SO24 9JH, UK
office1@jhpbooks.net
www.johnhuntpublishing.com

For distributor details and how to order please visit the 'Ordering' section on our website.

Illustration, design: József Vémi

ISBN: 978-1-78279-858-3
978-1-78279-857-6 (e-book)
Library of Congress Control Number: 2014948049

A CIP catalogue record for this book is available from the British Library.

Printed and bound by CPI Group (UK) Ltd, Croydon, CR0 4YY, UK

Contents

About the Principal Author

Mária Sági holds a Ph.D. in psychology from the Eötvös Lóránd University of Budapest, and after seven years research she received her C.Sc. degree (Candidate of the Hungarian Academy of Sciences). She was scientific collaborator of the Academy's Institute of Sociology and currently serves as Science Director of the Club of Budapest Foundation in Hungary. She is the founder and director of the former Körbler Institute Hungary, with more than 20 years healing practice in information medicine.

Mária Sági is the author and co-author of eleven books and some hundred and fifty articles and research papers on topics as varied as social and personality psychology, the psychology of music and art, as well as healing and information medicine, some published in English, French, German, Italian and Japanese.

Foreword

by Ervin Laszlo

A revolutionary development is under way today in the health sciences: the discovery that information is basic to organic functioning. This means that correct information is basic to correct functioning – that is, to the maintenance or re-establishment of health.

This discovery is the basis of the emerging field of information medicine. The book in the hands of the reader provides the foundations of an important method for the effective practice of information medicine: a new complementary – rather than categorically alternative – form of up-to-date health care.

Information in Nature

In the course of the last decade scientists in various fields of science have discovered the paramount role of information in the phenomena they investigate. Nature, it appears, is not like a giant mechanism, but more like a giant information system. It operates on information in the sense in which an information system or network does: information is the factor that determines the way a given network or computer behaves. A traditional typewriter does not have a program: when the key 'a' is pressed it activates an arm that types the letter 'a' on the paper. This is a mechanical and not an informational process. On the other hand in a computer, typing the letter 'a' activates a variety of responses as determined by the program of its software. The system's response is not a one-to-one mechanical reaction, but a programmed response based on information. It is in this sense that scientists are discovering the role of information in nature.

In classical science the information that governs action and interaction in the world is considered to be the effect of laws of nature: phenomena are said to 'obey' the laws. The set of all known and yet to be discovered laws constitutes the information we can assume is 'programmed into' nature – the information that codes the universe.[1]

In the 19th century the information responsible for action and interaction in nature was ascribed to the Newtonian laws of motion: causal connections between any 'x' and 'y' were to follow the laws of classical mechanics. In the 20th century the repertory of Newtonian laws has been vastly enlarged and in part replaced first with the laws of relativity, and then with laws derived from quantum theory. Information in nature proved to be more and more complex, and more and more divorced from the laws that seem to govern the behavior of things in our everyday experience.

In recent years further laws have come to light, entirely transcending the scope of classical mechanistic laws. These are in part probabilistic laws – such as those that describe the probability that an electron orbiting a given nucleus would be found in a given location – and in part laws of non-local interaction. The latter apply to instances where a given 'x' at point 'a' interacts with 'y' at point 'b,' where 'a' and 'b' are at a distance from each other that is greater than the distance light could have traveled in the time that elapsed between the observation of 'x' and of 'y'. These are the – not yet fully understood – laws of non-locality. Non-local events were thought to be limited to the quantum level, but they surfaced also at the level of life, and even at the scale of the universe.

There are classical causal relations as well as relativistic and non-local relations among things and events in nature. The information underlying these relations cannot be adequately grasped by the classical laws, and a full repertory of the relevant laws is not yet in sight. What has become clear, however, is that nature functions on the basis of information – highly complex information.

Complex information is the basis of the coherence of living systems. Genetic information is responsible for building the proteins and other basic building blocks of life, but there is more information in the functioning of the organism than the genetic and even the epigenetic information every cell, every organ and organ system is governed by information.

The most evident manifestation of the complex system of information that governs the living system is its coherence. 'Coherence' in this sense defines reciprocal relations among the parts of a system such that the coherent system acts as a single although complex entity. Its unity is the measure of its coherence, and its coherence is the indication of the adequacy of the information that governs it. Complex systems 'run' on information – complex information.

Information in living systems, and hence the coherence developed and maintained by information, has direct implications for the medical sciences. These sciences are, after all, the sciences of maintaining or re-establishing organic health, and that means maintaining, or re-establishing, organic coherence.

The organism is a highly coherent system – a system of which the coherence is assured by both classical and non-classical interactions. The human body consists of 10^{14} cells, and each cell produces 10,000 bio-electrochemical reactions every second. Every 24 hours 10^{12} cells die and are replaced. The co-ordination of this vast number of cells and their complex electromagnetic and chemical signaling is not ensured by physical and chemical interactions alone. The conduction of signals through the nervous system, for example, cannot proceed faster than about 20 meters per second, and it cannot carry a large number of diverse signals at the same time. Yet there are quasi-instant, non-linear, heterogeneous and multi-dimensional correlations among all cells in the organism, conveyed through highly co-ordinated organs and organ systems.[2]

Molecules, cells, and cellular assemblies resonate at the same or compatible frequencies whether they are proximal or distant. In terms of the biophysics of the organism, the same wave function applies to them. This holds true also in regard to the coupling of the frequencies of the molecules, cells, and cellular assemblies: faster and slower reactions accommodate themselves within a co-ordinate overall process: the respective wave functions coincide.

The coherence of the organism suggests that in some respects living systems are macroscopic quantum systems. This is supported by a number of findings in leading-edge biophysics, including experiments by Cornell, Ketterle and Wieman for which they received the 2001 Nobel Prize in Physics.[3] They demonstrated that living tissue forms Bose–Einstein condensates, which is a form of matter in which quantum processes occur at macroscopic scales.

A living organism is part of nature; a system that arose and is maintained in the context of local and non-local interaction with 'the rest of the universe'. Life is not a random occurrence or an epiphenomenon: it is part of the physical-chemical evolution of systems in the universe. This is a recent discovery; until now most scientists believed that life is a rare and perhaps accidental phenomenon. Living systems, it was said, can only come about under very specific conditions, and these are fortunate coincidences in the vast expanse of billions of galaxies. For life to occur, scientists pointed out, there must be a planet with the correct mass at the right distance from a main sequence G2 dwarf star; the planet must occupy a nearly circular orbit, and must have an oxygen/nitrogen-rich atmosphere, a large moon and a moderate rate of rotation; it must be at the right distance from the center of the galaxy and have liquid water on its surface; it must have a correct ratio between water and land-mass; and must be protected from asteroids by giant gas planets in the local solar system.

However, there is evidence that the substances necessary for life appear prior to, and independently of, these conditions. In October of 2011, a team of astrophysicists headed by Sun Kwok and Yong Zhang at the University of Hong Kong reported that organic molecules are created in stars.[4] To date some 130 molecules that constitute the basic building blocks of life have been found, including glycine, an amino acid, and ethylene glycol, the compound associated with the formation of the sugar molecules present in living systems. Exploration with NASA's space telescopes disclosed that water, methanol and carbon dioxide coat dust-particles around stars 420 light-years away in the constellation Taurus. They show up in interstellar dust clouds and in planet-forming discs around stars. At various stages of their evolution active stars eject organic compounds into interstellar space, thus distributing the complex molecules over vast planet-containing and potentially planet-forming regions.

Life is not a random or exceptional event in the universe: physical processes in stars produce the basic building blocks of the evolution of biological systems on planets. Only the higher forms of life – complex biochemical systems capable of metabolism and reproduction – call for conditions that are likely to be statistically rare in the universe.

The universe is a coherent system in its own right, even if it also manifests indeterminate processes that need to be mapped with chaotic attractors. Information is a basic factor in the universe, and it is a basic factor in the coherence of the systems that evolve in the universe. There are no categorical differences between living and non-living systems, between the living world and the physical world. The differences that obtain are differences in the information that codes the given systems.

New Perspectives for the Health Sciences

The implications of the role of information in natural systems are fundamental for the health sciences. As just noted, the maintenance of health in the organism is above all a matter of maintaining its coherence, and this depends on the information that codes the organism. Organic malfunctions are indications of a flaw in that information. Experience shows that correcting the flaw in the information can be more effective than interfering with the biochemical processes resulting from the flawed information. A new kind of medical science appears on the horizon: 'information medicine'.

The Austrian scientist Erich Körbler was one of the most important pioneers of the new information medicine. Possessed of an inquiring mind, a great aptitude for devising experiments, and an uncanny sensitivity to subtle energies, Körbler discovered that the human nervous system reacts precisely and dependably to the flows of information in its surroundings. He devised a simple instrument, the one-armed Körbler dowsing rod, that renders the organism's response clearly visible to the naked eye. The 'K-rod' amplifies the subtle involuntary movements produced by the subject's nervous system, enabling practitioners to perform an entire series of tests to demonstrate the response of the organism to the inputs and influences that reach it in its milieu.

Körbler codified his findings in the form of a basic 'vector system' that situates the observed movements of the K-rod within a sophisticated system of co-ordinates. Observing the precise movements of the rod provides indications of the compatibility or non-compatibility of a given input or influence in regard to the subject's organism. Beneficial effects resulting from inputs that are compatible with the healthy functioning of the organism are indicated by one type of movement; various degrees of less-than-beneficial up to seriously harmful inputs are indicated by a different set of precisely codified responses.

Dr. Mária Sági, the author of this remarkable book, encountered Körbler in her search for an effective screening method to protect her in view of her sensitivity to water veins. As she recounts in the Preface to this book, in Vienna she bought a bedsheet with a remarkable screening property developed by Körbler. Her experience using that sheet led her to look up the inventor himself: Erich Körbler. When she met him, she found to her delight that the screening method is only one element of a complex healing system developed by Körbler. He could diagnose and modify with his vector system bodily malfuntions, and all types of radiations in the surroundings. She wanted to know more, and she soon acquired the basics of the system Körbler called 'New Homeopathy'. This system represents a major therapeutic method–an embracing corpus of information medicine. Before long she has successfully promulgated Körbler's system in her native Hungary.

A deep friendship developed between Erich Körbler, and Maria, and her brother Istvan. They first became Körbler's disciples and then his esteemed collaborators. After Körbler's sudden death, Hans-Joachim Ehlers, the editor-in-chief of the German avantgarde health magazine *Raum und Zeit,* asked Mária and István to hold teaching seminars on New Homeopathy at the first, second and third level at 'Gasthof Gut Schlickenried' in Bavaria. They accepted and, beginning in the fall of 1994, conducted the seminars for physicians and natural healers for over a year and a half. Many of those who participated in these seminars adopted Körbler's system in their own medical and healing practice. As I already had the pleasure of meeting Körbler in person, I agreed to give the introductory lecture, on the scientific background of New Homeopathy.

Complete teaching materials were developed during this time, based on Körbler's articles, the Bavarian seminars, as well as on the three courses held for physicians in Budapest. The school that was founded at this time continues to function today, offering a Certificate based on eight weekend seminars and a concluding examination.

New Homeopathy is an empirical healing system, based on the reception of information by the organism. Unlike classical medicine, and many other branches of information medicine, the expanded system of New Homeopathy is not only local, sense-perceived information, but also non-local information beyond the scope of the bodily senses. Dr Sági's praxis offers clear and convincing demonstration that basically the same diagnosis and the same healing-effects can be achieved whether the patient is next to the healer or in another house, another city, or even another continent. In this introductory book (to be followed by a second volume focused on the individual application of informational and homeopathic remedies in proximal and remote healing), she presents the basics of this complementary healing method, destined to expand and revolutionize Western medicine in the coming years.

In studying the pages of this book the reader will be acquainted with a vast range of diagnostic and therapeutic methods, and the writer of this Foreword can testify to their effectiveness. He had the opportunity of witnessing several controlled experiments examining the physiological coordinates of practicing this method, demonstrating that the EEG (electroencephalograph) patterns that appear in the brain of the experimenter are reproduced in the brain of the patient in the absence of all sensory and physical contact between them.[5] This writer also had the good fortune of being treated by the author for the past twenty-five years with results that leave no doubt about the efficacy of the treatment. He can therefore commend this path-breaking work to the attention of everyone who is either professionally or personally interested in new developments in the art and science of healing. This is the cutting-edge of the next development: the integration of information medicine in the theory and practice of modern medicine.

Preface

My collaboration with Erich Körbler began in the fall of 1990. I found him 'by chance' – if there is such a thing. When I stepped into his Vienna study I was overcome by the feeling that I needed to know everything he knew. How did this come about?

This was a time when various energy-screening techniques were not yet widely known in Hungary. I was spending the summer in our thatched cottage in Balatonudvari by Lake Balaton and, as in so many previous summers, I never got a relaxing night's sleep there. I would wake up with big black shadows under my eyes that would then disappear later on during the day in the sunlight. I experimented with a mirror placed face down under the bed, but to no avail. Father Lajos, the old priest reputed for his knowledge of herbal and other natural healing methods, advised me, 'My child, you will have to part with that house.' I checked with my pendulum, and found many water veins running under the house and in the garden. Just to be on the safe side, I called in a specialist who said, 'Your measurements were as good as mine', meaning that he had found the same as I had.

For the next seven years I studied natural medicine with various healers in Vienna, while at home Father Lajos was my master in natural healing, and Mr. and Mrs. Kushi my teachers in macrobiotics. I combined the information on natural healing with healing through macrobiotics, and practiced my new skills. I asked one of my Viennese friends what he knew about screening water veins. He said he knew a reliable method but he could only acquire the thing needed for that in the fall – he was talking about a screening sheet. We agreed that I would buy one on my next visit to Vienna.

This is what I proceeded to do. One Friday night, at the place where I was staying in Vienna, I tested the sheet I had bought. That same night I experienced some very special sensations – as if I was levitating and there were two lamps heating me up. When I woke up in the morning I felt even worse than at Balaton – I was quite feeble. I went down to the street to make a telephone call, even though I knew I had little hope as my friend had gone away for the weekend. The phone just rang and rang. I returned to the apartment and took out the packaging for the sheet. On the cover I found a telephone number. So I set off once more to the telephone booth. I dialed the number and a man answered. He said he had something urgent to do at the moment but he would be free at about 3 p.m. the same afternoon and I could go and see him. He gave me directions. I couldn't even recall his name but I had his address I got on a streetcar, and at 3 o'clock in the afternoon I knocked on his door.

He had a large, oblong-shaped office, at least 10 meters in length. The front door was open and the vast room extended from an entrance hall of about 1 square meter. I knocked, and through a glass door I could see that he was sitting by his desk at the far end of the room. He stood up and started walking toward me as I stood there in the doorway already overcome with the magical conviction: *I want this knowledge.*

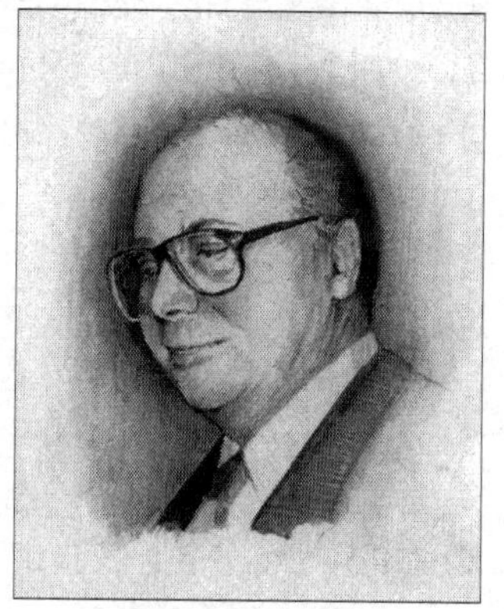
Erich Körbler (1938–1994)

We introduced ourselves – I was seeing Erich Körbler (1938–1994), the inventor of the 'magic sheet' I had tried out the night before. He received me most amicably. I was still feeling quite uncomfortable, which he transformed into a pleasant feeling with a single move: he kept two fingers on the top of my head for a few seconds, and turned my hairclasp from horizontal to vertical. (It turned out later that this was to connect the flow of subtle energies on the top of my head between the two hemispheres and free up my psychomeridian. (See Chapter 12.) In the conversation that followed he answered many of my questions.

He gave me his dowsing rod and encouraged me to try it. He saw that I was a practiced hand in the use of the pendulum. Next, I was rapidly introduced to some parallel lines I noticed on the wall behind his desk. There was also a piece of paper with five parallel lines – some of them dotted. In response to my question he explained that this served to screen unfavorable radiation from the sides. After the experiences of the previous night I had not a shadow of a doubt about this. The cause of my discomfort after that night was also soon revealed. He explained that in the case of such sensitivities the screening sheet had to be introduced gradually over about six days – first only up to the ankle, then up to the knee, then to the waist and only then under the head.

Once inside Körbler's laboratory, wherever I looked I saw something that made me want to ask questions. On a long table, for instance, I saw some small rocks. This was a sample series of zeolite pieces in different sizes. He told me that he used them for healing: he used his dowsing rod to select the right size of zeolite for the patient, put it in a small jar, and proposed wearing it in a shirt or a trouser pocket depending on the targeted part of the body, until improvement set in. This is a good way of acting on, say, tinnitus. I also found that this served not only to screen earth radiation but also to heal a whole range of different disturbances. I spent about an hour and a half with him.

Of all the things that I saw in his study, there was only one that did not fit his image in my view. On a table there was a series of bags and boxes of sugar – icing sugar, refined sugar, sugar lumps, all with different brand names. Seeing my questioning look – I no longer dared to bombard him with further questions – he suggested that I test the different kinds of sugar. After a number of unfavorable responses from his dowsing rod, one bag produced a positive reaction. I was surprised, as I had experienced nothing of the kind during my macrobiotic praxis of the previous seven years. I was holding a bag of rough-ground brown *Vollzucker* (unrefined sugar). Körbler told me that this sugar had a history. Before its production even began, the field that grew the sugar beets was enriched with minerals and transformed into high-quality organic soil. The objective was that the sugar beet should contain the necessary minerals. As regards the factory procedure, the production line was modified in such a way as to preserve the minerals in the sugar. All of this was devised and created in Austria based on Körbler's experiments and plans.

My idea of Körbler gained more and more depth. At first I thought I was getting advice on how to neutralize water veins but instead I found myself in a complex and well-equipped healing workshop. I found a number of radical innovations for various areas in life, such as diet. I saw no instruments, only symbols drawn on papers and a range of substances prepared for testing; a great many minerals, crystals, foods, vegetable extracts, homeopathic remedies, colored papers. In the middle of all of this was Körbler's rod, his version of the classical dowsing rod. It was part of a complex and coherent system which was extremely appealing to me for being so natural and simple, but I had no idea what formed its basis.

My time for my first visit was up. I bought a Körbler rod (I still have the receipt he gave me after all these years) and while Körbler was writing the receipt, I gathered my courage and asked him whether he thought it would be possible to make his healing method known in Hungary. I offered to be his ambassador. He said yes.

I had lots of work that autumn – I had to complete the final report on an international comparative research project on European identity and get it into print. I had little time left for other assignments, but even so, I took as much of my free time as I could in order to experiment with the dowsing rod. My Vienna encounter continued to fascinate me. A month later my research work took me to Vienna once more, so Körbler and I used this occasion to meet again. I recorded our conversation. Körbler told me that he was using the term 'New Homeopathy' to denote his healing system. He also talked about the role of electromagnetic waves, even though at this time he did not write these thoughts down, but was only in the stage of developing them.

A few weeks later Körbler visited Budapest and met my brother István. He proposed that while I was busy and we were still learning the use of the dowsing rod, Istvan could join him in the practical side of his efforts. At the time he was looking for a textile factory to produce his energy-transforming bedsheets.

Eventually, the Goldberger Textile Works in Óbuda became our business partner. They had to adhere to some very strict regulations in manufacturing the sheets. It was important to use 100% pure cotton raw material in which the threads ran vertically to each other. Körbler chose the necessary red pigment from a wide range of different shades from Germany. We mixed the pigment required for the pattern in big wooden tubs and, to improve its information content, added mineral zeolite. Zeolite carries information which is positive for the human organism. This operation could only be carried out in Istvan's presence. Before the pigment could be printed, Istvan tested it following Körbler's methodology. The greatest challenge was that the raw material – the textile – had to be stretched and threaded in such a way that the right angle of the fiber exactly matched the pattern of the printing cylinder – crosses of equal lines. If the pattern slipped even a little bit, they needed to start all over again.

During these efforts, a spirit of harmonious co-operation developed between Körbler and István, accompanied by profound fondness and trust on both sides. Each time we met, Körbler took the occasion to teach us. We, for our part, continued to practice until the next meeting two or three weeks later. Each time, he gave us exciting and new exercises and introduced us to different subject matters. By the end of the year I had also finished my project report and finally had time for new challenges. I talked about my new experiences to my healer friends, sharing my enthusiasm, and many of them seemed seriously interested. When they tested our first energy-transforming sheets, their initial curiosity deepened into active interest.

In January 1991, we traveled to Vienna with the crew of a television program called *Close Encounters of Type Zero* and recorded a series of shows, four parts of half an hour each, about Körbler. I acted as interpreter during the shooting. The first part was broadcast in February, followed by the others. It raised intense responses both in favor and against. A well-known Hungarian physicist invited Körbler for a 'duel' on television, and indeed the two of them turned up for this challenge at the appropriate studio in Budapest. This time Körbler also gave an informative lecture in the Lecture Hall of the Culture Research Institute in front of an audience of about 50 people.

Our co-operation became more extensive each time we met. We were now competent at using the dowsing rod and also successfully applied the sine curve as a healing symbol on a number of occasions. Back in the spring, Körbler had given me, for testing, a large sheet of wrapping paper with large figures of about 60-80 cm, drawn in red. It was a combination of Ys (ypsilons) and +s (crosses). He asked me to place this new combination of symbols on my bed under the sheet overnight, about where my spine lies, and then to report my experiences. I tried the method during my few days in Vienna and the result was pleasant, relaxed sleep.

Based on my experiences with the energy-transforming sheet, Körbler had thought I would be a good experimental subject to test the new, energy-building sheet. This is indeed what happened. I went home with the new combination of patterns. Once at home, as an experiment I painted the new pattern in waterproof ink on some textile to serve me until the first printed copy came out.

My physician friends and I organized a course to disseminate the Körbler method in Hungary. Körbler gave the first course in Budapest for physicians on New Homeopathy in June 1991. This was attended by 18 doctors who were specialists in acupuncture. Thanks to Dr Elvira Babindak and Jenő Kalo, the entire course was recorded on video. The transcript was made by Dr György Rados. Körbler did not ask for honorarium, only to reimburse him for his travel expenses. During his stay in Budapest, he was a guest of my brother, István.

The first course for doctors also brought a radical change in my personal life. At that time I lived in Óbuda, an ancient town district of Budapest, in a 51 m^2 apartment, on the third floor of a four-storey building. One side overlooked the Hármashatárhegy. It is a mountain at 495 m (1624 ft) above sea level, with digital radio / audio broadcasting systems. The apartment above, on the fourth floor, was occupied by a radio amateur with a full broadcasting and reception station and other technical equipment. Ten years before that, when I moved in, I asked one of the best radiesthetic experts in those times to come and test the apartment. My bed proved to be in a good position as regards underground water veins and radiation hubs. The testing was repeated several times over the year and they always found the same favorable results; still I woke up every morning with a headache which would only abate after two or three hours, after I took a shower, did some exercises and transcendental meditation (TM). I tried sleeping with my head the other way round – no improvement. In 1990 I finally consulted a well-known acupuncture specialist and asked for help. I started going for treatment twice a week, on Tuesday and Friday mornings.

The result was as follows. On Wednesdays I woke up fine, on Thursdays fatigued, with a headache which went away after a shorter period of time, on Fridays the same as before. After Friday's treatment the situation would be the same – Saturdays fairly good, Sundays the same as Thursdays, Mondays and Tuesdays just like in the past. After ten treatments the doctor said to me, 'Please, try to change something about the way you live. I cannot help you; I will not carry on treating you any longer. I have never had a patient whose condition remained unchanged after ten treatments.' I came away in tears and kept wondering what I could change. The doctor must be right – those words echoed in my ears. I was almost feeling guilty and hoping beyond hope that I would find what I needed to change.

After the first day of the training course for doctors, I took Körbler to my home where I was hosting him for his stay. This was his first visit there. Directly after we arrived, I went to the kitchen to make tea and he stayed in the room. A few minutes later he called out in excitement, 'Maria, wo ist die Rute? Wo ist die Rute?' (Where is the rod?) I could not possibly imagine what could have happened in such a short time! He had been sitting on the piano stool in front of the piano and underwent an experience the like of which, he claimed, he had never had before. His head grew heavy, he soon fell asleep and when he woke with a start, he felt a curious aching sensation about his heart. He told me that he had never in his life fallen asleep at that time of day (it was 5 p.m.); even when he had been up all night, he had not felt particularly tired.

He feverishly set to work with the dowsing rod, only hastily drinking his tea. He soon managed to ascertain that there was a combined beam of radiation arriving from the direction of the broadcasting tower to where my piano stool and indeed my bed stood – exactly the spot where my head was usually positioned. He worked hard for an hour until he finally identified how he could screen off these rays. In fact he was usually very quick to diagnose, taking only a minute or two with any person or living space. He used to teach people this quick operative technique, to help us avoid mistakes. He was of the opinion that working with the dowsing rod must be guided by intuition and this meant very swift decision-making (see later where we discuss the diagnosis).

Eventually, he stretched the sheet on which I had painted crosses and Ys as a screen at the appropriate height and angle, in one corner of the room. On the walls of the apartment which faced the hill, he nailed energy-transforming sheets from floor to ceiling, in several layers, and on the windows he drew large Ys in soap. He conjured up a completely new home for me. From the next morning onwards I never had a headache when waking up. This was surprising as it is believed that even getting used to good things takes time for our organism, particularly after extended exposure to something harmful. This usually takes two-three weeks. (Later on we built a canopy over the bed in the bedroom, to neutralize the radiation coming from the fourth floor.) The radiesthetic expert had also been right in saying that the radiation was not caused by an underground water vein or other earth radiation hub, but he did not think of the possibility of a harmful beam of radiation coming from the side. Perhaps he himself was not sensitive to it, and this is why it did not occur to him to test it.

One's own experience is the best master. Körbler's insistence that holistic medicine must always look at the living organism made more and more sense to me. The organism, whether human, animal or plant, must always be viewed as part of its environment, together with its electromagnetic resonances. The immune system can only counterbalance unfavorable influences from the environment up to a limit, beyond which the organism will start signaling. If we do not change the causes that provoke the response, no treatment can be of any use. My doctor gave the right advice when he told me that I should change the way I lived. But who would think of an external circumstance in a case like that?

During those years, studies about experimental testing of harmful environmental factors were on the increase both internationally and in my own country. Körbler pointed out many of them, and I translated or reviewed many of them for the periodical *Természetgyógyász Magazin* [Natural Healer's Journal]. What attracted most attention was the damage caused by electrosmog in households. Considerations of this kind were quite unknown in home design at the time. Although people having problems if they lived near high-voltage cables was already known, in the crowded living conditions of the metropolis few would have thought that electrosmog produced by the fuse box was the cause of their ailments. (Most commonly, the fuse box and the electric meter would be on one side of a wall while on the far side of the wall a neighbor would be struggling with headaches and with low energy levels as a result of poor quality sleep.) This was also the time, about 20 years ago, when the number of cell phones was sharply on the increase in Hungary, and this also meant an increase in the electrosmog produced by the phones. This triggered a whole series of debates.

Körbler was concerned simultaneously with eliminating harmful environmental influences and with healing. This is no wonder as his research activity in this direction had been inspired by his personal experience. On one occasion he was working on some low-voltage electricity measurements when he felt like eating an apple. The moment he picked up the fruit the needle of the instrument moved, and the screen of the computer also showed a different figure. He put the apple down; the needle returned to its previous position. He picked up the apple once more – the instrument reacted again.

He began to explore the cause of this phenomenon, and his professional path led him to co-operation with scientific research institutes in physics and biochemistry. He experimented in the Vienna Institute of Nuclear Physics, at Innsbruck University, at the Ludwig Maximilian University of Munich, and at the Children's Clinic of Vienna. Further, he made experiments in the field of healing. In co-operation with Professor König from Vienna, the greatest Austrian authority on acupuncture, Körbler examined the healing effect of symbols – of what he referred to as 'Geometrische Formen' *(geometric forms – referring to the shape and structure of an object).*

Whether he worked in physics, in biochemistry or in healing, he always looked for the simplest possible solution to make sure that his method could become available to the broadest public.

From 1989 onwards he published regularly in the German periodical *Raum und Zeit* [Space and Time]. Here, too, he encouraged his readers to repeat the experiments he described and report their findings. Readers sent much valuable feedback to the editorial office. Körbler's writings centered on two subjects – one was the environmental influences and the related experiments with the dowsing rod; the other was the internal environment, i.e. the healing of the organism. While we kept on practicing and continually experienced the efficiency of his system of healing, each time we met we were introduced to yet another of his inventions, whether they were in an experimental stage or in a finalized form.

These were the months when he created his high-potency informed water he named 'Himalaya water'. This indicated that it was analogous to the water which in natural circumstances was found in the Himalayas at an altitude of about 5000 m – representing a clean and powerful energy. Any urban tap water can be energized by adding two to three drops of Himalaya water.

He did serious work on water, regarding it not only as the cradle of life, but also as the information-mediating substance of the human organism, since 'informed water' was one of his chief means of healing.

During our entire co-operation I found his work so versatile, complex, so quick in practice and yet simple, that it was pure pleasure to work with him, even if, lacking an understanding of quantum physics, I found his explanations hard to follow. Körbler gave me a doctoral dissertation in physics written at the Vienna Institute of Nuclear Physics – it was not an easy read. He gave summer seminars in Raabs, Austria, with some members of the Hungarian team of doctors attending. We all practiced New Homeopathy, each at his or her own level of competence. Körbler had entrusted Istvan and me to represent his method in Hungary. It was our job to supply all those interested with devices, and with information, and to help with the application of the method.

Körbler received several awards for his research achievements. In 1989, in Brussels, the Innovative Research EG Centre gave him a Eureka Gold Medal, a De Chevalier diploma and the gold cross for the discovery of his systemic principle and for inventing the dowsing rod. On this same occasion he was awarded the medal of distinction of the Guglielmo Marconi Academy of Sciences in Rome. Two years later, the Association of Austrian Inventors gave Körbler a gold medal for research regarding information on operating in high-frequency zones. The head of the association lauded his activity in the presence of the representatives of several ministries and emphasized that these investigations were of great significance for the health and environmental science of the future.

Between 29 February and 1 March, 1992, we offered the second training course for doctors in Budapest that was recorded

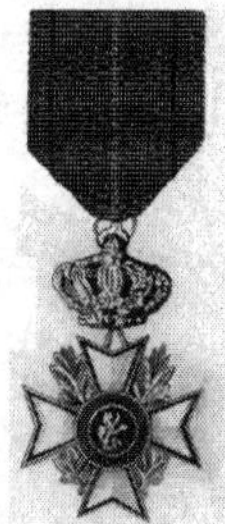

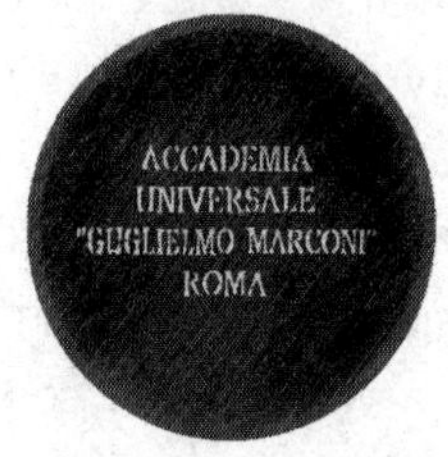

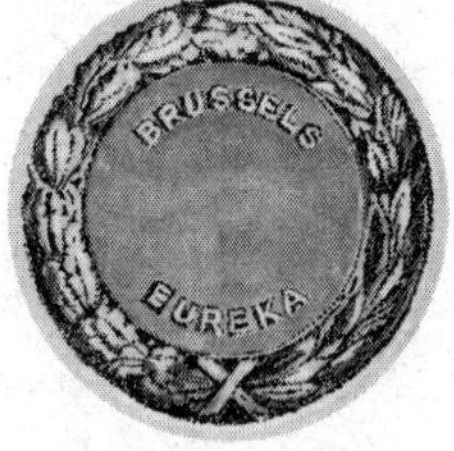

Körbler's awards

on video. By this time we were also talking about starting a clinic of natural healing in Budapest. Dr Elvira Babindak was a member of the Organizing Committee and, on the Committee's behalf, requested that Körbler be in charge of screening the clinic from harmful environmental effects. The foundation stone was laid in October. Körbler travelled to Budapest for the occasion and took the chance to collect information about how electric equipment for the wards could be purchased in Hungary. We went to the showroom of the Tungsram factory. At Tungsram they gave us a warm welcome and they surprised at the results of our information-collecting tour. I was the experimental subject during the tests, and Körbler tested all the light sources on display, including the traditional Edison-type light bulbs, the different variations of neon-lights, and a great many halogen lights. The results were far from promising. Besides the traditional pear-shaped bulbs, he could not find any light source which had a favorable effect on the human organism. The others merely varied in their degree of harmfulness, depending on the distance recommended from these objects once they are lit (for details see Chapter 17).

From the spring of 1993 onwards, events concerned with information transmission grew more frequent in Hungary. Starting in April that year we launched a new series of articles on New Homeopathy in *Természetgyógyász Magazin.* In 1993 we published four installments, in 1994 the following three parts came out, and at the same time we began to offer new training courses. The courses were given by Istvan and me as co-trainers. At the same time we were successfully treating a number of patients. The method was continually gaining in popularity.

Between 20 and 23 May, 1993, the Second International Conference on Natural Healing was held in Budapest where Körbler was an invited guest. He arrived at the conference on a Friday afternoon, stopping by on his way at Balatonudvari, where he helped me to screen our weekend cottage against environmental and electrical influences.

We started a renovation yet in February. We tried to take into account what we had learned thus far. The main problem was not water veins, although those, too, were significant. The electric cables and counter were in one corner of the room over the bed. The combination of the underground water-vein and the electrosmog certainly did not serve good health nor did they produce a good sensation. During modernization, an electric cable was laid underground leading to a fuse box on the back wall of the house.

When Körbler arrived in May, we placed an equal-armed cross of brass, 80 cm × 80 cm in size, on the ground in the courtyard to neutralize the entire area, then in order to shield the interior of the house, Körbler made equal-armed crosses of the same material as the dowsing rod, and we had them plastered into the wall.

By this time I had spent about two weeks in the house under reconstruction, regularly doing test measurements, still the results were poor. I presumed this was the result of my lack of sleep and all the hassle to do with the works. I telephoned Körbler and asked his advice on how to get refreshed, but he did not know. He knew that by now I was using the dowsing rod with assurance and in the right manner, so he could not tell why it was not working for me at the building site. He proposed that on his way to the conference he would stop by and examine the area.

As a first step, he set to work with an instrument called a 'trifield meter' (which measures the strength of electric and magnetic fields) and instantly solved the mystery. There was a utility pole about a hundred meters from the house. Körbler discovered that the power cables on the pole were connected the wrong way, causing a constant hazard to the five nearby houses connected to this pole. Had there been a power outage, this could have been life-threatening. This was the first and only time I have ever seen Körbler angry. We immediately went to the local electrician, arguing that they are not to leave people with a life-threatening electrical connection – what irresponsibility! But the electrician had finished work for the day and said, 'We'll do it on Monday… Anyway, if it's urgent, why don't you phone the Regional Electric Supply Company and get them to help you?' We only reached the emergency call service. Our case was not considered an emergency, so we were left to hope that nothing disastrous would happen until Monday, and we set off for the International Healing Conference in Budapest.

Luckily, nothing happened, and based on our complaint, they righted the electric connection on the coming Monday. When I returned to the house the following week, I was once more able to work with the dowsing rod.

Körbler's appearance at the conference was a great success. In his talk he described the basic working mechanisms of New Homeopathy and described the results which had been unknown to Hungarian audiences. After his talk, at the desk for New Homeopathy, patients were lining up to meet Körbler.

I also gave a talk at the conference, presenting cases of patients I had cured with the Körbler method. My results were particularly impressive in the case of children with allergy. Lots of parents with small children came to me with dozens of medicines and foods to test and asked me to help their children who had been suffering from allergy for one, two or even three years without improvement. The disease itself was usually neurodermatitis, with rashes on the limbs or the entire body.

Körbler himself only experimented with allergy treatments among friends, as his own patients were far more serious cases. He was usually sought out by people in an incurable condition, who had been suffering for years, were paralyzed or walking on crutches. By this time he was a widely known healer and although he did not have a practice anywhere, news of his near-miraculous healing spread like wildfire, so patients found him in the end. When I asked for his advice regarding the treatment of allergy, he told me that in addition to the *in-formation* treatment, I should treat according to my own experience. Körbler's in-formation treatment is the following: the patient uses his or her left index finger and middle finger to form a Y, and holds his or her right hand one or two cm above the right hemisphere of his or her brain, while for four minutes repeating rhythmically the name of the food that caused the allergy, and also looking at that food, if possible. This method, however, cannot be used with very small children. With babies and children below the age of one or two, we placed a piece of the allergenic food into a bottle which we sealed, and then drew the symbol Y on the bottle. The children were given the bottle to hold in their hands and play with, among their other toys. After about two weeks we would test the foods in question again. Skin complaints improved at a surprising rate simply by withdrawing allergenic foods and medicines from the children's diet. Rashes that had prevailed for a year or two vanished in five–seven days.

During the course of these treatments I realized, thanks to the indications of the dowsing rod, that with small children I needed to draw a symbol over the organ for a certain period of time. Sometimes this was over the colon, sometimes over the small intestines, at other times both, or over the liver. I used the dowsing rod to measure accurately the position of the sine curve or the place and size of the four lines. At first I checked my patients every one or two days. The symbols proved necessary for a long time, and sometimes needed to be applied for two or even three weeks before the child's condition became stabilized. Each child responded to a different diet and different treatment. Patients arriving with almost identical complaints required completely different therapy, proving that every person is unique.

Körbler was very pleased with my results. He encouraged me to write about what I had achieved up to that point. It was in the autumn of 1993 that I wrote a study on the new homeopathic treatment of allergic conditions published in Hungarian in the January issue of Volume 5 (1994) of *Természetgyógyász,* while in German it came out in issue No. 70/1994 of *Raum und Zeit*. Based on the principle of 'practice makes perfect', we became 'the allergy specialists'. The parents of my patients, and even I myself, looked on these quick recoveries as almost miraculous. The practice of the past 20 years has shown that this method really does bring a simple, sure, rapid and gentle relief from allergies.

In the spring of 1993 Körbler established a training center in Mönichkirchen, Austria, where during the summer months he offered intensive courses on New Homeopathy. This spacious place, a former inn, could comfortably house 15–20 participants, and the training took place at different points of the venue in a pleasant setting. When the weather was clement, lessons were offered in the garden. In the foyer Körbler created a permanent exhibit for students to illustrate how New Homeopathy works at the level of physics while in the garden he demonstrated the presence of various types of geological radiation. At a fish pond in the garden he showed us the difference between the radiation of live water and the radiation of underground water vein. All of this was only meant to provide background knowledge for practicing New Homeopathy, and was not meant to deliver a course on radiesthetics, even though it would easily have passed for one. In a room he had set up what he called a spine bed – a bed that lets the spine really rest and regain its original form. Students have taken turns to use this bed for the length of time needed.

On the last day of the Conference on Natural Healing Körbler invited István to Mönichkirchen to join him as his assistant at the training center. This was an honor for Istvan for a number of reasons – professional, moral and emotional alike.

Körbler had provisional talks with a candidate for an assistant, but eventually decided that if István was willing to live at the venue permanently until the end of September, he would be his preferred choice. During a co-operation of three years the two men had developed a profound friendship. Körbler once said that he loved and trusted István so much that he would willingly put his life in his hands. In late May István happily set out for Mönichkirchen. They set up the exhibition together, and though the building was not finished yet, the training began in June, and from that time on, it was offered every weekend, running in separate cycles for beginners, intermediate and advanced groups. There was always something interesting happening in the house. Several of the students came for extended periods of time and spent the time between courses practicing.

I myself arrived in Mönichkirchen in mid-August and stayed there almost a month. These were exciting times. I studied and practiced with a number of colleagues who were doctors or healers. I remember that all participants had some instrument lying in front of them on the table. They measured everything that could be measured from an energetic point of view. They compared our results – indeed, it was a true exchange of learning, and a great experience for all of us. István and I did not have any kind of instrument so I asked Körbler which instrument he would recommend to me if I had a chance to buy one. He answered, 'None of them. The dowsing rod can do everything; the only thing to consider beside the dowsing rod is a radionic device.' Later that year, Körbler was given such an appliance by Peter W. Kohne, the head of the Pronova Energetik company.

As regards my own learning, it was in Mönichkirchen that I fully understood the principle of neutralizing Disturbance Zones. Even though earlier I succeeded in neutralizing the bedrooms of all my patients and solved various problems of radiation at our summer cottage, it was only in Austria that I 'got' the whole picture and every element fell into place.

There I have learnt a great deal more. I have learnt a broader and finer application of the vector system, as well as the wonderfully complex web of connections in our organism, and the uniqueness of every organism. Körbler did not use a set material to teach – he had so many new cases and new inventions that day by day, and weekend by weekend we worked with a different patient. We were able to experience the healing system of New Homeopathy through many examples and cases, and this complex, holistic way of healing, thinking, and taking action became second nature for us.

Hardly had we got home from Mönichkirchen when it was time to hold the third training course for doctors in Budapest. Körbler trained us on the first weekend of October. Enriched with new knowledge, we went about our tasks with even more enthusiasm. A study based on our experiences of treating allergy sufferers was completed yet in autumn.

In late February 1994 Körbler made an appointment with Istvan and they agreed that they would meet in Körbler's office on the third of March. Istvan arrived at the agreed time but found the door locked. He went to Körbler's apartment, and there he learned that the previous afternoon, soon after arriving home his friend died unexpectedly of a heart attack.

In early April I received a telephone call from Ehlers, who said he would visit us in Budapest. He came on the morning flight and was leaving the same afternoon. I could not guess the purpose of this visit, but I did not have to wait long.

We received Ehlers at István's apartment. He invited us to lecture on New Homeopathy at levels I, II and III in Gut Schlickenried, Germany. We agreed. Starting in September 1994, we lectured for a year and a half. There were some 55–60 students in each seminar – doctors and healers.

Very soon our students became lecturers and stepped into our places. As we have learnt, the organizers prepared a set of teaching materials based on my courses given in Hungary and

Germany, taking over the whole curriculum, and using Körbler's writings that had been published in *Raum und Zeit*.

The school that started at the Gut Schlickenried property is still in operation today, granting certificates to those who complete a series of eight weekend seminars and a final test. Those who were interested in getting back to the original source have kept visiting us for more than 20 years by.

Körbler's death brought a fundamental change in our lives. This placed a huge responsibility on our shoulders: besides our work at home we needed to compile study materials, to lecture, and to see a host of foreign patients. We rose to the task. The 'miracle' never failed to take place for any of our patients. Even today, after so many years, I still marvel at how quickly the body responds to this gentle treatment method.

Although we have published more than 50 articles in this field, the time has now come to share with the public the knowledge of New Homeopathy and the experiments necessary for acquiring the method in a book. This book will be followed by another on information medicine, developed on the basis of the remote healing I have practiced over the past 20 years. But for this 'everyday miracle' to take place, everyone needs to start at the beginning. I wish the reader the best of luck!

Dr Mária Sági

Part I
Principles and Theories

Chapter 1

The New Way of Healing – the Transmission of Information

We are surrounded by a reality which we cannot perceive with our sensory organs. It has no flavor, no smell, you can't see it, hear it or touch it, and still it exists. It informs our brain, our nervous system, and our immune system; every bit of our body absorbs it. It is known to our spirit and, through extrasensory perception, it is also known to our consciousness.

In a holistic world-view, ancient civilizations, as well as tribal people living in natural settings, found it quite self-evident that man is an organic part of his environment, connected with the outside world in constant interaction and communication with all things. This is why they did not stifle the subtle-level resonances which they received through extrasensory perception.

The perception of what are called 'subtle energies' was a part of their experience, and thus their consciousness also worked with this factor. It was also self-evident that nature consisted not only of physical matter – that man's material body was only one dimension of the living organism. The energy of the spirit which permeates the entire world constituted an organic and indeed guiding part of everyday life.

As Hermes Trismegistus puts it in one of his tablets, 'As above, so below'. People were a part of the ecological unit of the Earth and nature. They knew and lived with subtle energies, both on the natural and the supernatural plane. They accounted for spiritual, emotional and energetic dimensions, and systematized their knowledge about this sphere no less than about the parts of the material body. They took care to heal the spiritual dimensions as much as to heal the material body. Indeed, often they attained the recovery of the body through the healing of the spiritual, emotional and energetic dimensions.

Ancient cultures gave various names to the field that carries information and energy. In Japan, Shintoism calls it *ki;* Chinese Taoism calls it *chi.* In ancient Hindu philosophy it was called *prana,* while in the traditional Judaism of the Near East it was called *chaim.* In Europe, Pythagoras among the ancient Greeks called it 'the central fire'. The alchemists of the Middle Ages spoke of *azoth.*

Ancient cultures viewed the world in many different ways, but one thing they shared is that they had not separated philosophy from their belief systems. Starting from the Middle Ages, while the Christian church retained, indeed, increased its hegemony, developments took a fresh course. After the invention of the telescope and the inception of the natural sciences in the time of Giordano Bruno and Galileo Galilei, the church could no longer retain its monopoly and so the natural sciences became separate from the moral sciences (philosophy and theology). As Galilei said in his *Natural Phylosophy* 'Primary is that which you can measure (weight, distance); secondary is that which we can perceive with our consciousness (color, beauty).' From that time on, the natural sciences were only concerned with exploring matter and measuring. As a consequence, people's perception in the Western world also became transformed and they ceased to care about the subtle-resonance information arriving through extrasensory perception. Even if some people had experiences of that kind, they considered it insignificant. The development of technology moved in in the same direction.

About 300 years ago Newton laid the foundations of modern thinking by establishing the laws of physics which seemed to offer a satisfactory explanation of the surrounding world. Over the past 300 years this material way of thinking went through a rapid and intense development. According to this kind of thinking, the world is organized on a purely material level. By examining matter, we can achieve practically everything and do not need to mix subtle or spiritual energies with the material approach. Belief in energies in spiritual dimensions was people's personal business.

In the modern period, medicine was the area where the concept of life-energy resurfaced. In the 18th century, Anton Mesmer called this force 'animal magnetism'. In the early 20th century Sigmund Freud called it 'libido' and Wilhelm Reich termed it 'orgone energy', to mention just a few examples.

In the technological, materialist civilization of the West, over the past 300 years, science took over the role of religion. Healing no longer formed part of the spiritual aspect of man's life, but was accorded a place among the natural sciences, and its development progressed at an amazing pace.

Most recently, however, scientific research has returned to the examination of subtle energies. This development can be seen as an upward spiral. On the bottom level we find the cultures of antiquity where man still formed a close unit with nature and perceived its subtle energies. As we move up the spiral, two types of development became increasingly distanced and the materialist side developed more intensely. As we move further up, we find that materialist technological civilization reached a level where, by using the methods of new physics, people could access subtle energies on the basis of scientific research. Although, Einstein already said fields govern the behavior of particles, it was only the research of the last 30 years that could access the subtle energy fields that people had sensed for thousands of years but were unable to study and explain for lack of adequate instruments.

Today, however, the latest findings of physics prove that we have transcended the materialist thinking of the last 300 years. The latest research shows that the universe consists not only of matter but also of what is called 'energy planes', energy that radiates in the form of waves. Indeed, organisms are variously dense wavefields. At the same time, by virtue of the fact that different types of waves emanate from the same energy field, all creatures connected with each other.

For a scientific explanation of this phenomenon we shall quote briefly from the work of Ervin Laszlo. Laszlo,[1] like a number of other leading scientists, suggests the concept of *quantum vacuum* to resolve the anomalies of Darwinist biology and psychology. The quantum vacuum is the primordial phenomenon of the cosmos and can account for the remarkable connections that are otherwise inexplicable by science.

The quantum vacuum contains energy of an amazing density. Wheeler estimated its matter equivalent at 10^{94} gram per cubic centimeter, which means that the energy contained in the vacuum is not only equal to the total quantity of energy in the matter but, according to calculations by David Bohm, exceeds it by about 10^{40} times.[2]

The quantum vacuum is not empty space. It is a significant element of the universe and it may be expected that in some way it should participate in all processes of the universe. The effects of the quantum vacuum appear in all the fields of the universe.

Fields exist in a curious form: their impact is observable, but they themselves are not. In this respect, they may be compared to a superfine net. If the threads of the net are finer than is visible to the naked eye, you cannot perceive the net itself. You might, however, be able to see the knots where certain threads intersect. It appears as if there were knots hovering in the air, even though they are connected by threads. Thus if one knot moves, the others shift as well. Therefore if we notice that the movement of one knot is related to that of the others, we must assume that they are connected by an extended net.

Fields can also store and transmit information. The above mentioned anomalies indicate that there is lasting information storage in nature. An effect (information) which has once emerged in one place and time, re-appears in other places and times. In physics, this is called 'temporal non-locality'. This means that the universe has memory. This, however, cannot exist in a vacuum: in empty space.

Laszlo claims that the subquantum field stores and transmits information in a holographic manner. In this way the memory of nature presupposes a holographic field for storing and transmitting information. Thus the vacuum is a connecting holo-field. The existence of this field resolves the anomalies experienced in physics, biology and other natural sciences.

Laszlo first called the subquantum field 'psi-field'; and then he called it the Akasha dimension. The Greek letter Ψ (psi) refers to the factor that complements Schrödinger's psi-function. At the same time, it refers to the connection between organisms to each other and to their environment. It connects people's consciousness as discovered in psychology and the epistemic sciences, including the mysterious connections known as 'psi-phenomena'. See Laszlo's books *Science and the Akashic Field*[3] and *The Akashic Experience.*[4]

The Role and Transmission of Information in Living Organisms

The importance of the role of information is evident throughout the living world. Bruce Lipton[5] described how the operation of the brain and the nervous system creates high-level connections among cells. Experiments prove that the brain is capable of emitting parallel impulses simultaneously from different cerebral regions. The synchronization of these impulses is extremely important. Scientists have investigated how fast we can co-ordinate the different areas of the body. Results have shown that when our mind begins to work and starts emitting waves, they are sent at a higher speed than cells could transmit through neural connections. The experiments have shown that the brain communicates beyond the level of neurotransmission in the nervous system.

Dietmar Cimbal[6] claims that the human body is a conglomerate of information organized within an energy field. This energy field is composed of scalar waves and it stores a tremendous amount of information. It is with the help of informational fields that the regulation of the body and its cells becomes possible. The human organism functions with the help of these informational fields.

According to the new scientific concept, the functioning of the human body is based not so much on the biochemical co-ordination of molecules, cells, tissues, organs and systems of organs, as on the exchange of biochemical, electromagnetic and quantum information.

Every organism has its own, localized information field connected with the localized fields of all other organisms in the world, just as all quanta are in instant connection with all other quanta. This is what spatial non-locality means in science. Living organisms are in contact with each other not only externally, but intrinsically. They are manifestations of a unified holographic field.

The holographic field is the internet of the natural world. Contact between healer and patient occurs through the transmission of quantum-level information. Thus the distance between healer and patient has no effect on the information transfer. Remote healing is physically possible.

The Role of Information in the Functioning of the Living Organism

The organism consists of particles which cohere to form atoms and molecules, which, in turn constitute cells, tissues and organs, and finally the living organism. Every part of the organism has both a material and an informational aspect.

In regard to the material aspect, quantum particles conglom-

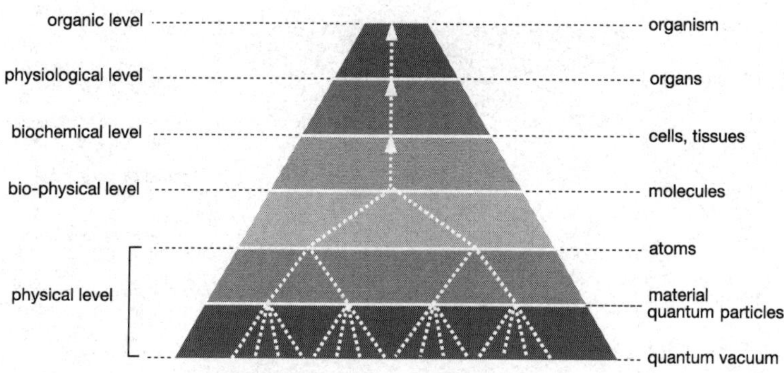

Figure 1. The material aspect and hierarchy of the emergence of the living organism

erate into atoms, atoms into molecules, cells into tissues, these into organs, and the organs into organisms *(Figure 1)*. In regard to the informational aspect we recognize that on the various levels of organization self-organizing processes take place as wave-frequencies of the components enter into phase. In this way coherence is created on multiple levels. According to Folker Meissner,[7] this coherence is a vast information system in which the exchange of information among every single cell guarantees that every cell knows what is happening to all the other cells. If this coherence fails to come about, the organism falls apart. Death is the disintegration of the coherence of the organism.

The decisive role and the importance of information increases at each successive level of organization. On the physical level, for instance, the role of the kind of information that connects quanta to atoms is far smaller than the role of the information that ensures the coherence of the level responsible for interconnecting organs into the living organism. *(Figure 2)*

Biology and classical medicine study the physical and biological processes that ensure the coherence of living organisms. The informational sciences, however, also examine the kind of information that governs biochemical and physical processes.

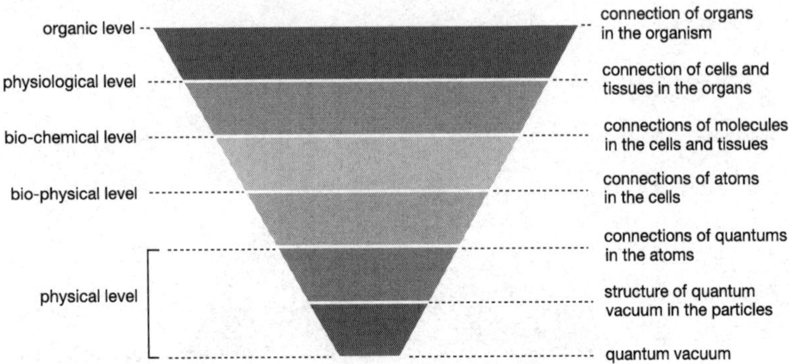

Figure 2. The decisive importance of information in connection

Just as on the internet you get the information that you used on entering the system, also molecules and cells are organized according to the information encoded in them.

Every living creature has its own unique character in terms of the information that governs it. Within this information we distinguish different layers, including the general information characteristic of the species. Within the organism, organs are governed by the information characteristic of them, and by the information characteristic of the individual. It is the general information that allows, for instance, for organ transplant, but at the same time it is also what causes difficulty because, due to the individuality of information, the body can reject the organ that has been transplanted.

The biochemical mechanisms of the organism are governed by information. Researchers realized this when they saw that giving a living organism different information makes it function differently. The biochemical process can be changed by information. For instance, as regards cancer, it has been pointed out that the problem is caused by the way in which the cells communicate with each other, i.e. by a block in the information flow. Dr Pier Mario Biava[8] discovered that cancerous cells can be transformed into healthy cells if the cancerous cells come in contact with proteins that carry the right kind of information.

What Happens If a Living Organism 'Breaks Down', i.e. Becomes Sick?

In order to answer this question, the medical sciences that developed over the past 300 years on the basis of biology and chemistry examined biochemical processes and identified their shortcomings. The information sciences, in turn, examine the connections that sustain life-functions through information in the organism. When something is not working properly in the living organism, classical medicine treats the molecule itself through allopathic medications. These alter and rectify the operation of the organs with the help of biochemical substances. Information medicine does not interfere with biochemical processes but merely changes the information that organizes them. In the case of functional disturbances, faulty biochemical processes can be changed in this manner; it is not necessary to address the biochemical molecule itself. Today, a number of researchers and healers (Fraser, Lipton, Cimbal[9]) claim that disease is merely an insufficiency of the information flow in the information system – it is flawed information. If we can access the appropriate information, we can eliminate the disease.

Every method of information medicine assists healing by rectifying the problems of information caused by pathogenic processes. Of all the innumerable methods of information medicine, I mention classic homeopathy as an example, as it works on this principle. In the case of high potencies, the homeopathic remedy introduces the information of the molecules into the body through a carrying substance. The healing information may be carried by water, an alcoholic solution, a sugar tablet, etc. (It must be noted, however, that the biochemical materials which are responsible for the nourishment of the body – in other words, the material aspect – do need to be introduced into the body: food cannot be replaced by the information on food.)

To use a metaphor from information technology, if something in our computer is not working properly, there are two possible solutions. One is that we take out the hard drive and replace it with another that is intact. In this case we are acting like a surgeon because after this operation the electrons run through the printed circuit in the modified way. The other solution is to rewrite the program. The program represents the information. When we rectify the program we are 'merely' changing the information; we don't need to take the computer itself to pieces.

There are multiple levels through which we can co-operate and interact with a complex system. There are material or physical interventions and there are informational interventions. There are cases where the computer is chronically malfunctioning which means that we need to replace the hard drive. In the case of a living organism this is when people say you need to cut out a cancerous growth or transplant an organ. At other times, when there are minor functional difficulties, no such intervention is required; it is enough to change the information, in other words, to provide the kind of information that restores normal functioning *(Table 1)*.

Table 1. A comparison of the elements of traditional and information medicine

Modern mainstream medicine	Information medicine
Examines and treats connections constituting life-functions through biological units	Examines and treats connections constituting life-functions through the information of biological units
Disease: faulty structure of biological systems	Disease: the fault of the information connecting biological units
Treatment: cure sick biological units by applying biochemical substances	Treatment: strengthening the immune system and rectify sick, faulty information

Subtle Energies and Information

The effect of subtle energies has been known since ancient times. Different cultures have used different types for purposes of healing and gaining strength. These include minerals, metals, the symbols of ancient cultures, physical movements representing symbols, the shape of rune powers, sounds, colors, acupuncture or, to take some methods from the modern age, homeopathy or Bach's flower remedies. This list is, of course, far from complete.

The action mechanisms of these symbols have not been studied in the past with the scientific methodology we use today, but people did work out and apply experiential methods that worked perfectly well. If we classify the methods according to the information carrier, we find that there are material substances (precious stones, stones), plants and shapes, body exercises, and impulses exercised on the body, such as stimulating reflex zones or acupuncture, and there are methods of a mental nature, such as positive thinking, prayer, and meditation.

What these methods have in common is that they convey information that corrects the flawed information causing disease and thus strengthens the immune system and activates self-healing processes that then lead to cure.

As Körbler has noted, it took a long time before the subtle-energetic resonance of substances was accepted by science. The science of the modern age did not focus on explaining these phenomena, as it lacked the instruments which could have measured information on the level of subtle energies. This is despite the fact that Le Bon demonstrated over a hundred years ago in France that all substances exposed to light emanate specific waves. He pointed out that this radiation behaves in the same way as radiant heat, light and electricity. His discovery inspired research in a number of countries until some months later another Frenchman, physicist Becquerel, announced a discovery that 'refuted' Le Bon's claim. Becquerel used stilpnosiderite in a mine that had never been exposed to sunlight, and found that the same radiation was present– he discovered hard rays. After this no one was interested in Le Bon's discovery: the fine information found in light and ultraviolet (UV) rays. Leading physicists have been active in nuclear physics and studied hard radiation. In the field of healing, research by Carl Ludwig Schleich, Georges Lakhoushy and Wilhelm Reich seen as mere chimeras, postulated the instruments needed for their measurement. It is worth mentioning the work of anatomist Carl Ludwig Schleich who assumed that resonances inside the body have their own information content. In his book *Vom Schaltwerk der Gedanken* [Connections of Thinking], published in Berlin in 1917, he described patients who could, by using mental powers and imagination, achieve what they wanted, for example, produce rashes or ulcers on their body within a matter of minutes, and could also make them disappear the same way. This led him to the conclusion that the malfunctions of tissues are caused by specific messages. Today we know that these phenomena are the result of communicational interactions above the physical level and belong to the psychosomatic sphere of medicine.

It was about 30 years ago that scientific development reached the point where an increasing number of physicists turned attention toward studying subtle effects. More and more began to ask what it was that is effective in homeopathic high potencies, even though over a dilution of D23 they contained not a single molecule of the original substance. According to one hypothesis, the pattern of the electric and magnetic fields characteristic of the original substance is transferred to a carrying substance (water + alcohol or lactose balls) and thus preserved.

In order to establish the scientific basis of the effect of homeopathy, scientists continued their investigation of dissipative, complex, open systems with high-sensitivity technical instruments. In *Scientific Foundations of Homeopathy, G. Resch and V. Gutmann*[10] describe the quantum structure of molecules and the way in which they may be influenced by information. Information is seen as 'indivisible, similarly to light and matter, rather than restricted to certain points or areas'. How material information affects the human organism was described by H. Klima, researcher for the Nuclear Institute of Austrian Universities at the March 1989 session of the International Academy of the Medical Sciences in Vienna:

> Living organisms (plant, animal or human) respond even to morphogenetically effective impulses of very low intensity and alter their coherent individual state. From a biophysical point of view, electromagnetic interactions are predominant in biological systems. This means that it is mostly electromagnetic signals that the organism registers as morphogenetic impulses. Thus, for instance, light as electromagnetic energy or in a chemically bound form not only transports energy to the plant or animal organism but also acts as a bioregulator. Even in small doses, depending on the wavelength, it can trigger germination or budding, cause cell multiplication or cell differentiation (even in human cells), stimulate or limit tissue growth, and influence the healing process in pathogenic conditions. Today we can show that in the course of immune defense reactions during the phagocytosis stage, the human organism emits low-intensity morphogenetically effective light in the 633 nanometer domain without amplification as visible light.[11]

Science today has reached the stage where it can measure and record the reactions of the human organism to subtle-energy inputs. Infrared radiation and thermography make it possible to measure the heat emitted by the human body as electromagnetic heat radiation in a space-time domain. This enables doctors to gain new information about the health of their patients.

The effects of medicines, drugs or anything that we come into contact became observable as well. The Institute of General Electrotechnology at Vienna University performed an innovative experiment in which Körbler himself acted as subject. He held the tip of his right index finger at a distance of 10 mm from a micro-heat-sensor specially developed for the purpose, and with the tip of his left index finger he touched a cigarette. Within a few thousandths of a second the instrument indicated an increase of 0.03 °C in body temperature. Similar experiments with other subjects and different instruments were equally successful. They showed that the human body responds even to extremely subtle radiations.

It also suggests how the healing methods of the past could be so effective; like healing powers of precious stones that doctors in India used for thousands of years, as well as the laying on of hands, and spiritual methods such as positive thinking, meditation, acupuncture, laser therapies, ozone, Singulette, oxygen and color therapies, Bach flower therapy, homeopathy, and a number of other methods. What all of these have in common is that they generate a radiation of a wavelength 633 nanometer in the body, and beyond producing a local effect, they regulate and stimulate the immune system.

It also proves that soft radiations can have unwelcome effects on the living organism. Certain geological radiations can increase the risk of cancer, and plants may affect people unfavorably. But how can we establish which of the subtle energies are useful and which are harmful for the organism? For this we need to define the content of the information carried by the substance.

Körbler focused his attention on the content of subtle-energy information.

The elements that surround us – earth, air, water, and living organisms, etc – all emit subtle energies in the form of high frequency terahertz waves. The reactions of our organism are complex and manifold. Körbler called it 'material information'. He started his research in the early 1980s and spent about 10 years on mapping out the regularities, influences, and their measurable features. At that time there were no instruments that could measure or graphically represent the contents of the information carried by such high-frequency domains.

Looking for methods to use, after many years of experimentation, Körbler found the 'magic wand' that was used for thousands of years. Applying sophisticated methods, he developed the wand into a sensitive hand-held tool, the dowsing rod. The movements of this rod give reliable indications of how harmful or how useful various high-frequency radiations for the organism are. He published his discoveries in *Raum und Zeit* as experiments that people could perform with the dowsing rod themselves.

Through further research and improvement of the dowsing rod, he found what he had been looking for: the vertical dowsing rod that provides data about the actual content of the information carried by a substance. This stand-up bio-indicator shows significant radial and transverse movements that come about while testing various substances, and this helps to decode the information content of high frequency radiations (see Chapter 4).

Körbler's next discovery was in the exploration of the electromagnetic field. He found that in the tremendously high frequency band, that is in the terahertz domain, even small differences in conductivity value become perceptible. A graphite pencil line has a different conductivity value than paper; a line drawn on a piece of paper works as an antenna for resonances, absorbing and emitting information.

If we draw a line on paper (or on the skin), we notice that it is surrounded by a typical field distribution. The ends of the line carry opposing polarities, and as a result, stationary electric and magnetic waves arise in the medium (i.e. the line on the paper), and this wave pattern continues far beyond the line. If we change the basic shape of the line, creating the letter L, the fields become correspondingly dense and thin around the angle and produce multiple similar shapes.

It soon became clear that Körbler had discovered a systemic principle for analyzing the distribution of fields and their polarity in both material substances and the organism. His experiments showed that the content of the information is defined by configuration, i.e. the molecular structure of the substances.

He also proved that in the domain of very high frequencies, symbols act as 'radiesthetic' connecting elements, and with their help we can purposively manipulate their information content. In this way we can enhance, weaken, or alter the effect of electromagnetic radiation on substances. By using this principle, Körbler developed the method named New Homeopathy.

Chapter 2

The Scientific Background of New Homeopathy

Körbler had spent more than ten years experimenting, researching, healing and lecturing before he finally set out to formulate and identify his healing method. A number of research institutions and leading scientists helped him with his experiments and exploring the impact of his method. These included the Austrian Society for Electromagnetic Bio-information of the Nuclear Institute of Universities in Vienna; Professor König, head of the Vienna Acupuncture Department; a research team headed by physicist professor Dr Beth at the Ludwig Maximilian University at Munich; the Max Planck Institute in North Germany, Professor Dr Hartmann and biophoton researcher professor Fritz Albert Popp, to mention only a few.

The name he gave to his method and its presentation in 18 installments is based on the research he carried out over the previous ten years. In the name 'New Homeopathy', Körbler referred to Hippocrates and Hahnemann.

Two and a half thousand years ago Hippocrates had summarized his observations in 60 medical treaties, claiming that 'most diseases could be cured through the same factors that caused their emergence'. This rule was confirmed 200 years ago by Hahnemann's discovery when he created the dilution system of homeopathy and, by doing so, introduced a method of treatment that proved effective ever since.

Körbler believed that Hahnemann discovered the electromagnetic transfer and impact mechanisms without being aware of it at the level of the science of his time. Hahnemann published his system of treatment in 1796; *Organon* appeared in 1810[1]; while the description of electromagnetic energies based on the experiments and theories of Faraday[2] and Maxwell[3,4] in the 19th century appeared between 1832 and 1873. Contemporary science clearly demonstrated the effect of electromagnetic (EM) waves on the living organism.

Körbler's method is based on the observations of Hippocrates and Hahnemann, but he went one step further and made it his point of departure that special electromagnetic impulses can be either pathogenic or healing factors for the organism.

This finding is the basis for distinguishing the effect of various EM impulses and information on the human body, identifying the types of radiation that can affect a living organism in a way that promotes its health and development, and those that are pathogenic.

The Role of Electromagnetic Waves

Körbler considered it important to draw attention to the fact that the laws of the theory of electromagnetism are of decisive importance for the functioning of the organism.

In the years after his death in 1994, classical electromagnetic theory has gone through a fundamental change. Experiments with measuring instruments have led biophysicists to conclude that the living organism reacts even to subtle impulses that cannot be explained by Maxwell's theory.

Some of these are weak impulses. According to the classical theory, cells do not respond to these impulses below their sensitivity level. However, the organism do respond even to impulses where electromagnetic waves are so flat that they are not believed to have impact.

Subtle energies are transmitted by *scalar waves* that have magnitude but do not convey *vectorial energy*.

According to the classical notion, an external energy source produces a flow in energies that affects all bodies. In other words, energy affects the body that absorbs it: A affects B, the law of cause and effect. When information is transferred the scalar wave outside the body enters into interaction with the wave emitted in the body. If the two waves are in the same frequency domain, *adaptive resonance* emerges between them, and the information stored in the external energy source is transferred to the wave field emitted by the body.

Distant interactions in quantum physics were discovered in the micro-dimansion and it was believed that they do not exist in the macro-dimension. In the past several decades, however, it was discovered that they occur not only in the macro-dimension accessible to us, but even in the cosmological dimension. What has so far been called the 'non-locality of quanta' exists also in the dimension of atoms, molecules, cells, organisms, and even in the astronomical dimension. This demonstrates a previously unrecognized level of coherence in all dimensions of the universe.[5]

According to the current view, the living organism is not a classical biochemical system but a non-classical, non-local, so-called macroscopic quantum system that emits constant wave fields and interacts with the wave fields around it. A macroscopic quantum system is not a passive object obeying external impulses, but like a radio transceiver, is in constant interaction with other systems around it. Of all these interactions, a measurable effect is produced by those that the ones resonate with the corresponding wave fields.

The discoveries made since Körbler's death have supported his discovery that the regulation of living organisms on the subtle-energy level takes place partly in the nanometer domain of EM waves. Such extremely high sensitivity can only be represented in quantum physics. Understanding and applying these laws has led to the emergence of a new methodology in medicine that is able to influence organisms through minute changes in wave radiations.

New Homeopathy has introduced a radically new practice in medicine. It takes into account the subtle energies, radiations and information that come from the outside and influence the organism, including its immune system.

The Thermodynamics of Living Organisms

Theories that look on development as the key to the unification of the different disciplines take note of the fact that over time nature builds into increasingly complex forms. Developmental processes are continuous, even though they can be abrupt and non-linear.

Elemental particles cohere into atoms, atoms into molecules, and molecules into crystals. The molecules then join to form macromolecules and these join to build more complex, cell-like structures related to life, and eventually cells build multicell organisms and these constitute social and ecological systems. It is not necessary and not even reasonable that all these organizational processes should obey separate rules. The same basic rules, acting as nature's 'algorithms' may create the dynamics of interaction on which complexity in nature unfolds from the particle level to the level of living organisms. These basic laws of development hold sway in all domains of nature.

In the 1950s, as part of his investigations, Erwin Schrödinger discovered the relevance of the Second Law of Thermodynamics. According to the Second Law, in a closed system the amount of heat represented by the movement of atoms evens out due to collisions in their movement.

In the terminology of physics, the processes taking place in closed systems are 'work'. Work can only take place in an energy flow. The flow ends when the processes that created it cease: when the differences in the levels become equalized. A system is able to do work when there is a difference in its heat or concentrations. These store the energy required for work. This can be defined in reference to entropy. Where differences in energy levels are maximal, entropy is minimal, i.e. the system is capable of performing work. Where the differences are equalized, entropy is maximal; there are no energy flows in the system and the system cannot perform work.

When a closed physical system performs work, it moves in the direction of the equalization of heat concentration and ultimately reaches a state of equilibrium. Living organisms, by contrast, do not 'stop working' since they replace their spent energy with free energy.

In 1947 Ilya Prigogine[6] wrote his doctoral dissertation on the behavior of systems far from equilibrium, and in the early 1960s Aharon Katchalsky and P. F. Curran developed the mathematical foundations of non-equilibrium thermodynamics.[7] They showed that classical thermodynamics cannot explain evolutionary processes in open systems. In the real world non-equilibrium systems develop in non-linear processes and are open to free energies from their environment. They absorb negative entropy (free energy) and emit or dissipate entropy. Such systems are the basis of life. As Schrödinger noted in the middle of the 20th century, 'life feeds on negative entropy.'

Since open systems far from thermodynamic equilibrium dissipate entropy while performing work, Prigogine called them 'dissipative systems'. Systems of this kind are in a steady state when the 'negentropy' [negative entropy] absorbed from the environment is equal to the entropy produced within, and they may also grow and become more complex – if the negentropy carried by their importation of fresh energy exceeds the entropy produced within the systems.

The living organism is a so-called open, dissipative system that dissipates the entropy it produces into the environment and absorbs free energy, i.e. *negative entropy*. This is only possible if there is a constant energy flow from the environment. On our planet this is granted by solar energy and forms the basis of life. The organism, although it performs work and produces entropy, replaces the energy it uses with free energy, so that its total entropy does not increase.

When the organism is growing, its entropy decreases. Körbler believed that besides food and air, electromagnetic waves in the nanometer domain also act as sources of free energy.

The Discovery of Chaotic Attractors

In 1963 the American meteorologist Edward Lorenz, in attemption to simulate the world's weather on a computer, in applying the formula 'Z2 + C (constant) = Z′ discovered the so-called 'chaotic attractors'. The science of digital non-linear systems was born. Then the way in which order and coherence appear organisms became clear. It became clear that under the slightest external change, a chaotic systems shifts from one condition to another at crucial points of bifurcation.

The easiest way to imagine a chaotic attractor is the following. Whirling water is turbulent and turbulence is one of the forms of chaos. Let us observe the movement of an object in a whirlpool, for example a leaf. If we shine a light on it, the leaf will show a circular motion in the water, and this we can capture for example by a time-exposure in a camera. The longer the exposure, the more accurately the many individually varying circular paths will conform to an overall pattern. That pattern is the chaotic attractor of the system. If we disturb the surface of the water, for instance by throwing a small pebble into it, the floating leaf may quit its trajectory and either assume a different circular trajectory, or may leave the whirlpool altogether. This models the sensitivity of a system governed by a chaotic attractor to even the smallest disturbance.

The human organism can be modeled by chaotic attractors, the same as all open systems. Systems of this kind are extremely sensitive: if the initial condition of the developmental process of the system changes, or the process is disturbed if only to an immeasurably small extent, the processes in the system will be measurably altered.

Chaotic attractors are also known as butterfly attractors, since the trajectory described by the world weather system modelled by Lorentz had the shape of a butterfly with spread wings. Even minuscule alterations in that system produced a shift of trajectory from one of the wings of the butterfly to the other, demonstrating the ultra-sensitivy of the world weather system to changes in the environment.

The Role of Information

As Laszlo shows in *The Connectivity Hypothesis*,[8] the exchange of information between living organisms and the outside world takes place in interaction with a complex field. Every particle of the body is capable of working as an antenna; it receives and emits waves. Since it is embedded in the body, we can change the reception and emission of waves by inserting a geometric symbol. This is the essence of New Homeopathy. Under the influence of the inserted geometric symbol, the wave emitted by the body assumes different characteristics.

This influence may create dramatic morphological changes in the system. The system may change in a positive or a negative direction. Small impacts occur either through direct contact or as a result of electromagnetic waves in the nanometer domain, or else by absorbing information beyond the electromagnetic domain. This is shown by the effect on viruses. Russian scientists proved over 40 years ago, by easily repeatable experiments, that electromagnetic waves can cause and spread disease. They separated two identical cell cultures with a thin sheet of glass, and they infected one culture with a virus that caused a pathogenic condition. The other culture also developed the pathology. The cause was not the virus itself but its information, namely the change in the electromagnetic wave. This shows that the primary component in the functioning of the immune system is the interaction between electromagnetic waves and information. The chemical reaction to the interaction only comes second.

The Principle of Coherence

Every living organism is a thermodynamically open dissipative system. During transitions from one phase to another, in a state far from equilibrium, the elements of such systems show co-operative behavior. Coherence in the system describes this behavior, this means the coincidence of the phase of the waves emitted in a system, or between diverse systems.

For a long time it was believed that in the macroscopic domains of the world there is no coherence of this kind. This is not the case. It has been discovered that the kind of coherence characteristic of quanta in the microscopic domain also exists among complex macromolecules, cells and living organisms. Experiments performed by Eric A. Cornell, Wolfgang Ketterle and Carl E. Wieman in 1995, which in 2001 won them the Nobel Prize in Physics, proved this fact.[9,10] The experiments show that under certain conditions separate particles and atoms can mutually penetrate each other like waves and create an interference pattern.

In 2007, Gregory Engel and his colleagues[11] demonstrated that the kind of coherence characteristic of quanta appear in the case of *Chlorobiaceae bacteria.* Just like an 'energy cable', the chromosome that collects light become connected to the reaction center of the bacterium. Without this wave-type transmission created by quantum coherence there could not be photosynthesis, the basis of all life on the planet. Living organisms could not have evolved, nor could they be functioning. The human body is built of approximately 10^{14} (100 000 000 000 000) cells, and in every cell 10,000 bio-electrochemical reactions take place every second. Every night more than 10^{12} (1 000 000 000 000) cells die and the same number are replaced. The concerted regulation of such an amazing number of cells in the organism and their supply with complex electromagnetic and chemical information cannot be explained by physical and chemical interactions. Information transmission in the human body is highly effective (for example, in the epigenetic system) but the propagation velocity of the processes and their information content exceed the range of physical and chemical interactions. Signals carrying information cannot travel faster in the nervous system than approximately 22 m/s. However, the cells of living organisms are in nearly-instant, complex, heterogeneous, and multilevel connection with each other. This suggests the quantum-thype coherence of the living body.

The Coherent Evolution of Living Organisms

The fact that biological organisms could develop on our planet indicates that coherence is a universal trait in the world. In the case of living organisms this also extends to the entire organism, including its genetic pool.

There is both statistical and experimental evidence to the effect that the genetic information encoded in the organism is in permanent interaction with the organism. Contrary to classical Darwinian theory, the genetic pool does not mutate randomly, independently of changes in the body. This is important because otherwise the chances for the emergence of complex organisms would be extremely low. The number of possible genetic recombination is so large, that the emergence of viable species through accidental processes would require far longer than the time that was available for evolutionary processes on Earth. The development of feathers, for instance, does not bring about the emergence of a reptile that can fly; it also calls for radical changes in muscle and bone structure. The development of the eye requires thousands of mutations finely tuned with each other. The likelihood of random mutations bringing about a positive result is negligible. Statistically, only one in every 20 million mutations is likely to produce a viable outcome, in itself, each mutation is more likely to reduce rather than improve the fitness of the species.

Another argument against accidental mutations producing viable organisms is the finding that complex organisms are 'irreducibly complex'. The parts of irreducibly complex systems are connected to each other in such a way that removing (or altering) any part of the system breaks down the whole system. For an irreducibly complex organism to mutate and remain viable, all parts need to retain their functional relationship to all the others throughout the entire process of mutation. According to microbiologist Michael Behe[12], it is highly unlikely that this could have been achieved by accidental mutations among the elements of the gene-pool of living organisms.

Chapter 3

The Conceptual Foundations of New Homeopathy

New Homeopathy belongs to the field of *complementary medicine,* and its method can be applied along with all other natural healing and curing methods. It examines the organism from a new perspective which even Western-type medicine is beginning to take into account, even if it does not apply it in daily practice. This new perspective is the reaction of the organism to the subtle-energetic impulses coming from its environment. Examining the communication of the organism on the level of subtle energies enables us to explain a number of traditional healing methods and suggests possibilities of combined application.

New Homeopathy does not aspire to replace Western mainstream medicine, since in the case of acute danger it is primarily the biochemical balance of the organism that needs to be restored. However, it does look for openings where a cure can be promoted more successfully by activating the self-healing processes of the organism based on communication on the subtle-energy level. It presents the possibility of altering information through the role played by the internal micro-formal structures of the organism and puts the use of external geometric symbols in the service of a cure. In order to understand the various aspects of curing by altering and transmitting information, we need to examine the mechanisms of absorbing information and transmitting information inside the living organism.

Körbler lead us step by step to an understanding of this mechanism. Out of all the commonly known biophysical and biochemical aspects of the functioning and metabolism of the cell, the smallest unit of the organism, he only highlighted the ones that he found important for an explanation and understanding of his method. These range from the subtle-energetic communication of cells to the coherent functioning of the organism.

How Information is Absorbed through Electromagnetic Waves

Körbler demonstrated:

- the definitive role of geometric symbols;
- the way in which cells absorb subtle energies by water molecules in the cell, transforming themselves into new geometric symbols;
- the role that electric processes play in maintaining optimal cell tension and, thereby, health;
- the role of electromagnetic regulation in body functions;
- the primary role of electromagnetic processes in the emergence of disease, particularly viral infections;
- the electromagnetic aspects of the operation of the immune system;
- the wavelength range of the functions of our organism between 1020 and 100 nm;
- the possibility of abrupt change taking place in this domain as a result of an energy input in the range of Planck's coefficient, i.e. *the quantum potential*[1];
- channels on the cell membrane that have been discovered to serve the transmission of information;
- the conditions for the impact to take place when the organism is in an unstable state, i.e. at a bifurcation point.

By demonstrating these things, Körbler has created a new medicine to complement Western mainstream medicine. Knowing and understanding these things is crucial if we wish to decide the level of intervention we need in the case of different pathologies. We need to decide how far biochemical support is necessary, if at all, and what kind of techniques need to be applied on the level of information and subtle energies. In the following section we will describe the most important teaching, considerations and methodological aspects offered by Körbler in the order in which he taught it at his Budapest seminars between 1991 and 1993.

Electric and Electromagnetic Effects in the Cell

For a deeper understanding of dissipative systems (i.e. open systems far from thermodynamic equilibrium) we will look at the changes which take place under a subtle-energy input to the smallest unit of living organisms, the cell. We will also look at the resulting electric processes.

The human body consists of cells, and cells consist of molecules. In each cell there are about 10^{12} water molecules. These are in constant electromagnetic contact with each other. Keeping the human organism alive requires constant absorption of information and energy. In the absence of these, and in line with the Second Law of Thermodynamics, the entropy of the organism will grow and life processes will sooner or later end. Atoms consist of particles which are sensitive to quantum effects. If the atom is hit by a wave of radiant energy the particles will react to it and the atom will enter an excited state. In other words, the trajectory of the electrons around the nucleus of the atom will be altered. In the living organism every single atom is in an excited state. This is why a constant absorption of energy is required, partly to sustain this state of excitation, and partly to transmit energy (radiation) and scatter it in the environment.

For a new chain of atoms, i.e. a molecule, to emerge, energy is required. A molecule can emerge if there is sufficient energy introduced into the free electrons around the atoms. Beyond this minimal energy requirement the cell requires the electromagnetic input for the tension in it to emerge and be preserved.

A cell is only able to reproduce itself if it is provided with energy from the outside, since its reproduction calls for zones of tension. The energy coming from the outside triggers dynamic processes inside the cell that take place with the mediation of water molecules. If conditions change, for example the temperature goes up, the thermodynamics of the molecules will also change and so will the specific vibration pattern of the cell. The new resonance pattern will create a new interaction between the cell and the organism. The new resonance pattern also needs to guarantee an adaptive resonance between the cell and the rest of the organism. In a healthy cell this does take place and contributes to the coherence of the organism. If this fails to take place then the survival of the cell itself occurs at the cost of damage to the organism; in other words, a pathogenic process is set off.

The Function of Water Molecules in the Cell

Water is the chief constituent of all living organisms. For instance, jellyfish and certain algae contain 98% water; the body of an adult human being contains 60% water; our blood contains 80% water, and 70–75% of our brain, muscles, and liver, and 20% of our bones are made of water. Water is actually a mineral that acts as a liquid within a certain temperature zone. In this state water molecules are very active. Structures within the cell are determined by dipolar water molecules. The water molecule consists of one atom of oxygen with a negative charge and two atoms of hydrogen with a positive charge. These constituents are at an angle of 104° to each other. The negative charge of the oxygen atom is stronger than the positive charge of the hydrogen atoms; therefore if a positive ion arrives in the water as a result of an external influence, the oxygen atoms will arrange themselves around the positive ion. If the charge of this ion is strong, water molecules will arrange themselves not in one, but even two or three rings, in a spherical form. Radiation coming from the outside, however, introduces not a single ion, but an arrangement of positive charges. Thus, the density of the water molecules arranging themselves around the positive ions will produce a varied array of formations, appearing as holes in Swiss cheese.

Some molecule connections are denser; others are sparser. Wherever the charge of the positive ion is not strong enough to bind the water molecules, the connection of these molecules will be unstable. Under the influence of a new impact from the outside, i.e. if the pattern of charges is altered, the water molecules will rearrange themselves in a new formation (these formations are called 'clusters'). A constant that is about 80 times higher than the 'dielectric' constant of air, the emergence of hydrogen bridges, and the resulting heat is the foundation of these gigantic 'chemical factories'. The change in the structure of water takes place at 37 °C because this is the temperature at which water molecules are least stable. Normal body temperature fluctuates around 37 °C. At this temperature it is easy to introduce new information into water molecules with minimal energy; through electromagnetic waves information can be introduced into the cells of the body.

The molecular structures that emerge through the process determine the influence of the radiation arriving at the cell from the outside, as they determine whether the electromagnetic and other rays do or do not affect the cell.

The role and significance of this quality of water molecules is shown by the fact that water makes up about 82% of the cells of the human body. Other components of the cell are the following: proteins 2%; fats 3%; complex carbohydrates 1%; small organic molecules 0.4%; and inorganic molecules and iodine 0.5%. In the case of protein molecules, for example, there are about 200,000 water molecules for every protein molecule. In other words, around every protein molecule there is a construction of water molecules. This structure becomes active under the influence of energy from the outside and grounds the electromagnetic conditions required for the chemical reactions in the cell.

The information content that emerges in the cells is based on the various formations of water molecules. It plays a crucial role in the immune system of the body.

Since Körbler's death there have been a number of biophysical research projects that have shown that water molecules of the living cell play a far more important role in life than it was believed in the past. The water in our organism is not identical with the 'ordinary' water existing outside our organism. Body water has a different structure and dynamics, and it is due to this special structure and dynamics that water significantly contributes to the coherence of the organism. This is why no living organism can exist without water. In the following section we describe the results of relevant researches based on explorations by leading researchers Emilio Del Giudice and his colleagues.[2]

For decades, liquid water has been considered a collection of molecules bound by static short-range forces, such as hydrogen bonds. This single-state concept of liquid water has been challenged in recent years: it appears that it can assume a wide variety of states. Alternative states can be generated by irradiation with electromagnetic waves by the introduction of inert materials, the dissolution of fullerenes (a form of carbon), as well as by exposing water to biological processes.

This finding is consistent with quantum electrodynamics (QED). QED foresees the appearance of diverse 'coherence domains' in water, each with a specific electromagnetic field. Water in the living organism has a specific coherence domain, and biomolecules in the organism resonate with the frequency of this domain. Every intake of energy changes the frequency of the domain, creating an effective coupling between water and its surroundings.

It appears that the ensemble of electromagnetic waves released during a biochemical cycle in the organism is imprinted in the water contained in that organism. There is a close interaction between the biochemistry of the organism and the electrodynamics of the water it contains. The organism 'informs' the water, and the informed water affects the whole organism (as well as normal water and various inorganic materials). This transfer of information occurs without the expenditure of any conventional form of energy.

The bi-directional transfer of information between the living organism and water within that organism harmonizes the phase of the frequencies of the various parts of the organism, thereby contributing to the non-local coherence of the whole organism. The findings coming to light in the biophysics of water, together with the puzzles confronting molecular and genetic determinism, corroborate Hans Fröhlich's bold hypothesis that all parts of the living system create fields at various frequencies that infuse the whole organism. Through informed water, the specific resonance frequency of every molecule and cell in the living organism is harmonized, and long-range phase correlations come about similar to those that occur in superfluidity and superconductivity.

The Electric Function of the Cell Membrane

The difference in electric potential between the interior and the exterior of a biological cell is the *membrane potential.* In a 'state of equilibrium' when all the forces are balanced out, the difference in the voltage between the inside and the outside of the cell is between -60--70 mV. It is called the resting potential. Internal electric processes must be in order for the required ion exchanges to take place.

A healthy cell membrane is an excellent insulator, better than anything humans could create. This means that fundamentally the structure of the cell is extremely resilient. The cell membrane can insulate voltage of up to 38,000 V. (If only we could create insulating material of such excellence, we could touch high-voltage cables with our bare hands.) This amazing insulating quality, however, depends entirely on the kind of electric information the cell receives.

If the organism comes in contact with a 'favorable vibration pattern', membrane potential will increase. If, however, the vibration pattern is unfavourable, the membrane potential decreases. For example, if the interior voltage becomes less negative (say from -60 mV to -40 mV), the cell will look like a punctured ball where the air is escaping and the surface can be indented. This is a sick cell that transmits negative information to the surrounding cells. As a result, the membrane potential of the sorrounding

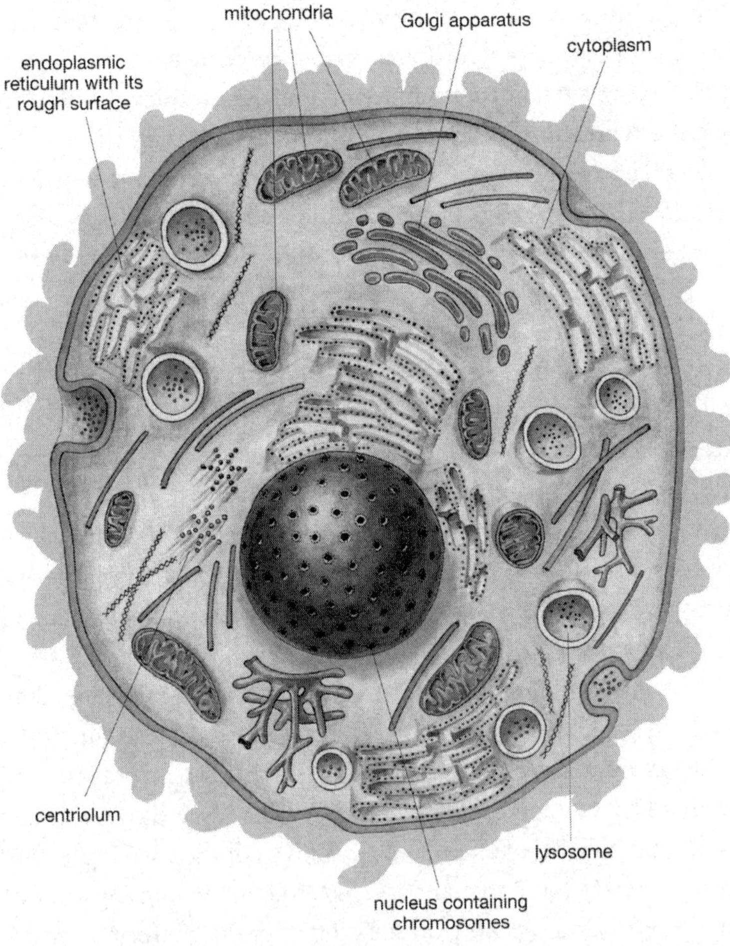

Figure 3. Image of a cell with reduced voltage

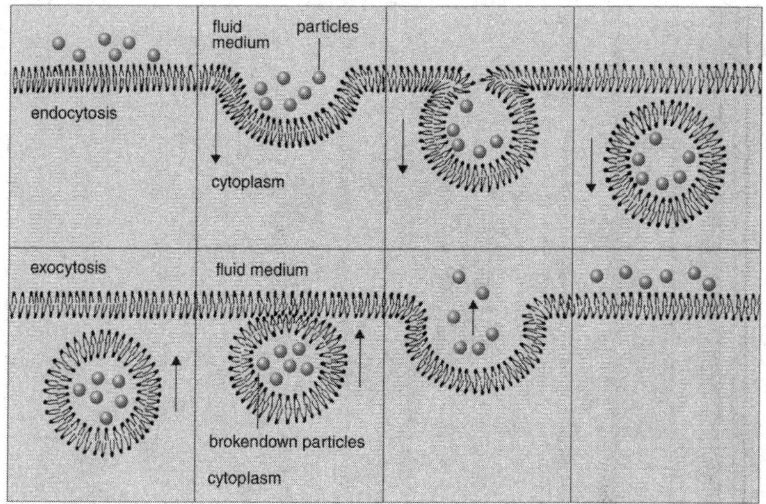

Figure 4. In-folds in the wall of a cell with reduced voltage

healthy cells also decreases, for instance from -60 to -50 mV, or even lower. In a case of serious diseases, the value of membrane potential can fall so significantly that the organism no longer proves viable. As a result, all along the cell surface invaginations appear and destructive organisms such as viruses can enter the cell *(Figures 3 and 4).*

The Model of the Electric Connection of the Virus to the Cell

The structure of the virus is the key to how the virus attaches to the host cell. It attaches to the cells along the invaginations of the membrane that appear when the membrane potential decreases notably. Once the connection has taken place, a protrusion appears at the point where the virus is connected to the cell. The charge of the amino acid chains in the cell changes and the chain disintegrates. Now it has become possible for the virus to introduce its own genetic information into the cell. Now the latter will pass on the information of the virus and serve its proliferation. This is the electric explanation of viral infections.

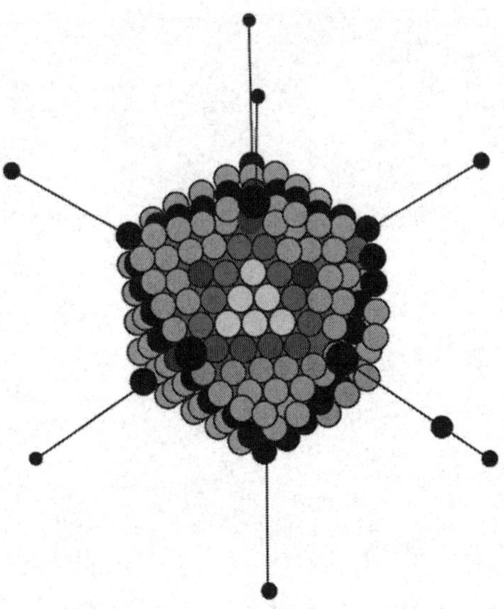

Figure 5. Sketchy representation of an adenovirus

In terms of geometric form, there are hundreds of thousands of types, but their basic structure is identical. As a result of antigenic drift and antigenic shift, viruses appear in different geometric forms – this is how they manage to escape from our immune system. But the way they attach to our cells is the same *(Figure 5).*

Viruses absorb the subtle-energy radiation of the environment through their 'antennae', but pass on their own information to the cell by penetrating the cell membrane with their own form and information. Once the virus is inside the cell, that cell ceases to exist as an effective component of the organism. The virus is always stronger than a cell.

In these cases New Homeopathy suggests that the cells surrounding the diseased cell need to be provided with favorable, constructive information to restore optimal membrane potential. This way the cell that absorbed the virus cannot gain more energy; it becomes isolated and the phagocytes will destroy it. Without such an intervention, cells containing viruses will proliferate because the cell with the virus passes on its information to other, enfeebled cells and thus the 'biochemical immune system' cannot intervene.

The Adaptation of Organisms to the Effect of Subtle Energy in Their Environment

In the development of living organisms we observe the following regularities: simpler cells can only evolve to form complex organs to the extent permitted by external conditions. On the other hand, the living organism protects itself against harmful influences from the external environment, including damaging factors on the level of subtle energies.

The capacity for self-defense is observable even on the level of single-cell animals such as a paramecium. A show called *Telekolleg*[3] on Bavarian television presented an educational short film about an experiment carried out on a paramecium. The animal was in a dish filled with liquid. Next, a drop of some 'incompatible' liquid was dripped into the dish, at a certain distance from the paramecium. The animal fled at lightning speed toward the more protected direction. When, however, a drop of 'compatible' liquid was dripped into the dish, the animal did not move. What is the explanation of this simple fact? As far as we know, paramecia have no sensory organs, but 95% of their cells is made up of water molecules. The molecules of the liquid in the dish immediately started to resonate with the molecules of the 'incompatible' liquid dripped into it. The paramecium 'sensed' the incompatible frequency and fled. This shows that resonance plays an important part in communication even in single-cell animals. Incompatible frequency provoked the paramecium to perform the fleeing behaviour. The experiment demonstrates that even the simplest form of life, like a single-cell animal, has a communication system. It is already intelligent information processing.

If we observe the development of a plant, we find that if there is a rock obstructing its growth, the plant will grow around it. The same happens if invisible obstacles occur on the level of subtle energies: for instance, the plant protects itself against underground water-veins in the same way – it will wind its way in a direction to bypass it, depending on the intensity of the subtle-energy flow.

Motile organisms, however, have to find other ways to protect themselves against harmful influences; they developed other defense mechanisms. The capacity for self-defense is defined by the information stored on the electromagnetic and quantum level within the organism. The most important elements of this are encoded in the geometric form specific to the development of the organism.

Figure 6 offers a summary of the frequencies, wavelengths and energy bands of electromagnetic waves ranging from cosmic radiation to radio waves. It gives us orientation about the radiations affecting our body, showing which wavelengths are harmful and which are not for our organism. The higher the frequency, the smaller the wavelengths and the more energy is carried by the photon.

In the high-frequency portion of the electromagnetic spectrum we find harmful ionizing radiations. When radiation transfers its energy to matter, ionization happens. The ionising radiation hits an atom, and the atom loses electrons. This turns the atom into a positively charged ion. Hard rays are the highest energy rays. They can traverse relatively thick objects without being absorbed. It means that they have short wavelength and great penetrability.

The next range contains the radiations characteristic of human bodily functions, from the non-ionizing far ultraviolet of the 100 nm range to the near infrared range of approximately 1020 nm, which also includes visible rays of around 320–700 nm. Radiations with a wavelength longer than 1020 nm, i.e. microwave, radar, satellite, television and radio waves, may be

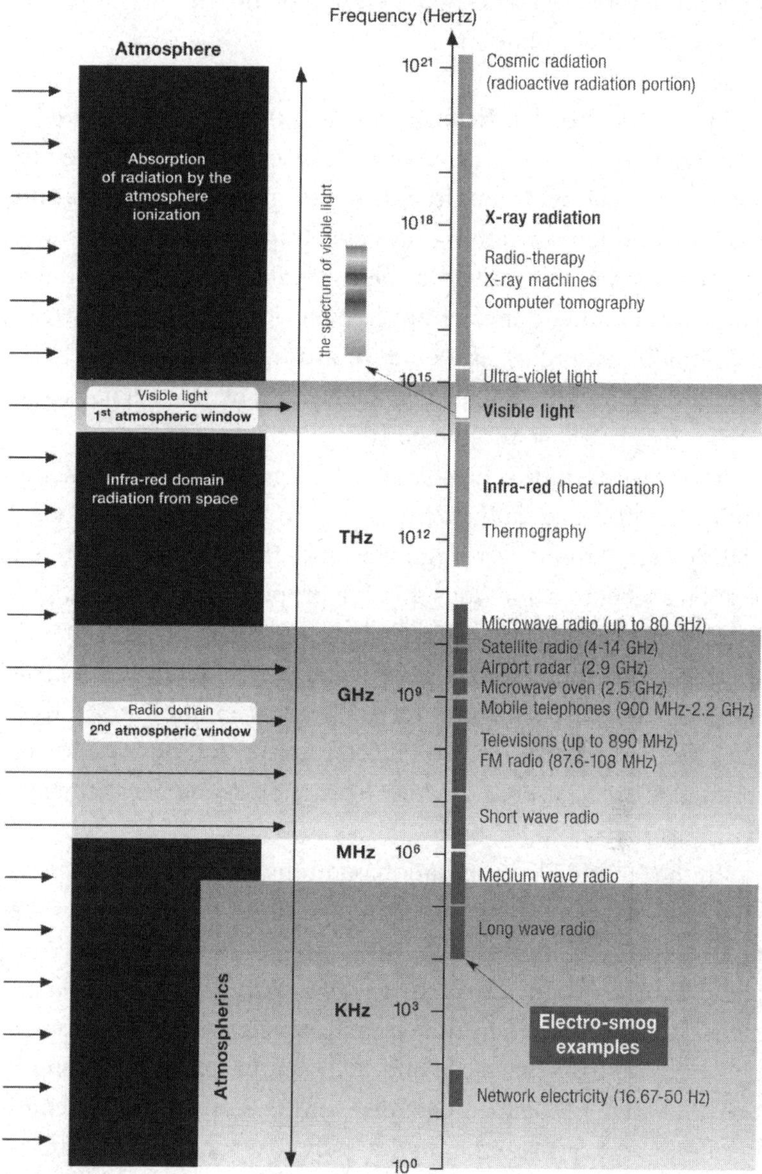

Figure 6. A summary chart of different types of radiation

harmful to the human body depending on how far we are from the source of the radiation.

The Effects of Radiation in the 100–1020 nm Range

If we wish to act in a targeted and effective manner, we need to know about the wavelength and the origin of the information reaching our body. Incoming rays penetrate into the organism to varying depths depending on their wavelength. This is equally true of coherent and incoherent frequencies of the non-ionizing UV domain (sunlight), as well as of infrared radiation. The redder the light and the longer the wavelength of the radiation, the deeper it penetrates into the body.

The reasons for this have to do, among other things, with the multiple reflections and fractures due to the non-homogeneity of the external tissues. The light becomes fractured and scattered as soon as it enters and does this at a proportionate rate of a $1/\lambda$ (lambda) grade 4 factor, which means that blue light is scattered 16 times more than red light. For instance, the depth of penetration into the skin is 0.1 mm for UV rays, 0.55 mm for red (633 nm), and 1.6 mm for infrared (1000 nm). While rays of a lower frequency cause a sense of warmth, higher frequencies only impart information to the body.

In the 100–1020 nm radiation band the *slightest amount of energy* is sufficient to bring about change in the functioning of the organism. This diminutive quantity corresponds to Planck's constant, in other words the quantum of action. If the radiation arrives at the cell at the appropriate wavelength, it may cause abrupt change (the butterfly effect). The appropriate wavelength is in the zone of water molecules, and this is what most commonly provokes a reaction in the body. The ideal wavelength is $\lambda/2$, and this value provides a frequency that is high (and low) enough to impart information.

Therefore, when the electromagnetic radiation reaches the cell, molecules inside the cell come into motion, and this specific energy penetrates the cell because channels in the cell membrane specialized for admitting energy become activated. In 1991 German biophysicist Erwin Neher and German cell physiologist Bert Sakmann received the Nobel Prize for Physiology and Medicine for their studies concerning the ion channels found in the cell membrane.

The Condition of a Critical Bifurcation

Cells react to external impact continually in time, but in varying ways. A strong stimulus can produce sustainable change if the organism is in an unstable condition; in other words, if it is in a condition of critical bifurcation. This is a point at which life processes can take one of two directions, and it is decided which direction they will take.

An organism comes into a state of critical bifurcations when one or more physical parameters in its environment changes abruptly and greatly; for example, if there is a major increase or decrease in temperature, or light conditions change sharply. Every cell in the organism reacts to a change of this kind; for instance, by an increase or decrease of energy in the cell components. Incoming stimuli cause the cell to change and to register new information. This is what happens, for instance, in the process of birth. The infant is transferred from a temperature of 37 °C which it experienced inside the mother's body to the cooler temperature of the ward (i.e. the outside world). Moreover, its life-giving medium also changes – from the fluid which surrounded it inside the fetal membrane the infant is transferred to open air which represents a new energy field and new information. These influences make a long-term impact on the newborn.

Electromagnetic Aspects of the Immune System

The immune system functions mostly through the responses of the electric, electromagnetic and scalar components of the complex holographic field (see Chapter 2). It responds to the energetic and information fields which affect the body, depending on the way in which these reactions influence the condition of the molecules; in other words, whether they make it more or less active. The chemical reaction of the immune system is a consequence of this process.

In order for the immune system to decide whether it needs to intervene, it needs powerful communication zones where it admits information on the subtle-energy level. These are found on the most remote extremities of the body – on the hands, fingertips, the soles of the feet, and the tips of the toes, as well as on the eyes, face, ears, and the top of the head. These are areas that contain a great number of nerve endings and tactile bodies. Radiation affecting the body will only find its way into the organism in areas where the nerve endings are very close to the surface of the skin, or are distributed along the surface of the skin.

During the operation of the immune system electromagnetic waves are produced with a dominant frequency of 633 nm even though other frequencies also activate a response from the organs. 633 nm is the wavelength of the color cherry red. It causes cells to reach a higher level of coherence. In the case of disease we can help by activating the sick organ or system of organs with coherent radiation of the wavelength of 633 nm. There are several ways to convey coherent radiation of a wavelength of 633 nm to the diseased organism – partly by methods which stimulate the body itself to produce coherent radiation of a 633 nm wavelength, and partly by methods which produce coherent radiation of 633 nm from the outside. An example of the latter is soft laser irradiation or laser acupuncture.

The Cell as Receptor

Stimuli arriving through our sensory organs are perceived not only by chemo-receptors – the organism perceives them in a complex manner. Each of the cells is also, in itself, a receptor which reacts, among others, to electric stimuli. Humanity has been using stimuli in pain reduction since ancient times without understanding the language of cells or their sensitivity to external electromagnetic information. The stimuli are produced, among other things, in traditional Chinese acupuncture, ritual bush drums in Africa, or the aroma and color therapies commonly used in our time. What these traditional healing methods have in common is that they influence the body in a complex manner through the stimulation zones and thus have a targeted influence on directing and regulating mechanisms. This is why it is possible to heal a sick organism by these methods.

Reflex Zones Representing the Entire Body

In a complex dissipative system every part represents the whole. This is also the case in the human organism. Our body has evolved to contain a system of points that ensure that the most important information is perceived at multiple centers on our body's surface. The various reflex zones (soles of feet, palms, face, etc.) and the meridian system represent projections of our entire organism, where the part stands for the whole.

One such area is that of the ears. Traditional acupuncture has long recognized this representative role. By stimulating or treating a representative section on the ear we may affect an organ, or even the entire organism. Treatment applied at these points, using extremely small impulses close to Planck's quantum of action, can result in radical changes in an organ, or in the immune system. This has been known to previous generations and has been used in healing for thousands of years, massaging the reflex zones of the face, soles and palms, and stimulating the various acupuncture points in the ears and along the meridians.

Körbler Discovered Additional Representation Points of the Whole Body.[4]

1. He discovered a projection of the spinal column on the top of the head, which he named the *spinal column meridian.* Testing it allows for a very rapid diagnosis. The spinal column meridian is a line found on the skin of the head which goes from the center of the top of the head to the hairline on the forehead. At the meeting of the forehead and the scalp we find the representation of the cross bone and at the top of the head that of the first neck vertebra. This offers information about the condition of the individual organs and through it we can also influence the organs.[5] The Chinese had known about the spinal column 2500 years ago but they were mistaken about the location of the first neck vertebra: they located it at the hairline, whereas in fact this area is at the top of the head. (The Chinese probably thought about it the opposite way because a map of the hairline, when spread out, looks like an animal hide.) Since by this method the reflex zone was not effective, its use was abandoned. Körbler, however, rediscovered and reversed it, and it is now functioning again. By stimulating the part which is at the top of the head you can influence the individual's general condition, just as by stimulating the 'third eye', the solar plexus, or the first dorsal vertebra.
2. Körbler also discovered the so-called *psychomeridian* which goes from the top of the head backwards to the point where the skull meets the spine. The psychomeridian gives us information about the condition of the psyche. By testing it one can test and even correct information from the past. Through the psychomeridian we can influence the psyche and intervene in the psychosomatic cycle.
3. Körbler found that examining the area on the inside of the wrists provides accurate information about inflammation

in the body and thus named this area the *inflammation point*.

4. On the left-hand side of the chest underneath the third rib Körbler discovered a point the examination of which give information about the degree to which the body is affected by mycosis; he termed this the *mycosis point*.
5. Körbler's *antibiotic point*. By examining this point underneath the ninth rib, below the right shoulder blade, center, it serves to inform us how heavily the organism is impacted by antibiotics and whether antibiotic treatment is advisable.

Testing the Coherence of the Living Organism

The living organism constitutes a coherent and co-operative system. It is an open dissipative system, surviving in its environment by all of its parts absorbing free energy from the environment in a co-ordinated manner. By doing this it re-balances the entropy produced by its functioning.

An open dissipative system needs to connect to its environment as an organized whole. In Prigogine's system,[6] this is what characterizes systems in what he calls 'the third state'[7]. In order to exist in this state, every part of the system needs to operate in a concerted way. We know that every cell performs over a hundred thousand reactions per second. These can only be aligned if there is a constant multidimensional, near-immediate information transfer between all parts of the body. This condition exceeds the bounds of the known processes of biophysical and biochemical information transfer. Therefore it may be assumed that the coherence of the living body is based on the resonance of quantum vibrations, in this way assuming the absorption of non-local information, which means that the body has a unified wave function. According to quantum physics, these effects occur when a particle is in the excited state – the state where information transfer becomes possible. In the human body this comes about due to the unified energy flow from the top of the head to the tip of the toes.

In the human body there are also electric manifestations of this coherence, partly because energy flow has a unified direction from the top of the head to the tip of the toes. The electric polarity of all particles and parts is the same. This guarantees communication among the body parts, as well as between the parts and the organs crucial for the coherence of functioning. If the polarization of a part is reversed in the positive–negative chain, the coherence of the electric current is broken; an energy blockage emerges. Methods of New Homeopathy can detect the disturbance in the electric communication of the organism even before the emergence of symptoms. In the case of energy blockages the affected organ or body part becomes isolated from coherent communication, a disturbance occurs between this part and the central nervous system, and it lacks the required supply of subtle energies. Therefore the most important task for New Homeopathy is to detect and eradicate energy blockages.

Thus, in order to preserve health, we need to strive toward sustaining the coherence of the body. The self-healing potential cannot operate unless this coherence is present, since all processes of the organism manifest in the resonance of cells and organs.

There are, however, also some disadvantages to the coherent operation of the organism. If there is a local lesion (injury) in the body, owing to the tendency for coherence, it will affect the adaptation processes of the entire organism – they become deformed and can result in disease and a bad overall sensation because the information of the injury is amplified in the body's information storage system.

In the course of testing for tolerability and intolerability, New Homeopathy explores how energetic and informational processes outside the organism affect the overall coherence of the body. It maps out these connections from the point of view of the extent to which adaptive resonances emerge between the body and the various frequencies from the outside world. The highest degree of adaptive resonance indicates perfect health. Every illness comes from disturbances of resonances between the outside world and the body. If we want to keep a person healthy, the most important thing is to make sure that the internal resonances patterns and external radiation are in balance.

According to New Homeopathy, the organism and its environment are connected by constant multilateral connections – this is true of interactions of all types of substances, plants, animals, humans, and the interactions of the natural world. This means that the living organism is affected by electromagnetic and subtle-energy radiations of a number of different intensities and qualities at the same time, which provoke specific reactions in the various zones of the body.

We distinguish effects that fundamentally benefit, or damage the organism. The changes in the energy condition of the body are shown by the dowsing rod. Information affecting various parts of the body may be recognized by the fact that the quality of the body's radiation changes. New Homeopathy can show how radiation that is harmful for the body can be identified and neutralized. In the same way we can transform harmful radiation into useful radiation for the living organism and thus improve the organism's capacity for utilizing subtle energies. New Homeopathy can also show how we can restore coherence in disturbed zones of the organism by using geometric symbols.

Chapter 4

Körbler's Dowsing Rod

What moves the dowsing rod? What causes its consistent patterns of movement?

In the 21 years since Körbler's death, science has made huge advances in explaining paranormal phenomena. In his lifetime, the very explanation of electromagnetic space was a novelty compared to classical biophysical explanations. Today's biophysical experiments are able to capture not merely the effects of electromagnetic radiation, but even the subtle-energy impacts of scalar waves and quantum fields.

The movement of a dowsing rod is the result of this highly complex system, perceived by the central nervous system. One aspect of this is exploring the impact of electromagnetic fields. Körbler's aim was to substantiate the effectiveness of his method by demonstrating the effects of such fields.

He found the way to experimental testing through a personal experience. In the early 1980s his daughter was two years old and suffered from an allergy to wash powder. Her skin was covered in rashes. Their pediatrician sat the little girl up on the examining bed, looked at her and spread his arms helplessly. Körbler felt there must be a way to find a treatment for her dauther's problem. What is more, he wanted a method accessible to all people. Ten years later, the dowsing rod was being used on a mass scale for home and for healing purposes. On one occasion, Körbler sent 600 dowsing rods to an area of India where there were not enough doctors and nurses, and medics were also trained to help in simpler cases.

The dowsing rod is a one-armed pendulum that is 64.5 cm (ca. 25.4 inches) in length. It consists of a wooden handle of 8.5

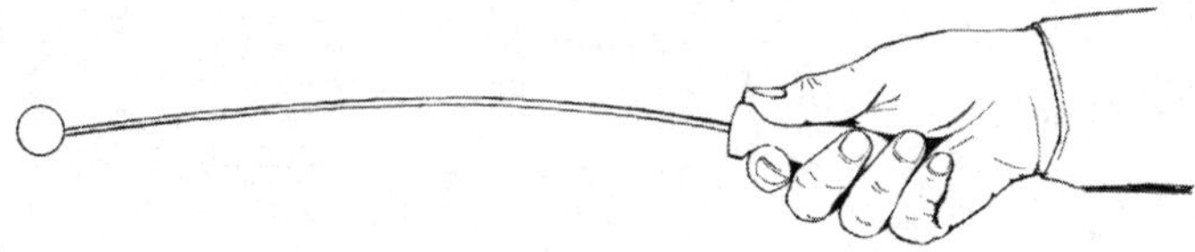

Figure 7. The dowsing rod

cm (3.35 in); a stick of 2 mm (0.08 in) in thickness and 54 cm (21.26 in) in length made of PVC enriched with copper ions; and a wooden ball with of a diameter of 2 cm (0.8 in) at the end. The length was calibrated by Körbler so that the pendulum would work in the hands of a person with average sensitivity *(Figure 7).*

This instrument works as a 'receiving' antenna that perceives the electromagnetic and other waves of the environment. The handle acts as an electric amplifier, the PVC stick enriched with copper ions provides the antenna effect, while the length of the stick with a wooden ball attached to the other end is to guarantee the sensitivity to oscillation. (The length of the stick is important. If, for example, we were to make a stick of the same materials but with a stick half the length, the instrument would show no movements at all.)

How does the dowsing rod work? Körbler offered the following explanation. 'This instrument senses the electromagnetic radiation in our environment. Its antenna shape causes it to have an automatic positive–negative polarization where one pole becomes the body of the person holding the handle; the other pole with the wooden ball is held close to the person or object under examination.

What is the purpose of a dowsing rod? Körbler developed the dowsing rod as an instrument specifically suited to indicate subtle energy phenomena, like low-voltage electric fields, electromagnetic (EM) waves, and other forces that cannot be measured by standard instruments. This measuring instrument can only be called an indicator or an examination tool, since it does not

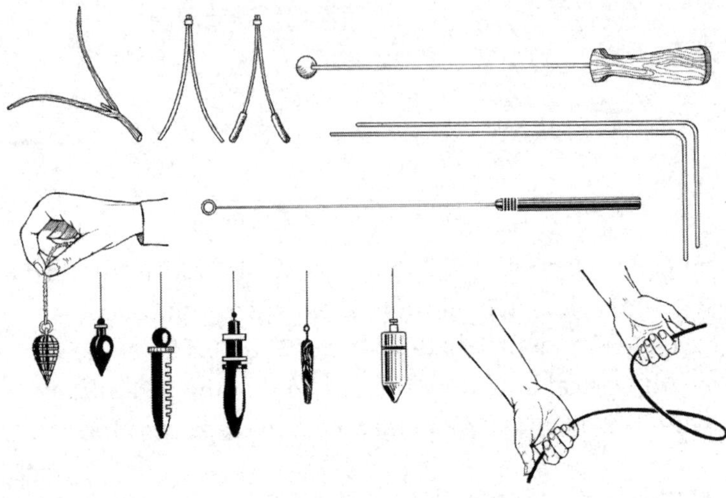

Figure 8. Different types of pendulum

satisfy criteria for measuring instruments in usual scientific practice. It does, however, show the subtle-energy interactions between the tester and the tested material, revealing to what extent the information of the tested material is favorable or unfavorable for the tester's organism. The first level in the use of the dowsing rod is when we test materials for ourselves. The material can be anything. As a next level we can start testing for others. Again, the subject of the test can be just about anything: living creatures, plants or animals, foods, or materials in the household. The third level is important for healers who – with the help of the dowsing rod – can establish the subtle-energy diagnoses of their patients and choose the indicated method of treatment.

Forerunners of the dowsing rod were the various versions of pendulums used in different periods. Pendulums for examining geo-pathogenic zones have a rich history, but their use required a special sensibility, sensitivity and practice *(Figure 8).* The relevant literature1 presents the different variations in detail. Use of such pendulums deservedly provokes the criticism of contemporary scientific practice. It is a subjective tool which only functions for a select few. People make use of subjective means when objective measuring instruments are not available. The phenomena, however, that they try to measure, may exist. This was true of the water or the treasure sought by some individuals in the past, and it is equally true of people with this kind of interest in the present age. The only difference is that the physical experiments of the present offer scientific evidence that the subtle-energy phenomena sensed by the body actually exist, even if we lack the instrument for perceiving and measuring them. We are left with subjective tools. The greatest drawback is that they are influenced by the thinking of the experimenters. This is true, however, of all human phenomena; we know the power of the human mind. In the operation of the human body, the power of our consciousness can even influence the behavior of biochemical substances. This is demonstrated by innumerable experiments.

There are two crucial points at which the dowsing rod differs from earlier versions of the pendulum. The first point is related to its subjective quality. Körbler took proper account of the subjective factor. He first invited us to focus on this factor and then, in order to enable us to use his extremely sensitive instrument, gave us all the recommendations which would help us exclude

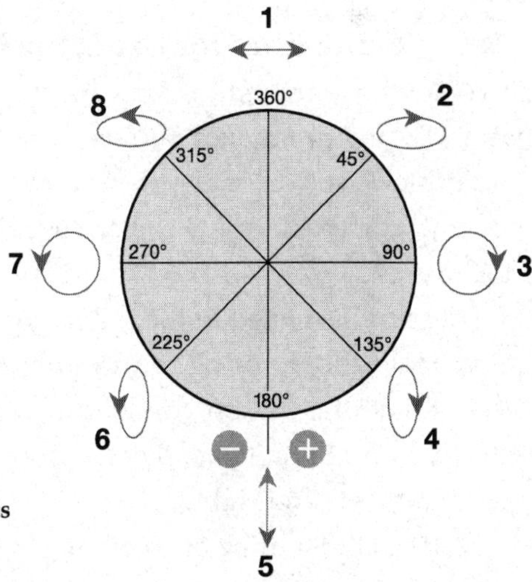

Figure 9.
The eight different movements of the dowsing rod

the disturbance of our thinking and reduce subjectivity in the testing to the minimum.

Another important factor where the dowsing rod differs from formerly used types of pendulum is that it operates along the 'system of eight vectors' discovered by Körbler. While examining living organisms (human, animal, vegetable), the rod shows one of eight possible kinds of movement, and these correspond to eight different energy levels in living organism *(Figure 9)*. Körbler described this system as follows:

> *In studying the indicative movements of the dowsing rod I discovered the regularities of the forces which cause the wooden ball at the end of the instrument held by the tester to make significant vertical, horizontal or circular movements. Since the direction of the movement depends both on the person of the tester and the type and quantity of the substance tested, it is clear that we are talking about very special information. Therefore I named my discovery the principle of the reversibility of systemic information. (See Chapter 6)*

This is the system which unfolds step by step during the experiments described below, starting from the simplest ones.

Guidelines for Using the Dowsing Rod

Anyone is encouraged to experiment with the dowsing rod but, naturally, practice makes perfect. How should one start?

Körbler used to warn people on every occasion that the movement of the dowsing rod can be influenced mentally, by our thoughts.

This may be tested in the following manner:

a) Hold the dowsing rod in front of you at eye height and think of a person you love very much. After a while you will find that the end of the dowsing rod swings horizontally left and right.
b) If next you think of a person you have problems with, the

end of the dowsing rod will move vertically up and down.

c) If you think of nothing at all, the dowsing rod remains immobile.

It is important that, while testing, we should be neutral, and accepting, and not influencing the result with our consciousness. If our attitude is negative, or one of rejection *('It is all humbug but I will try anyway')*, we may block or otherwise affect the functioning of the dowsing rod. If we anticipate the result or 'know-it-in-advance' *('I am sure this cake is good for me')*, the signals of the dowsing rod will be distorted, and instead of the real situation, it will reflect merely our wishes. Therefore, in order to eradicate intrusive thoughts, it is a good idea to ask ourselves, mentally or out loud, how the information of the substance to be tested would affect the tester *('Is this apple good for me?')*. This question is not addressed to the dowsing rod; it only averts other thoughts thus opening doors to a genuine test result.

Experience shows that for 85% of the testers the end of the dowsing rod swings horizontally, and this can be interpreted as a 'YES' while vertical motions indicate unfavorable effects or 'NO'. (The explanation of this will be discussed later.) For the others (15% of the testers) vertical motion means favorable and horizontal motion means unfavorable effects.

Let us find out which group we belong to:

First think of some great joy or a person you love very much, and speak the word or the person's name out loud a few times. If the dowsing rod moves horizontally, we belong to the 85% of the set of testers. If it moves vertically, we acknowledge it and work with the rod in that way until we find the cause of the phenomenon with the help of an expert.

As a counter-test, think of something terrible, and say the word a few times. In 85% of the cases, the end of the rod moves vertically, and for the others it will move horizontally.

Later, when performing tests, horizontal movement will

mean YES, that is a favorable answer, while vertival movement will mean NO, that is an unfavorable answer.

Preparation for testing

Since our measuring instrument is our body, we are only fit for testing if we are in an optimal physical and mental state. When we are feeling just a bit tired, the rod will show an imperfect answer. The result of the tested material (e.g. food) will appear as a non-optimal condition. If for example our condition is indicated by a vertical movement of the rod, i.e. movement in the vector position 5, it will show the same position even if it is testing something that is good for us.

In order to avoid such mistakes, before we start testing we must make sure to be in an optimal mental and physical condition, and in a general sense of bodily comfort. Examine your condition by placing the palm of your left hand over the top of your head and observe the movement of the dowsing rod. If it moves vertically or in a circular way, draw a few vertical lines over the nape of your neck starting from the top of the head and as far as the first vertebra. This action will free up the psychomeridian (see below) and make you fit for testing at least for a short time. Another method to make yourself fit for testing is to connect the two brain hemispheres with the thumb and the index finger of your left hand. Use both methods if necessary. Avoid practicing, learning and testing with the dowsing rod if you are short of sleep, too tired, hungry or thirsty. Any disharmony of your mental state will affect the signals of the rod. If you feel deep sorrow, if you have been affected by sudden grief or loss, or if you are tormented by negative emotions, this will all appear in your test results. No one except the most practiced testers should use the dowsing rod in a state like this, and even then only in cases of utmost necessity, if you must provide urgent help for yourself or someone. First, of course, you need to stabilize your own condition and only then can you proceed to help.

Testing with the Dowsing Rod

Since we start our work by testing a whole range of different materials, it is a good idea to write down your test results. Right-handed people need to hold the dowsing rod in their right hand, left-handed people in their left hand. Hold it horizontally in front of you, bent your arm gently, at the height of your navel. Your free arm must not touch your body. If you are standing in a place clear of disturbances, the ball of the rod will stand still. If not, find a place free of earth or other electromagnetic radiation.

1. **Testing the EM information of food**

1.1. Take an apple in your free hand. If the information the apple carries is favorable for you, the end of the rod swings horizontally, left and right. When the rod moves vertically, it means that now it is not favorable for you to eat this apple. The reason can be the type that – at the moment or usually – would not have a favorable effect on your digestive system. Or the apple is unripe, or it has been influenced by chemicals. Do the experiment with other foods. *(Figure 10)*

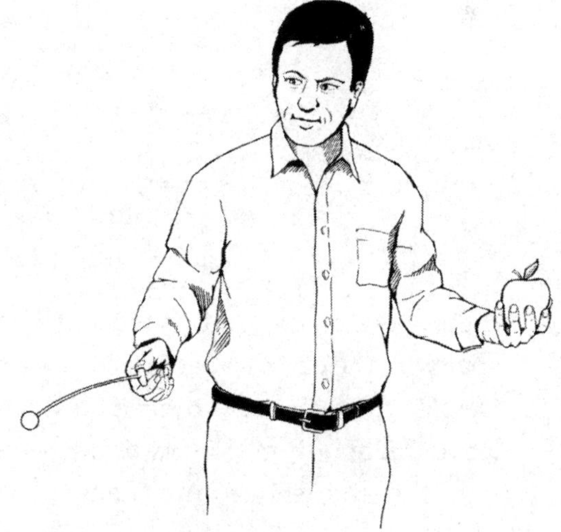

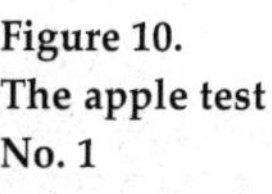

Figure 10.
The apple test
No. 1

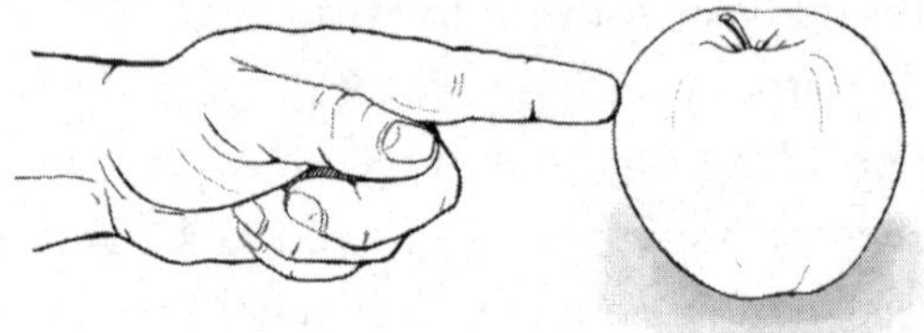

Figure 11. The apple test No. 2

1.2. Now put the apple on a table and touch it with the index finger of your free hand. Ask the question, 'Is this apple good for me?' After a few seconds the dowsing rod will swing horizontally if the answer is favorable. Instead of touching, you can hold the palm of your hand about 5 cm above the apple. The rod gives the same answer. Perform this experiment with other foods. *(Figure 11)*

2. Testing the healthy and the flawed part of a fruit

2.1. Take an apple which is flawed on one side. Put it on the table and use your index finger to touch alternately the healthy and then the flawed part. At the healthy part the dowsing rod will swing horizontally, at the flawed part vertically. *(Figure 12)*

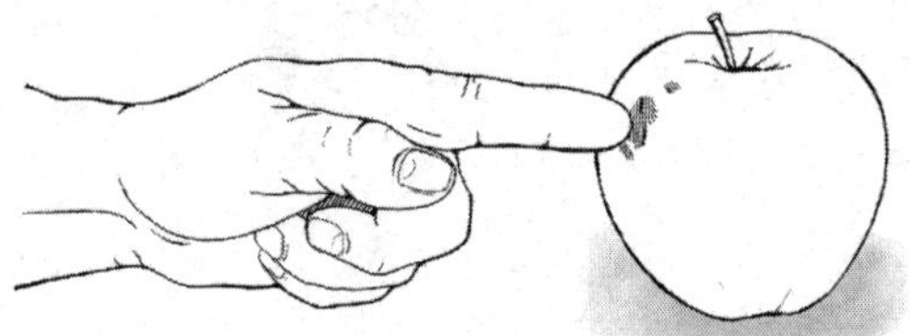

Figure 12. Testing the flawed part

2.2. If the speck on the apple is too small, touch the flawed spot with the tip of a short piece of wire, or of a needle. Despite the fact that you have used a transmitting object (a piece of iron, copper or other metal) while testing, the rod shows the same answer as before.

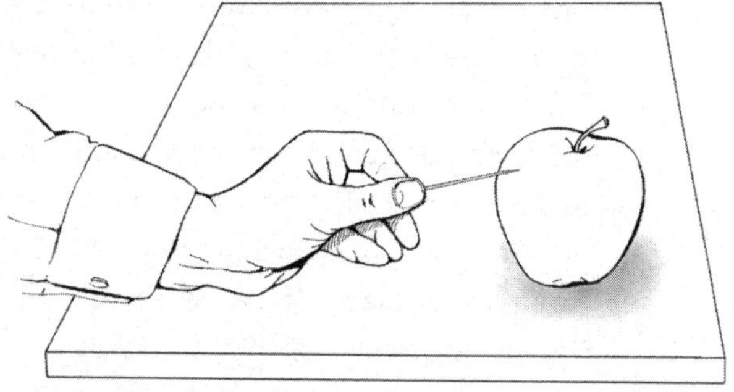

Figure 13. Testing with a sound

Regardless of what fruit or food we test, the rod swings horizontally for the healthy part of the tested material, and vertically for the flawed part. *(Figure 13)*

3. Testing quantities

3.1. Place a packet of sugar in your free hand. The dowsing rod will swing vertically up and down. If you now pick up just a pinch of sugar between your thumb and your index finger, the ball of the dowsing rod will swing horizontally. Choose other spices, herbs, or any kind of food in different quantities and observe the end of your rod. Initally, test only foods and other substances that you use on a daily basis but never poisons or drugs. *(Figures 14a and 14b)*

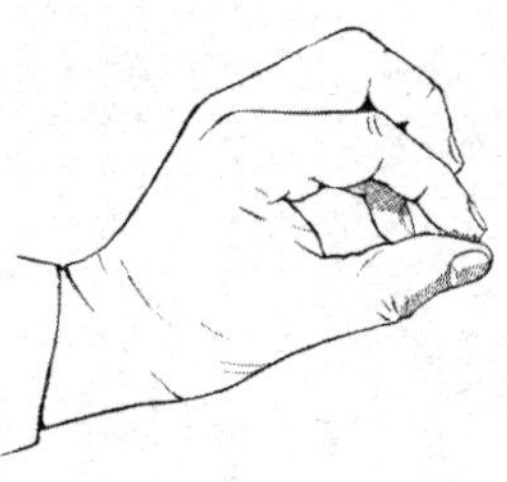

Figures 14a and 14b.
Quantitative testing with refined sugar

4. Testing the favorable and unfavorable EM information in personal belongings and household articles

4.1. Take a clean underwear out of your wardrobe, hold it between the tips of your thumb and your index finger, and test it with the dowsing rod. If the fabric is favorable for you, you will experience the dowsing rod hovering horizontally. If, however, it is moving vertically, the fabric or color of the underwear is unfavorable for you, or there are vestiges of wash powder left in it. You can test your clothes or bed linen in a similar manner. *(Figure 15)*

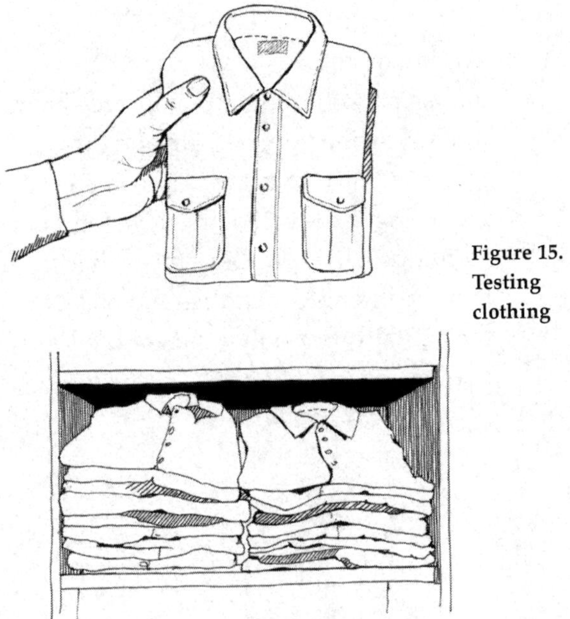

Figure 15. Testing clothing

4.2. Test your toiletry, cosmetic articles, detergents and rinsing substances used in your household.

4.3. Touch the top of the table in your room with the tip of the index finger of your free hand. In a favorable case the dowsing rod will swing horizontally. If you experience the opposite, it means that either the quality of the wood or the treatment used for the surface of the table, or the chemicals used in the course of its production, such as anti-fungus treatment or glues, are unfavorable for you.

4.4. Place a set of different minerals on the table and examine their compatibility with the help of the index finger of your free hand. It is quite likely that for some of the minerals the dowsing rod will swing horizontally. Note that different minerals may prove to be favorable or unfavorable for different people. *(Figure 16)*

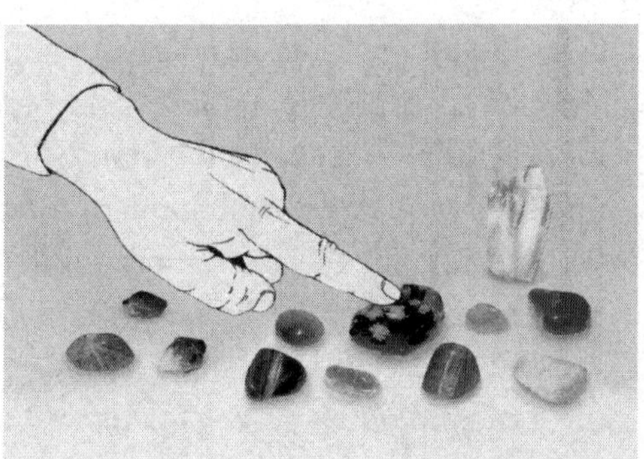

Figure 16. Testing minerals

5. Testing the EM information of metals

5.1. Prepare three pieces of the same type of metal. This can be, for example, three keys. Hold and test each key, one after the other. The end of the rod will swing clockwise if the substance is iron, copper, brass, silver or gold. *(Figure 17)*

5.2. Now walk around your room and examine all metal objects, touching them with the index finger of your free hand. The dowsing rod will always swing clockwise.

6. Testing for others

Testing for other people we do essentially the same way

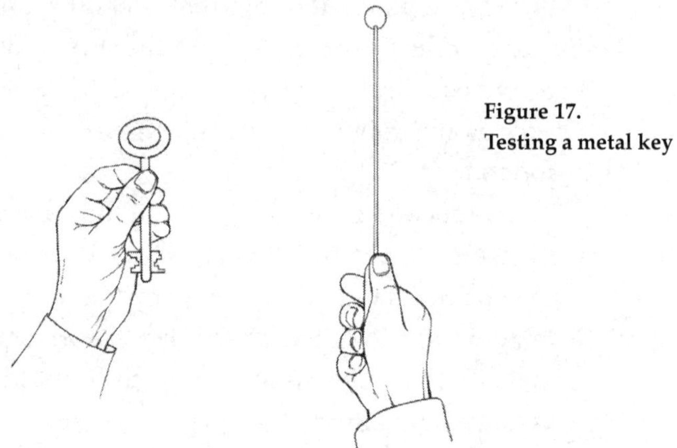

Figure 17.
Testing a metal key

as we do for ourselves. Experience shows that for most right-handed people the left hand perceives the information (this is always the hand holding the object under testing, or the right hand of the person under examination) and the right hand emits the information (this is where you hold the dowsing rod).

6.1. Put the object under testing (apple, medicine, etc.) in the left hand of the other person, and take the person's right hand in your left hand. Perform the test. *(Figure 18)*

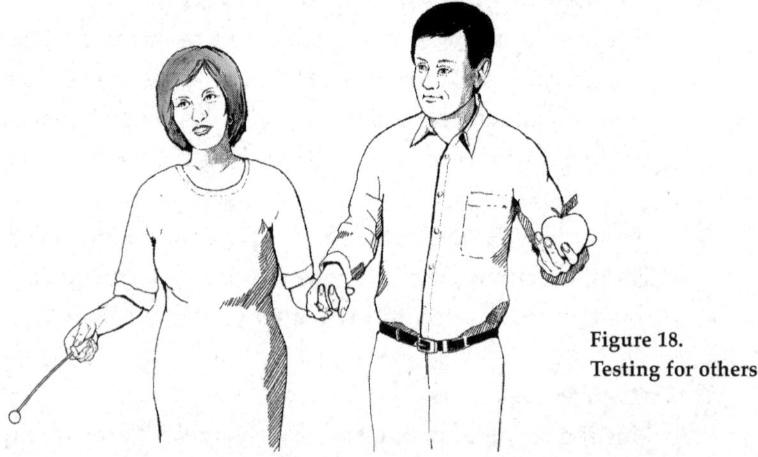

Figure 18.
Testing for others

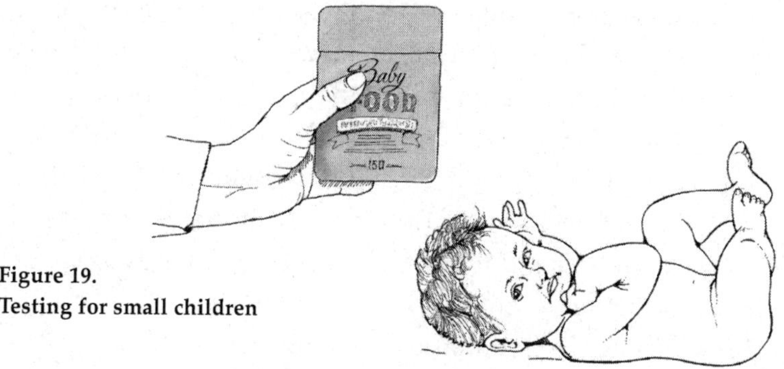

Figure 19.
Testing for small children

6.2. When we test for small children, we hold the food or medication close to the head of the baby sleeping in its cot. *(Figure 19)*

7. **Testing the body**

The dowsing rod can also be used to test the subtle-energy of our body. You can proceed in the same way as you do in regard to material things. If the condition of your subtle-energy is good, the dowsing rod moves horizontally. If our condition has in any way changed, the bio-indicator will swing vertically along the disturbance zone in the hand of a beginner tester. At the beginning you must content yourself with this much. For experienced practitioners the various changes in the condition of our body's subtle-energy system will be shown by one of the eight possible kinds of movement. We describe the details in Chapter 7 on Healing.

7.1. Testing the aura

Take your dowsing rod in hand and hold the palm of your free hand facing toward your body, about 10 cm away from your stomach. The dowsing rod will now move horizontally or vertically depending on the condition of the organ. Test other parts of your body, for example, near your heart or your liver.

Every organ and every organ group has an electromagnetic radiation pattern, an aura of its own environment that changes according to the condition of organ.

7.2. Testing the organs of the body
Now touch the different parts of your body with the index finger of your free hand. While holding your rod, try to find and test the energetic boundaries of the organs of your body.

7.3. Testing the boundaries of energy zones
Repeat experiment in paragraph 7.2. in such a way that during testing you slowly pull your index finger along your skin. Observe the end of the rod: the direction of swinging will change from vertical to horizontal, or the other way round, at the boundaries of energy regions of varying intensities.

7.4. Clothes carrying information of our body zones
Presume that during testing we find that the intensity of our body's liver area has changed. If we take e.g. a pullover that we wear for a while and test the area that was next to the liver, we can read the information just as if we would have tested the liver itself. Touch this area with your index finger. The dowsing rod will move vertically, in accordance with the disturbance zone. For a more accurate image we can wear an abdominal bandage made of cotton for a few hours, and then test this piece of cloth.

7.5. When examining other persons or domestic animals we act similarly as when testing our body. Hold your palm or your index finger about 10 cm away from your subject or touch the relevant body parts or zones with your index finger.

8. Testing the EM information of the electric power in your household

8.1. Establishing the position of electric cables in the wall
Use your left palm for an antenna. Where the end of the dowsing rod swings clockwise, there is an electric cable in the wall.

8.2. At hubs consisting of electric sockets or the crossing of other cables, the dowsing rod will circle to the left.

9. Testing harmful EM information in your environment

9.1. Testing geo-pathogenic zones
Just as we described earlier, the dowsing rod is held horizontally, at the height of the navel. The other hand does not touch the body. If you move very slowly around the room, you might find the dowsing rod starting to move vertically up and down. If this happens, stop and count the number of oscillations until the direction of the oscillation changes; it turns horizontal again. This is how we test for underground water-veins, or other geo-pathogenic zones. If you wish to define the individual pathogenic zones separately, you can use your left hand as an antenna in the following manner:

9.1.1. Finding the effect of an underground water-vein
Point your left index finger vertically toward the ground and wait until the dowsing rod starts to move. If it is swinging horizontally, there is no underground water-vein in the area you are examining; if it is swinging vertically, you must reckon with an underground water-vein. The intensity of the movement will show how powerful the effect is. If you count the number of oscillations, you will find out how many meters down the underground water-vein is. If you are measuring outdoors and find a puddle of water or a little pond on the surface, the dowsing rod will respond by hovering

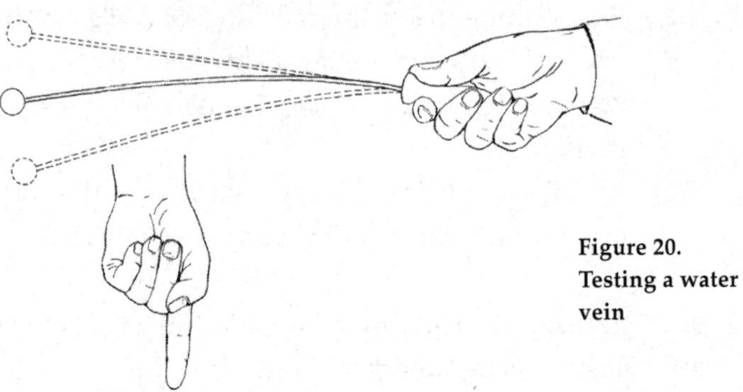

Figure 20. Testing a water vein

horizontally (provided that it is good, healthy water). *(Figure 20)*

9.1.2. Finding the effect of landslides and geological fault-lines

Spread the fingers of your left hand and hold them vertically toward the ground. If the dowsing rod hovers horizontally, there is no landslide in the place you are measuring. If the dowsing rod swings vertically or circles anti-clockwise, there is a landslide or fault-line at the place you are measuring. *(Figure 21)*

9.1.3. Finding the effect of Hartmann and Curry's slides

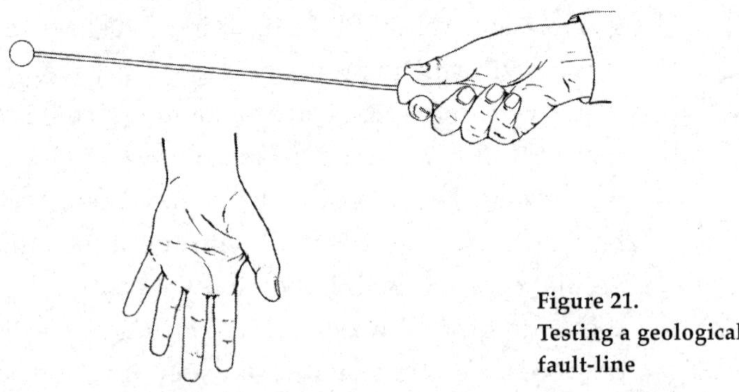

Figure 21. Testing a geological fault-line

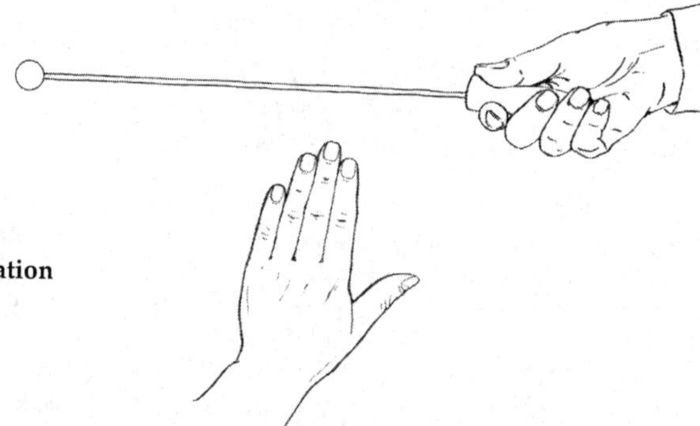

Figure 22.
Testing lateral radiation

You use your left palm as an antenna. Turn your palm toward the surface to be tested and move it slowly up and down, and then at various angles. Wherever the dowsing rod shows vertical movement you have found lateral radiation. *(Figure 22)*

9.1.4. Finding the effect of radiation crossings and hubs
Clench the fist of your left hand and hold it with the little finger down. Move your fist slowly laterally and lengthwise. Wherever the dowsing rod shows a circling movement to the left, there is a radiation hub. In this case you use the above described methods to examine what sort of radiations the hub consists of. *(Figure 23)*

9.2. Finding the effect of a broadcast satellite

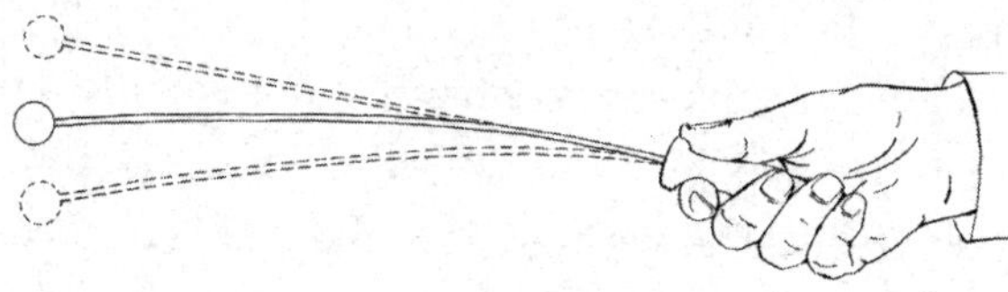

Figure 23.
Testing a radiation hub

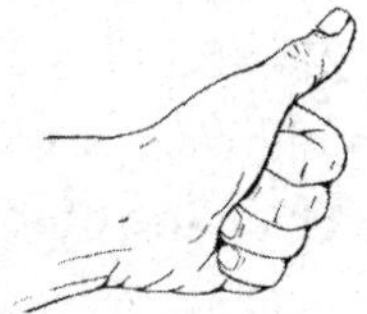

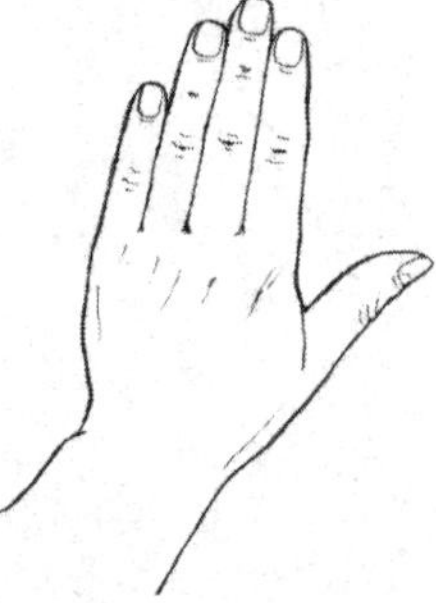

Figure 24. Testing the radiation of a satellite transmitter

Hold your left index finger toward the ceiling and slowly move it laterally and radially. Wherever the dowsing rod shows a circular movement to the left, you have to reckon with the radiation of a satellite station. This kind of testing will also enable you to orient an antenna you are about to mount. *(Figure 24)*

The Supported Vertical Dowsing Rod

So far we have seen that the hand-held dowsing rod shows whether the EM information carried by a substance is favorable or non-favorable for our body. We have also learnt that food, object or anything else that is good for one person may well be harmful to another. But what is the reason for this? Körbler created another experimental instrument, the vertical dowsing rod that enables its user to get closer to the answer.

The vertical dowsing rod also consists of a PVC rod with a wooden ball at the end.

However, instead of a handle, it is set into a pyramidal base. The rod is flexible, and with the wooden ball at the tip, it can move freely. The vertical dowsing rod is also easy to use. Hold the test object in your left hand, then - squeezing gently - get the stick of the rod between the thumb and the index finger of your right hand at about 2 cm high above the tip of the pyramid. Now count the number of each kinds of movement the rod makes. *(Figure 25)*

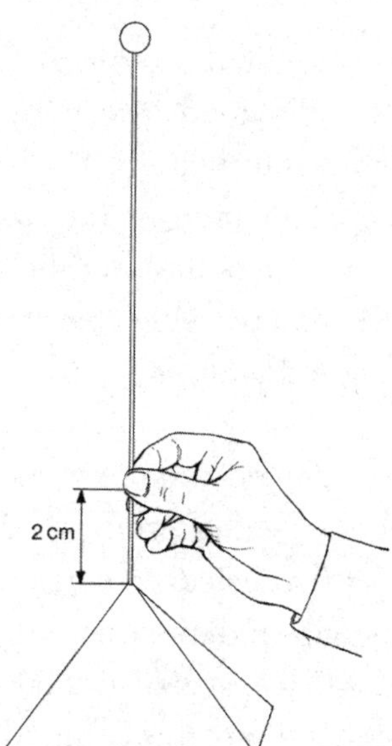

Figure 25. The vertical dowsing rod

If your hand-held dowsing rod tends to swing horizontally in response to an apple, the vertical dowsing rod responds to the same apple by swinging toward and away from the body of the tester: Körbler called this a *radial motion.* After that, the vertical dowsing rod makes a few circles, and then it swings diagonally: to one side of the tester's body – Körbler called this a *transverse motion.* This is the *movement pattern of the apple* in the mirror of the testing person's organism.

Experience shows that radial motion means 'approval', which means the information the testing object carries has positive effect on the tester's organism, while the *number* of transverse motions shows the *extent* of the 'harmful' effect.

When comparing the hand-held and the vertical dowsing rod, radial motions of the vertical dowsing rod correspond to the horizontal movements of the hand-held dowsing rod, while transverse motions correspond to the vertical movements. The circular movements of the vertical dowsing rod also inform us about the favorable and unfavorable communication between the test object and the tested person.

Regarding the tests with the vertical dowsing rod we can say that all substances carry 'good', meaning favorable, and 'bad', meaning unfavorable, information. The two different dowsing rods show the effect of the information carried by the test material in a different way. While the hand-held dowsing rod shows that the test material is favorable or unfavorable for the body, the vertical dowsing rod *presents details about the extent of the effects.*

How do we evaluate the number of the three kinds of movements the vertical dowsing rod shows? When testing an apple, that is favorable for the tested person's organism, the vertical dowsing rod starts with radial motion, then makes a couple of circles, and switches to transverse motion. Here, the count of radial motion is higher than the count of transverse motion. Whereas, when the effect of the tested material is unfavorable for the tester, the vertical dowsing rod starts swinging diagonally showing unfavorable effects; and the number of oscillations will be higher than the number of the favorable swings.

Körbler found that on examining an object made of gold, the vertical dowsing rod made 63 radial and 63 transverse oscillations on all occasions, and between the two kinds of movement, it made six circles, clockwise. The movement pattern of greater celandine *(Chelidonium majus)* extract was 63 radial and 40 transverse swings.

If we test a metal object with the vertical dowsing rod, we experience an interesting phenomenon. The number of radial and transverse oscillations are always equal, and they are separated by a certain number of 'circles'. While, as mentioned before, the hand-held dowsing rod makes circular movements when testing metals.

It is important to know that the swing pattern we get is always individual. It is a number that changes not only by person but also from time to time. It shows the relationship between the test material and our body. If, for example, the same apple is tested by several people, the number of oscillations will differ, because every person's organism reacts in its own way. This information is highly valuable for the tester, because the movement pattern of a *disturbance zone* of a body can give us ideas about a possible diagnosis, and it helps us to choose a treatment. Thus, with the help of the vertical dowsing rod we can find out the quality of the tested material through the movement pattern, naturally, always in the mirror of the tester's organism. The number of radial and transverse motions depends on the condition of the testing person and is in that sense unique to the individual.

We can use the system of the vertical dowsing rod for testing drugs. Körbler examined hundreds of materials with the vertical dowsing rod and classified them by their movement patterns. He tested the radiation of different zones and points of the human body. He found that in the cases of disturbance zones, which he registered with an accuracy going to the millimeter, and in the cases of diseases, the numbers of transverse oscillations are high, while the numbers of radial oscillations are low. Movement patterns of remedies like homeopathic substances and herbs, on the other hand, always consisted of a larger number of radial movements and a lower number of transverse movements.

Chapter 5

Further Experiments and Findings

The Information Content of Various Substances

The information content of various substances is determined by the geometric forms found on the molecular level of the substance. Our organism in fact responds to the forms of the material structure which may be examined through electron microscopes. This can be tested in the following manner. If you touch the electron microscope image of a silicon crystal, i.e. its molecular structure, and with your right hand you hold the fixed, vertical dowsing rod, you will observe a certain number of radial and transversal movements. If afterwards you touch a real piece of silicon, you will get the same result. If you now proceed to change the structure of the silicon with pencil lines on a print-out of that structure, the test result will be different from that of the real silicon. *The information carried by a substance is determined by the geometric forms found in the structure of the molecule.*

Figure 26 shows the electron microscope image of an object made of gold, which will enable you to perform the above described experiment with a gold object. *(Figure 26)*

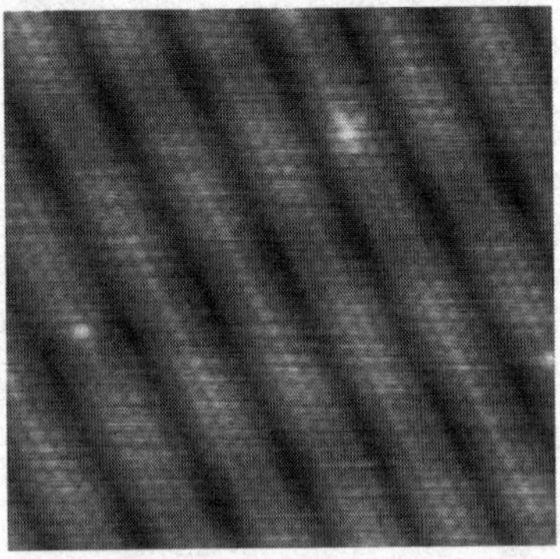

Figure 26.
Electron microscopic image of an object made of gold

Place your left index finger on the illustration of the structure of gold, and you will find that the dowsing rod shows the same kind of movement pattern as if you were holding a genuine piece of gold in your left hand. You will experience the same phenomenon in all substances if you replace the substance with an image of its structure.

Transferring Information to Various Substances

Körbler discovered that if we hold an object or substance in our left hand, our body can act like an antenna. It transfers the 'information of the object' from our left hand to our right hand in an unmodified form; in other words, our body carries out the information transfer. *Körbler named this phenomenon the 'left–right meridian'*. This is an extremely important phenomenon since the information transfer happens in an open dissipative system where the information passes through unaltered. This way the information carried by a substance can be transmitted to a *mediating substance* like water or stones. The medium that thus becomes informed may then be used for healing purposes.

The following experiments demonstrate the existence of information transfer in the body:

1. Fill a glass full of water and hold it in your free hand. If it is a good-quality water, you will notice horizontal swinging. Now place the glass on the table and take a piece of metal in your hand. As mentioned before, the dowsing rod will make a circular motion. After the tests, out down the bio-indicator and pick up the glass of water, and with the water in your right hand and the metal in your left, wait about 4 minutes. After that put them on the table again side by side and test the glass of water. You will observe a circular motion of the dowsing rod. Your body has transferred the information of the metal to the water.

   The water will retain the information of the metal even after it is poured into a new container. If you pour away part of the water, and replace it with tap water and stir the 'mixture' repeatedly, the water you added will also assume the information of the metal from the informed water. The water will retain this information until you introduce new information to it or neutralize it by boiling the water. The explanation is that over 55 °C the effect of the previously introduced information is erased.

2. Now pick up a piece of metal and examine it with the dowsing rod. As usual with metals, you will experience a circular motion. Then put it down and pick up an apple. The test shows horizontal swinging. Put down the rod, pick up the metal with your right hand. Hold the metal and the apple for 4 minutes, then place them on the table and test them. As you touch the piece of metal with your index finger, instead of circular motions, you will observe the ball swinging horizontally. The information carried by the apple has been transmitted through your body into the metal. Repeat the experiment with any optional substance. Let your imagination soar. Transfer information from a chamomile flower to a pebble or from a cabbage to a coin, etc.

Verifying the Transfer of Information with the Vertical Dowsing Rod

With the help of the vertical dowsing rod, as we count the number of oscillations, we can confirm that, indeed, the information of a substance has been transferred to a medium, like water or stone. Let us see how all of this happens in practice.

Hold a piece of gold in your left hand and a glass of water in your right for 4 minutes. Put the gold down, and take the water in your left hand. Test it first with a hand-held dowsing rod, then with the vertical dowsing rod. Both will respond as if you were holding a gold object – the hand-held dowsing rod will make circular movements, while the vertical dowsing rod will show the movement pattern characteristic of gold objects.

Next, hold the glass of water infused with the information of gold in your left hand and in your right hand, hold pure water in another glass for 4 minutes. Testing the second glass will provide the same results as in the first case. You may repeat the experiment any number of times and you will get the same result.

If you place the index finger of your left hand on the electron microscope image of gold and hold another glass of water in your other hand for 4 minutes, upon testing the water you will get the same result as before: *the water 'absorbed' the information of gold.* No matter what substance, crystal or herb you take, information transfer will happen.

Testing the Functioning of the Dowsing Rod

Körbler devised some experiments to demonstrate how the dowsing rod produces the different movement patterns in accordance with the different degrees of compatibility of the test object. He also worked out test controls to rule out misinterpretations regarding the operation of the dowsing rod.

The following experiments require a few apples, some leaves of savoy cabbage, a few sheets of blank, unruled paper, a pen or pencil, transparent sticky tape, a pair of pliers, and a thin and possibly lightweight wooden stick of approximately 50 cm (this can be a reed or a long piece of straw).

Experiment No. 1

Draw a line of about 10 cm on a piece of paper and lay the paper in front of you so that the line is lying at an angle to you. Now place the dowsing rod in your right hand if you are right-handed or in your left if you are left-handed. With your free hand, pick up an apple that makes the dowsing rod move horizontally. Now, hold the apple while you touch the left end of the line: the direction of swinging will remain horizontal. Then touch the right end, and the dowsing rod will swing vertically.

Ask someone to sit down at the table facing you. Place the paper in front of your partner, again at an angle. Pick up the apple again and, and just like before, proceed with the tests. You will observe the dowsing rod swing vertically at the end of the line at *your left,* and it will swing horizontally at the end of the line at *your right.*

This experiment suggests *the reversibility of systemic information.* In the first experiment, the line, which works as an antenna, was within the bounds of your aura and the rod took on a certain polarity. In the second experiment, the line was in your partner's energy field. *The line's magnetic poles reversed.*

Repeat this experiment so that push the paper step by step toward your partner testing the line ends after every step. This way, you can measure the bounds of your aura versus that of your partner.

Experiment No. 2

Place the same paper in front of you so that one end of the line points toward your body. Hold the apple while with your index finger you touch the end of the line pointing toward you – the direction of swinging will remain horizontal, corresponding to the apple. Now touch the further end of the line – the direction of swinging will change to vertical.

Double the length of the line and test it as you did before: the results will not change. Regardless of the length of the 'antenna', its polarity behavior remains unchanged.

Experiment No. 3

Now, place the 50 cm wooden stick in front of you on the table, with one end pointing toward your body. Experiment as you did in the previous instance: and again, the result will be the same. An object also acts as an antenna and is subject to the same regularities. We should recall that our body perceives information in the traditional sense of non-conducting substances. This

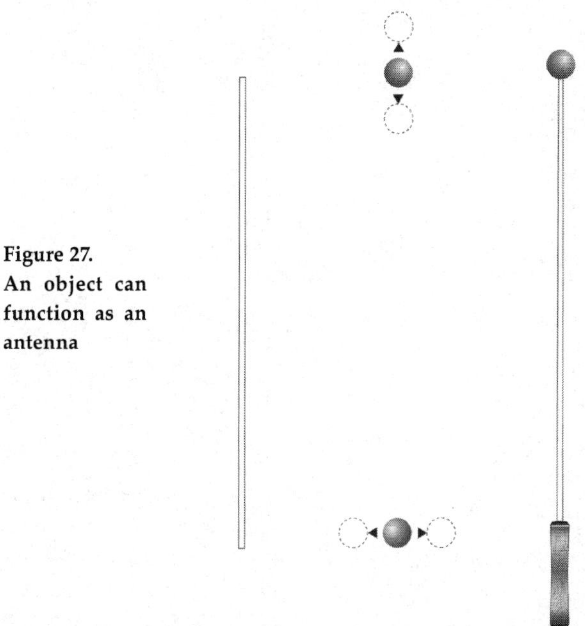

Figure 27.
An object can function as an antenna

information passes through the terahertz domain, which is the tremendously high frequency portion of the electromagnetic spectrum. Owing to this, all substance have a certain conductivity, and therefore, act as an antenna. *(Figure 27)* Given that the dowsing rod and the stick have the same geometric structure, they have the same polarity, and so they act in the same way. Their polarity will remain unchanged regardless of whether you hold them in your hand or put them on the table. The polarities indicate one specific electric condition of the dowsing rod. A state of equilibrium emerges between our own potential and the charge of the air surrounding the tip of the dowsing rod. The weight on the end of the dowsing rod (the ball) produces an additional pre-voltage. Now, if the electric condition in our body changes, or the electric condition of the air does, this will cause the tip of the dowsing rod to be diverted, and this will cause it to swing.

The movement of the rod is determind by the electrical charge of your body and the electrical charge present whereever the test is carried out.

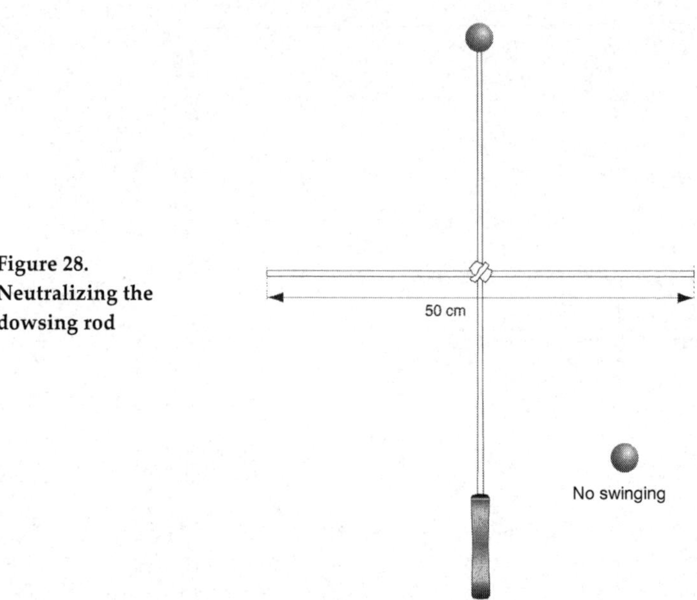

Figure 28. Neutralizing the dowsing rod

Experiment No. 4

This experiment demonstrates how you can neutralize the dowsing rod by using an electric connecting element (e.g. a stick). Draw an equal-armed cross of any size on a piece of paper. In this symbol, the electrical charges are equal but of opposite signs, and their just opposition neutralizes any flow between them. Now pick up the apple and the dowsing rod. Hold the apple about 10 cm above the cross and watch the tip of the dowsing rod. The cross neutralizes the electrical charge in its area.

Next we attempt to neutralize the dowsing rod. Fix a 50 cm long stick across the rod to form a cross. Now carefully pick up the dowsing rod so that its position remains horizontal and test the apple – we will see no movement. Test other objects, as well. No matter whether you hold the tested object in your hand or you hold the dowsing rod over it, there will be no movement. *(Figure 28)*

In the following experiments, where we shorten the 'cross-stick' step by step (see experiments Nos. 5–7), we avoid testing metal objects because these create a circular movement.

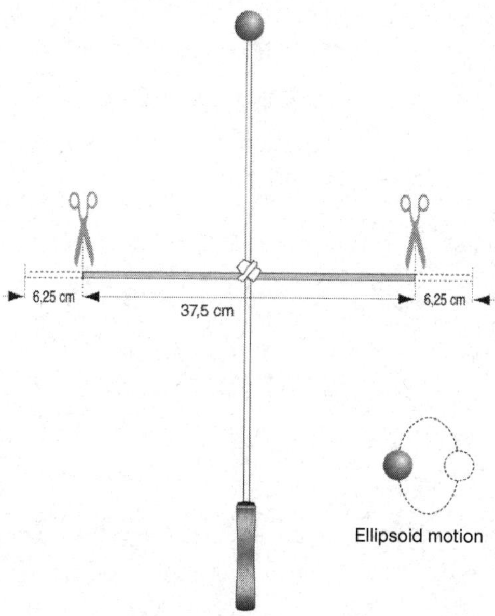

Figure 29.
A modified dowsing rod No. 1

Experiment No. 5

Shorten the stick that you fixed to the dowsing rod by 6.25 cm at each end and test the apple again. The dowsing rod will move along a vertical ellipse, clockwise. Now, if you are testing a substance that is intolerable to your organism, the dowsing rod will move horizontally clockwise, describing an ellipse. By shortening the cross-stick we have changed the electrical characteristics of the dowsing rod. There is still energy flow but it is in accordance with the conditions of the modified dowsing rod. *(Figure 29)*

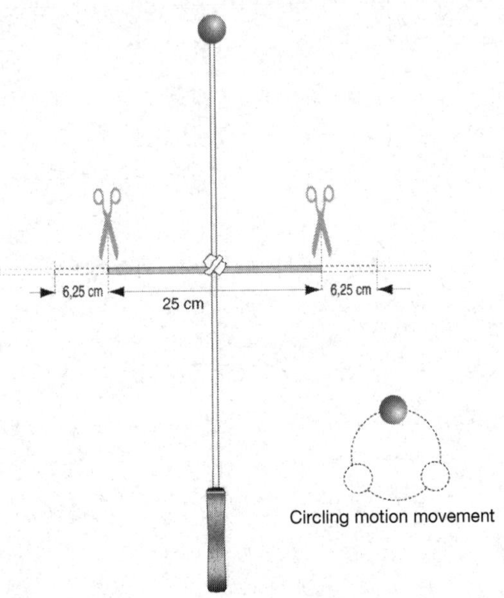

Figure 30.
A modified dowsing rod No. 2

Experiment No. 6

Shorten both ends of the cross-stick once more by 6.25 cm, so that the total length of the stick will now be only 25 cm. Test the apple – the dowsing rod will make a circular movement, clockwise. The direction of rotation reveals whether the effect is favorable or unfavorable for your organism. Clockwise motion means favorable, anticlockwise means unfavorable effects. *(Figure 30)*

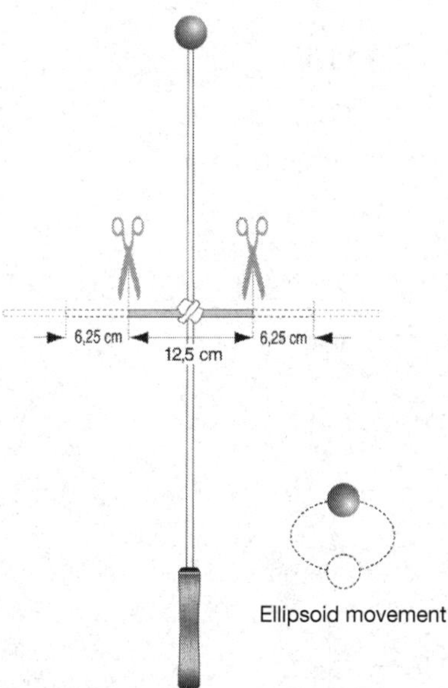

Figure 31. A modified dowsing rod No. 3

Experiment No. 7

Shorten both ends of the cross-stick by a further 6.25 cm at each end. Repeat the test – the swinging movement will again be elliptic. When testing the apple, again, the dowsing rod will move horizontally, clockwise, describing an ellipse. Finally, remove the remains of the cross-stick. Test the apple, and the dowsing rod will once again move horizontally. *(Figure 31)*

These experiments have demonstrated that the swinging of the dowsing rod depends on the form of the rod since it is that which defines the current distribution of the electric fields.

Neutralizing the pendulum and the magic wand

The above principle holds true for all magic wands and also the sideric pendulum. In the case of the sideric pendulum, the string or chain acts as an antenna, while the form of the weight is not relevant in its operation. The pendulum can also be 'switched off' if you use a piece of wire the same length as the rope, applied

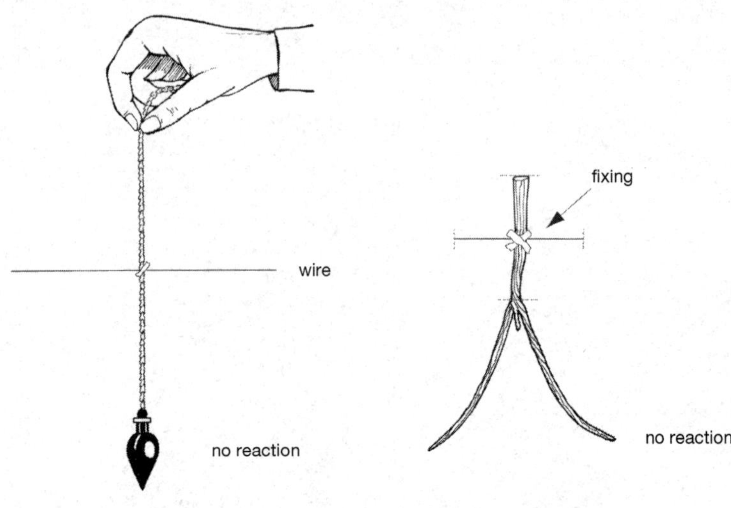

Figure 32.
Neutralizing the pendulum

Figure 33.
Neutralizing a magic wand

in a cross shape. To neutralize a Y-shaped or fork-shaped magic wand, you need to fix the cross-stick in the middle of the straight part, diagonally across. *(Figures 32 and 33)*

These experiments have shown that magic wands and sideric pendulums operate due to the antenna nature of the electrical charge present where the test is carried out. In other words, they move according to the type of electric condition that our body mediates to the testing instrument.

Testing the Reliability of the Dowsing Rod

Experiment

Now that we have come to understand the secret of the dowsing rod, we shall test its reliability. Place a few leaves fresh and a few leaves of yellow savoy cabbage on the table. Draw a 2-cm-line on a piece of paper. Pick up the fresh and then the yellow cabbage leaves and hold them about 3 cm above the middle of the line. In the case of the fresh and healthy leaves, the dowsing rod will swing horizontally; while with the yellow leaves, it will swing vertically.

On another sheet of paper draw two parallel lines of 2 cm each. The distance between them should be around 0.2 cm. Similarly, draw a cluster of three, then four, and five parallel lines on separate paper each. Lay the sheets side by side on the table. Now pick up the yellow cabbage leaves and while holding your outstretched index finger at a distance of about 3 cm above the middle of the two parallel lines, do the tests: the dowsing rod will move vertically shaping an ellipse.

Now hold your index finger over the middle of the three parallel lines: the dowsing rod will move in circles, anticlockwise.

Test the four parallel lines: the dowsing rod will move horizontally, describing an ellipse.

If you test the withered cabbage leaf over the middle of the set of five lines, the dowsing rod will move horizontally.

If you become doubtful of the results while testing, repeat the tests one by one, starting with the one-line test and ending with the five-line test. If in the five-line test you register movements contrary to the one-line test, you are sure that your testing is correct. *(Figure 34)*

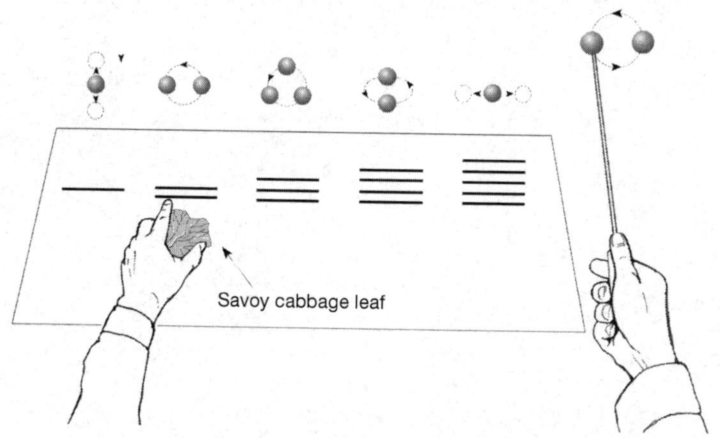

Figure 34. Testing the reliability of the dowsing rod

Distribution and polarization of electric and magnetic fields

Experiment No. 1

Draw a line of 10 cm on a clean, unruled sheet of paper with a pen or a pencil. Put the dowsing rod in your right hand (or left if you are left-handed) and in your other hand hold a small object which causes the dowsing rod to swing horizontally. Hold this object in hand while with your index finger you touch the left end of the line: the dowsing rod will move horizontally. Now touch the right end of the line: the dowsing rod will swing vertically. Touch the middle of the line: the dowsing rod will stop moving.

Now, following *Figure 35,* touch the spots above and below the line in your drawing. Motions of the dowsing rod are as shown in the figure:

- In the area marked **'a'**, the direction of swinging is the same as in the area marked **'A'**, i.e. the left end of the line.
- In the area marked **'b'**, the direction of swinging is the same as in the area marked **'B'**, which is the right end of the line.
- At the middle of the line at 0, there will be no motion.

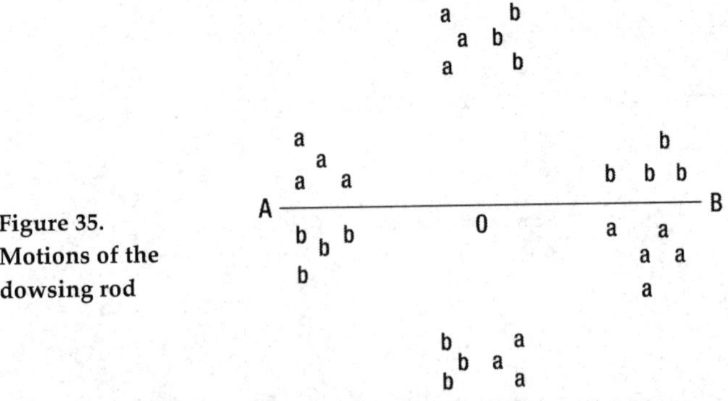

Figure 35. Motions of the dowsing rod

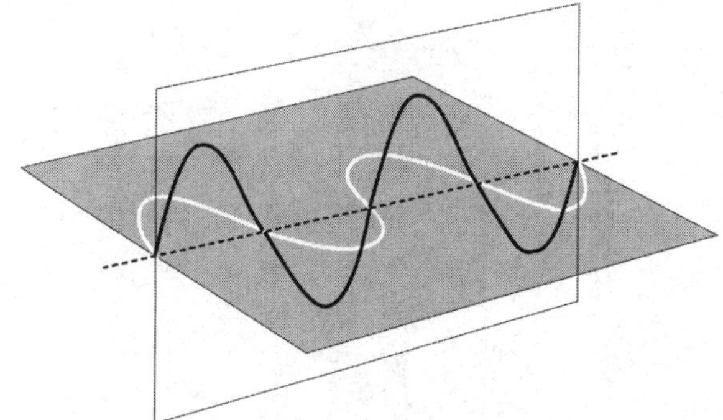

Figure 36

In the previous experiment, by means of the dowsing rod, we experienced a type of electromagnetic field where electromagnetic waves exhibit polarization as a result of the waves oscillating with more than one orientation. *Figure 36* depicts the *distribution of the electromagnetic fields around a line, where the line behaves like a 'superconductor' that captured the waves causing them to become standing waves (See Chapter 3 'The function of water molecules in the cell' for superconductivity).* The electric field is in a vertical plane and the magnetic field in a horizontal plane. The fields are in phase and at 90 degrees to each other. *(Figure 36).*

Now rotate the paper so that the line points toward your body. While performing the test – see *Figure 37* – in each case you will find that the end of the line closer to you exhibits the same polarity as all the left-hand-side end-points did before.

Depending on the position of your line, fold the long or short edge of the paper back 4 cm, and place it on the table so the line 'stands' vertically in front of you. Test the ends of the line as before. You will find that the end of the line pointing upwards has the same polarity as the ones on the left side or the ones close to your body had just before. Touch all the spots as shown in *Figure 35*, as well: the result will be as expected: a = A, b = B, etc. In this experiment we gained three-dimensional information about a line with respect to its electromagnetic field, and also its antenna-type behavior. We were particularly mindful of the distribution of the fields.

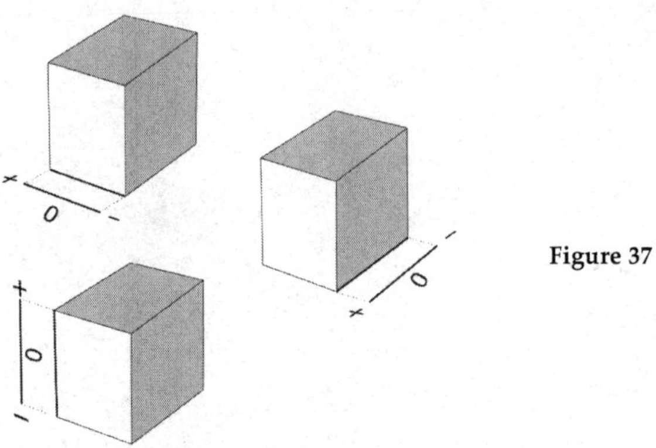

Figure 37

In the next experiment we will test a spherical object, such as a ball or a globe *(Figure 38 and 39)*. Observe the distribution of the fields while performing the tests.

Experiment No. 2

Use the index finger of your free hand to touch the left-hand side of the object. The dowsing rod will swing horizontally. Touch the right-hand side of the sphere – the dowsing rod will swing vertically. Touch the point ont he surface of the sphere nearst to you – the dowsing rod will swing horizontally. Test the most remote point of the surface – the dowsing rod will swing vertically. Now try to reach the bottom-most point on the surface of the sphere – the dowsing rod will swing vertically.

On a sphere, identical polarities are found on the left, front and top. On the right, bottom and at the back we find the opposite. The zero point which is known to be inevitable with different polarities is not to be found anywhere on the surface. This means that it must be inside, in the center of the sphere.

Mark a point on the 'equator' of the sphere and start a set of experiments with a simulated 'sunrise'. Observe as the distributions of the fields are changing on the sphere. Repeat the tests until you reach the mark. The 'north pole' and 'south pole' will remain identical throughout the spinning. At the other points, the distribution of the fields will keep shifting *(Figures 38 and 39)*.

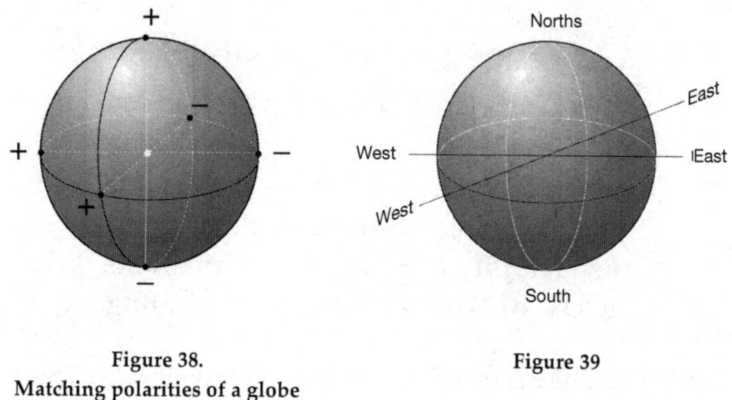

Figure 38.
Matching polarities of a globe

Figure 39

Should you wish to compare the conditions you have just experienced with those that obtain on our Earth, there are a few other factors you will need to take into account. The electric system of the Earth is an existing reality. All we can influence is its effect, i.e. the distribution of the magnetic field. The Earth is in interaction not only with the energy of the Sun, but also other energies, such as the energy of the Moon, as well as its own energy and its spinning energy. The weather and its positive or negative charge also heavily influence the distribution of the fields at all points except the polar zones.

Chapter 6

Experiments for Transmitting Healing Information

Körbler's Principle of the Reversibility of Systemic Information; the Use of Geometric Forms in Healing

The experiments described so far allow us to notice how consistently the hand-held dowsing rod shows favorable and unfavorable information – in the former case it moves horizontally, in the latter, vertically. This indicates that communication between the biological system of the tester and the tested substances takes place according to a shared language; it is like a universal language understood by all. This language enables cells to communicate with each other and with all substances they come into contact.

The multilateral connections of subtle-energetic resonances of substances and biological systems determine our lives as elementary principles. This is why Körbler's discovery, 'the principle of the reversibility of systemic information', is of outstanding importance. This principle applies to the tremendously high-frequency band. In this domain all forms act as secondary antennas and all objects (substances) have some form of electrical conductivity. It is the ability to carry the flow of an electric current. A given substance responds to an applied electrical field. The electric field around the substance becomes polarized according to the geometric forms of the substance that comes in contact with it. This means that due to the influx of information, when we apply a geometric symbol to the substance, a corresponding charge pattern is produced in accordance with that symbol, and it is that pattern that is conveyed. This is the basic tenet of New

Homeopathy which Körbler named 'the principle of the reversibility of systemic information'.

Since the above phenomenon is caused by a difference in conductivity, any form constituted by any object, such as a pen line on paper, or a geometric form made of wire or of wood, or even a ray of light of a given form, will generate a change in the subtle-energetic information of the substance when it is in contact with a living organism. Experiments also suggest that it does not matter whether the line is of 10 cm or 1 cm long: the polarization will be opposing at the two ends of the line. It means the quality of the information carried by the form is independent of the dimension of the form being applied. In case of equal-armed crosses, notwithstanding variations in size, the information they carried is always the same. However, the distance at which the effect is manifested depends on the size of the cross.

The use of geometric symbols is based on the principle of reversibility of systemic information, both in the case of healing and of averting or eliminating harmful radiation. The geometric symbols used by New Homeopathy in healing, such as the equal-armed cross, a Y, a sine curve, Körbler's vector system, are suitable for changing the information content of electromagnetic waves coming from the outside or from inside the body. In this chapter we describe the properties of these symbols.

In the following section we present a series of experiments that will allow you to experience how objects and forms behave as secondary antennas in transmitting and transforming information through the terahertz range. During the experiments it also becomes clear how the healing information is transmitted while using the symbols, i.e. how the information of the living system changes in line with Körbler's principle of the reversibility of systemic information.

Experiments related to the magnitude of the line as a geometric form

Experiment No. 1

Draw a line of about 20 cm on a blank sheet of paper. Pick up the dowsing rod in one hand, while in your left hand you hold an object that causes the dowsing rod to move horizontally.

Test this object so that you first touch the left end of the line with the index finger of the hand holding the object, and the dowsing rod will continue to swing horizontally; then touch the right end of the line and the rod will swing vertically. As usual, touch the middle of the line with your index finger – the ball at the end of the dowsing rod will stop moving.

Repeat this experiment with any substance – in every case you will note the change in the direction of swinging and also how the dowsing rod stops when over the middle of the line *(Figure 40).*

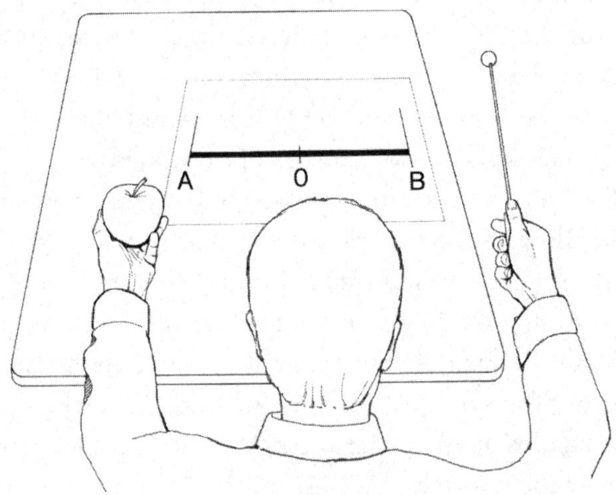

Figure 40.
The line as an antenna

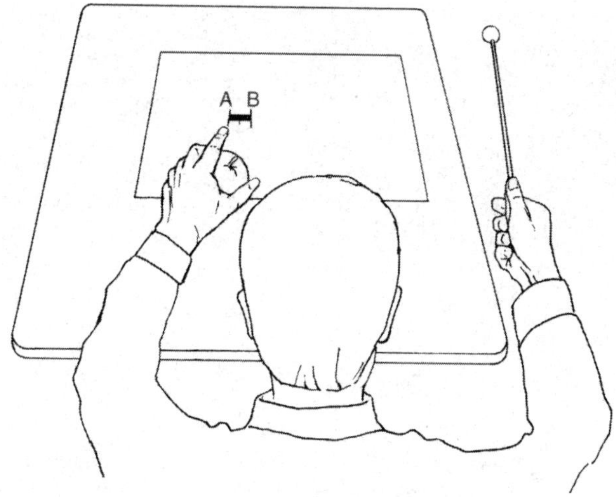

Figure 41.
The antenna effect is independent of the length of the line

Experiment No. 2

The next experiment explores how the size of the secondary antenna, i.e. the length of the line, influences the transformation of systemic information. Draw a line of 1 cm. Touch the left end of the line with the hand holding the apple – the dowsing rod will swing horizontally. Now touch the right end – the dowsing rod will swing vertically. Touch the middle of the line – the dowsing rod will stand motionless. This demonstrates that the principle of the reversibility of systemic information operates in every case, regardless of the dimension, even in the smallest dimensions such as on the level of molecular structure. *(Figure 41)*

Experiments to identify the effect of the wave amplitudes

Experiment No. 1

Draw a wave curve of growing amplitude on a blank sheet of paper. Touch the following points with the index finger of the hand holding the tested substance:

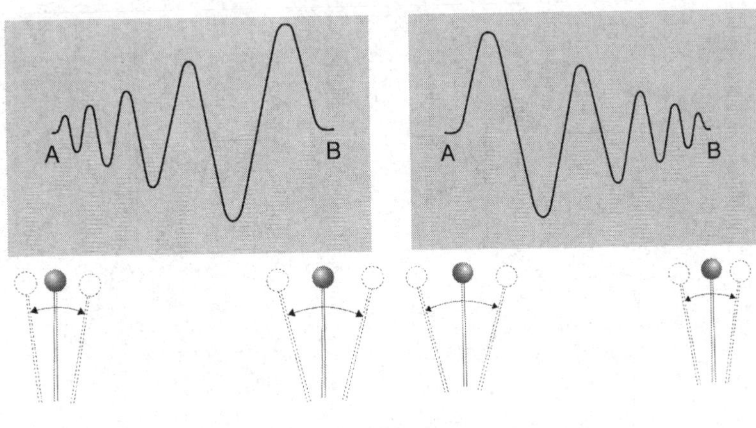

Figure 42

Figure 43

Point **A** – the intensity of the movement of the dowsing rod remains unchanged.

Point **B** – the intensity of the swinging of the dowsing rod will increase. *(Figure 42)*

Experiment No. 2

Take the above figure and lay it out in front of you with the waving line decreasing from left to right. Now touch point **A** – the dowsing rod will swing intensely;

touch point **B** – the intensity of the swinging will decrease. *(Figure 43)*

Basic Symbols in New Homeopathy

Anthropological research shows that peoples living at the most remote points of the Earth have been using the same geometric symbols since ancient times. Without having knowledge of each other's activity, they used them to keep themselves healthy and vigorous and to recover from disease.[1] These basic symbols are the following: symbols consisting of 2–9 parallel lines, the equal-armed cross, and the Y symbol.

Interestingly, these symbols are completely identical to the basic symbols used by New Homeopathy. If we add the sine curve, we will have the full range of the basic symbols applied by New Homeopathy. Knowledge and experience gained in the fields of electronics, and the latest findings in quantum physics and in theoretical physics of chaos revolution guided Körbler to introduce these symbols into the healing practice. The antenna-like structure of these symbols makes them ideal for eliminating disharmony in the body – e.g. a disharmony in the functioning of an internal organ; in other words, a disharmony in the electromagnetic charge pattern of the corresponding area.

Below we present the basic geometric symbols, opening each section with an experiment by Körbler. These experiments reveal how the Körbler symbols work as 'secondary antennas'.

The Equal-armed Cross

The first basic symbol in New Homeopathy is the *equal-armed cross.* In the following experiment you will gain a step-by-step experience of how the electric field emerges and then restructurs itself between the arms of the cross.

Experiment No. 1

This experiment will require two pieces of wire – or any thin straight piece of material, such as metal or wood – 10 cm each. Lay one of the pieces crosswise in front of you. Pick up an apple – you will see the dowsing rod move horizontally. Now touch the left end of the wire with the index finger of the hand holding the apple. The rod will continue to swing horizontally. Now touch the right end of the wire and the direction of swinging will change to vertical. Touch the wire in the middle. The dowsing rod will stay still. Now lay the other piece of wire across the first one so that you get four equal arms. Test it as before. No matter where you touch the cross, you will experience no motion. Where the wires cross each other, the opposing electric fields become superimposed; they neutralize each other's effect, i.e. they block the flow of energy. Thus the wires block information flow and cannot act as a 'secondary antenna'.

Experiment No. 2

Draw a line of about 20 cm. Name end-points **A** and **B**, as in *Figure 44*. Mark the middle with **0**. Touch the various points on the paper with your index finger and compare the results with the ones in *Figure 35*.

Touch point **A** – the dowsing rod swings horizontally.

Touch point **B** – the rod swings in the opposite direction.

Touch point **0** – there is no motion.

Touch points **a** – the direction of swinging is the same as at point **A**.

Touch points **b** – the movement is the same as at point **B**.

Touch point **0** – there is no motion

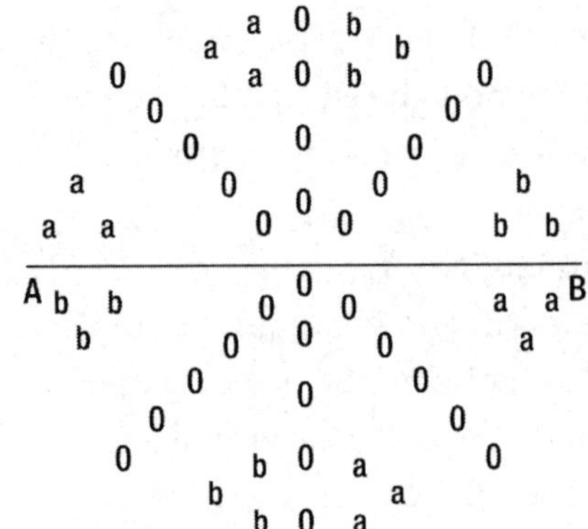

Figure 44

Naturally, this phenomenon takes place in three dimensions. Once you become adept at performing these experiments, you can repeat the tests so that you do not touch the paper but you hold your fingertip at about 1 cm above the marked point. The further away you hold your finger from the paper, the less vigorously the rod will move; i.e. the weaker the information flow will be.

Put your paper in a position so that you have an oblique line in front of you. The end of the line closer to you will behave in the same way as end-point A in *Figure 44* before. Further reactions change in accordance with this.

Experiments related to transforming information with the equal-armed cross

Körbler demonstrates through various experiments on information transference how we can test the power of the equal-armed cross to block information flow.

For these experiments, you will need a metal key, and another object that you previously tested with the vertical dowsing rod to establish its information. You will also need a white sheet of cardboard and a felt-tip pen. In this series of experiments Körbler used a homeopathic remedy of D23 dilution.

Experiment No. 1: If you hold the key in your left hand and the homeopathic remedy in your right hand for 4 minutes, the information of the homeopathic remedy will change, since your body will have transmitted the information of the key to the substance.

Experiment No. 2: If you hold the key with a folded-up sheet of cardboard and repeat the experiment this way, the information of the key will be transmitted again into the homeopathic remedy.

Experiment No. 3: If, however, you draw equal-armed crosses on the outside of the cardboard with the felt-tip pen and do the experiment that way, the information of the key will not be transferred to the homeopathic substance.

At the end of each information transfer, the quality of the homeopathic remedy can be identified with the help of the vertical dowsing rod.

The equal-armed cross in information medicine

The above experiments demonstrate well that the equal-armed cross blocks the information flow. Körbler explained this phenomenon with the principle of the reversibility of systemic information. He published the results in *Raum und Zeit* 'Universalrute III Special 3, pp 11'. *1990–93.*

Transplanting these qualities of the equal-armed cross into practice and exploiting the protective function of this symbol in all fields of life played an outstanding role in Körbler's work. After years of experimentation and a long study in anthropology, he developed the most practicable devices. The *energy-transforming sheet* has a pattern of equal-armed crosses to neutralize geopathic zones. Körbler mainly used it to clear harmful radiations from sleeping areas, although he also applied it under carpets or nailed it to walls, etc. Wherever a transforming sheet could not be applied, he used equal-armed crosses outdoors and indoors to neutralize geopathic zones.

An interesting instance of synchronicity is that the protective role of the equal-armed cross surfaced in a number of different contexts in 1990–91 in Austria (Vienna and the Ötztal Alps), Hungary (Budapest), and in Germany, in *Raum und Zeit.* In 1990 Körbler obtained a patent on the transforming sheet. Production of the sheet according to the strictest instructions was launched in fall 1990 in cooperation with the *BUDAPRINT Goldberger Textilművek Rt.* in Óbuda, Budapest, Hungary. As we mentioned in the Preface, the various stages of the work were supervised and the product tested by my brother, István Sági. (We preserve to this day the printing cylinder with the cross pattern we were given as a present when BUDAPRINT was closed down in 1997.) Körbler presented the new invention in *Raum und Zeit, Special 3* 'Endlich ein Bettuch gegen Erdstrahlen', pp 29-31. 1990-93.

Körbler studied the use of the equal-armed cross among primitive peoples and reported that members of the Huichol Indians living in a remote region of the Sierra Madre mountains in

Central Mexico still use the equal-armed cross to protect themselves from harmful influences. It is used in healing and to provide geopathic and spiritual protection for the living areas. Cross-shaped body ornamentation is used to protect their health. Crosses of a few centimeters are worn on the body, while large crosses of about 2 m are used to protect larger spaces.

Körbler offered an explanation for this phenomenon: the effective range of equal-armed crosses depends on the size of the cross, since that is what determines the size of the wave emitted. His experience showed that placing the crosses is most effective with one arm oriented to the North, because this is how the partials and secondary waves are strongest, granting maximum chance for the exact replica of the original wave to spread further.

Optimal placement of the equal-armed cross is something we practiced and tested continually in Hungary, in an attempt to neutralize harmful geopathic radiation in homes. Körbler used this method wherever it was necessary. At a school in Vienna, he placed an equal-armed cross at a turn in the stairs where children very often used to fall over. After the cross was introduced, the children ceased to stumble or fall over. (In the final chapter we will discuss in detail the options for using equal-armed crosses to neutralize geopathic zones.)

In fall 1991 news began to appear about Ötzi – a human body found by an Austrian tourist in the Ötztal Alps, 60 meters from the Austrian–Italian border, on the Italian side.[2] A mummy with brown-coloured skin was found frozen in the glacier, bearing parallel lines on his back, legs and wrist, and an equal-armed cross on his knees. Next to it they found a stone knife, a bronze axe, a bow and some arrows. Thorough examination and an autopsy revealed that there were adhesions corresponding to the parallel lines. The frozen body was established to be approximately 5000 years old.

In Issue No. 55 of *Raum und Zeit,* published in January 1992, in an article called 'Neue Homöopathie VI', Körbler gave a detailed analysis of the significance of the equal-armed cross and parallel lines found on Ötzi's body. Earlier, in 'Neue Homöopathie II', he had already explained that in ancient cultures, besides the use of medical herbs, healing was also practiced by drawing parallel lines and equilateral triangles on the body. They did so, although they probably culd not explain the secondary antenna effect of geometric symbols in the terahertz regime. Based on Körbler's system, the same geometric symbols are now used in healing with the assistance of the dowsing rod. The equal-armed cross is used, for instance, in cases where tranquilization is called for.

In his article 'Neue Homöopathie II'[3] Körbler analyzed the electromagnetic protective function of the Christian cross, which is less potent from an electromagnetic point of view than the equal-armed cross. This aroused my interest and I began to study crosses that appear on Catholic sacred objects and fabrics. To my surprise, in most places I found equal-armed crosses. The splendid patterns of chasubles widely used equal-armed crosses, either in an ornamental form or in an ornamental setting. Most chasubles showed an equal-armed cross on the back, even in the case of monochrome chasubles. The cloth covering the chalice also shows an equal-armed cross, and the list could go on much longer.

Around this time I witnessed the following scene in the Opera House, during a performance of *Tosca*. 'On the right-hand side of the stage an aged priest is praying, with a huge cross suspended from his neck. Suddenly, the devil appears to him in the form of a man. With a quick, instinctive flash of a gesture, the priest grabs the cross with his right hand, covering up just enough of the longer member for the rest to produce an equal-armed cross. Hiding behind the huge cross, he holds his arm right out in front of him, and calls out the usual spell, 'Be gone from me, Satan!' The scene was truly impressive and breathtakingly dramatic. All of this leads one to ask the question whether Christian culture might not also recognize and use the equal-armed cross as a sacred symbol and a protective instrument.

The subject was thoroughly researched by Dr Róbert Csiszár who explored the various cultural manifestations of the cross as a healing symbol and its application in healing.[4]

The Y

The second basic symbol in New Homeopathy is the Y symbol. In the experiments described below we shall see how this symbol influences the electromagnetic information of the test object.

Experiment No. 1

Use a pencil or pen to draw a Y of about 10 cm on a blank sheet of paper. Pick up an apple and during your testing touch the drawing at any point: the dowsing rod will always swing horizontally. *(Figure 45a)*

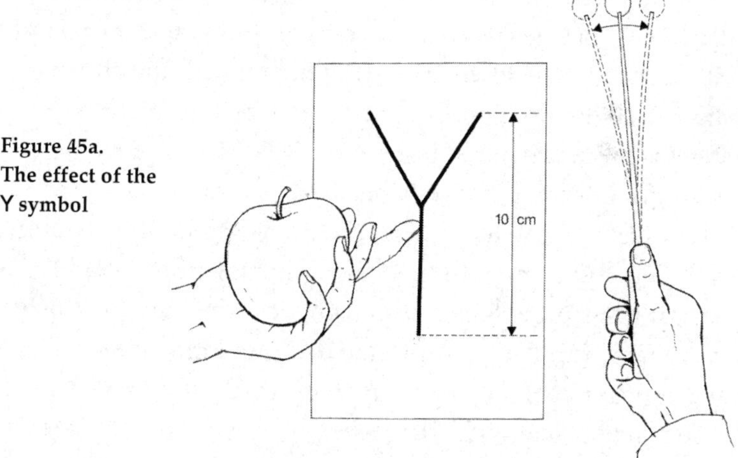

Figure 45a. The effect of the Y symbol

Now test a packet of salt. The dowsing rod will move vertically, indicating that this amount of salt is unhealthy for you. With the hand holding the salt, touch the drawing at any point – the dowsing rod will start moving horizontally *(Figure 45b).*

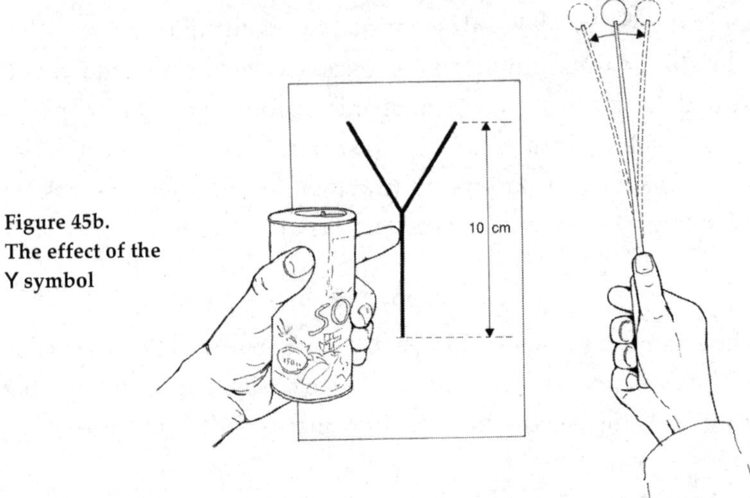

Figure 45b. The effect of the Y symbol

This means that the electromagnetic information of the packet of salt has turned favorable under the influence of the Y symbol.

If you test a packet of refined icing sugar, you will find that it is unhealthy for you. This means that when we put the sugar in our mouth, its electromagnetic information will represent an extra hazard besides its chemical reactions. If you keep a packet of icing sugar close to your body, soon you will find that its radiation is so intense that its electromagnetic information is perceived as an unfavorable resonance. This can be prevented by drawing a letter Y on the outside of the packet.

We must make a distinction whether we are testing an object or a living organism with the Y symbol. In the case of a lifeless object, it transforms the electromagnetic radiation of the object to a tolerable form but, naturally, it does not influence the chemical composition of the object. In other words, if you treat a poisonous substance with the letter Y, you only change its electromagnetic radiation but the substance itself will remain poisonous.

The same rule applies if you treat freshly picked fruit with the Y symbol. If a fruit is unripe or has been treated with chemicals, the Y symbol will only change its electromagnetic radiation but the chemical composition remains unchanged. If it was unhealthy for our organism, consumption should be avoided even after treatment with the Y symbol.

Use of the Y symbol

Being aware of the role of letter Y as a secondary antenna, Körbler explored the areas where the *information reversal function* of the Y symbol can be useful for people. He examined its role in neutralizing geopathic zones, and as a result of the experiments, he devised an *energy-building sheet* with a pattern of a *combination of equal-armed crosses and* Y*'s.* This sheet serves to improve the subtle-energetic quality of any place.

Körbler found that the combination of these symbols neutralizes lateral radiation, and it also averts the harmful radiation of satellites. (In the final chapter we give detailed attention to the uses of the Y symbol in neutralizing geopathic zones.) If there are many different types of geopathic exposures, using the Y symbol can render the energy of the place tolerable or even favorable for humans. If the energy of a place was favorable even originally, combinations of symbols containing a Y symbol will turn it into a 'power place', which means that for humans it will serve as an energy field of the kind characteristic of noted cathedrals, churches, or places of worship. This is why Körbler advised that before examinations we ask the patient to lie down on a sheet of this kind for about 10–15 minutes, and only then we can start our examination. It is enough time to rebalance disharmonic frequencies coming from tiredness or fatigue, and the examiner receives valid information about the condition of the body.

The Y symbol in healing

In the natural universe we find a number of examples how the Y 'works'. In the world of plants, for example, the Y-shaped branch-off points of trees correct information that is harmful for

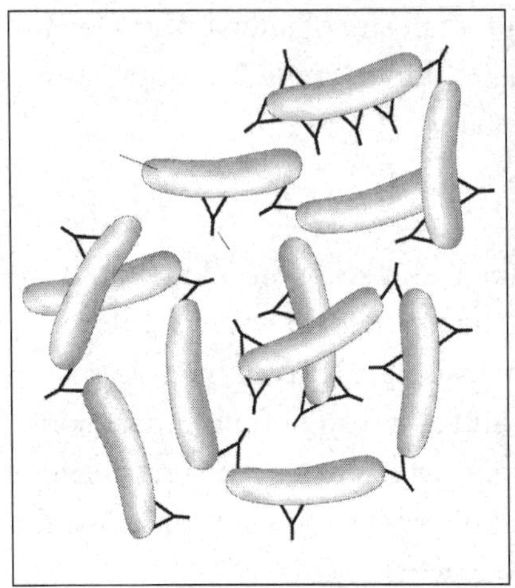

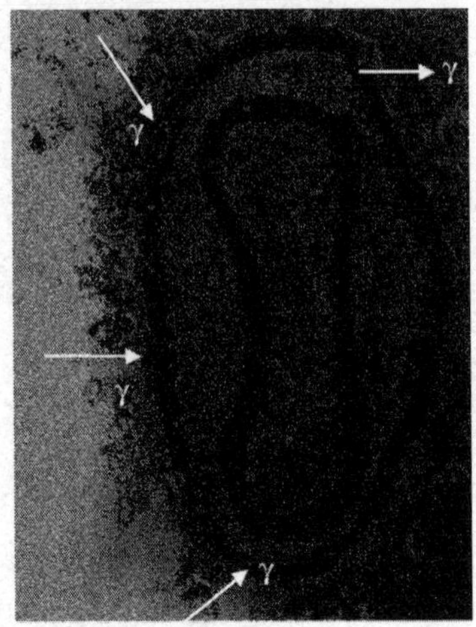

Figures 46a and 46b. Y-shaped antibodies

them. This is particularly salient in single-trunk trees. Another example: our immune system uses a geometric symbol against unwelcome invaders in the form of the antibody. This is a Y symbol whose role has been known for a long time. An antibody molecule consits of two group-specific heavy protein chains combined with two light chains. During an immune defense reaction these large Y-shaped protein molecules – also known as immunoglobulins – stick to the bacteria or form bridges between them causing them to precipitate *(Figures 46a and 46b)*. Electron microscope images of different viruses show clearly how one or more Y-shaped antibodies, a hundred times smaller than the virus itself, are stuck to it. The Y symbol alters the charge pattern of the virus, preventing it from multiplying, so it falls apart and is carried away by phagocytes.

In the case of a living organism, the Y form regulates and strengthens the energy circulation of any given place. It is very powerful. This form awakens and increases energy flow, either in favor of the organism or against it. Therefore it is used with the greatest circumspection in healing. When used, the effect must be monitored continually, because it may cause an overly intense flow of energy and launch an inflammation process, or aggravate an already existing one.

At one of our New Homeopathy courses in Budapest we had a student who had been struggling with an inflammation of the middle ear and had drawn a Y symbol at the base of her ear, after which her pains grew intolerable. This was the point at which she came to see us, asking what she should do. We examined her with the dowsing rod and proposed the use of a sine curve. As a result, her condition improved rapidly.

Use of the Y symbol is extremely useful in enhancing the energy flow in the body when it is insufficient. If, for example, it is necessary to improve venal circulation, then as a gentle method, it is a good idea to use the Y symbol.

If the lymphatic system lacks energy, using the Y symbol will stimulate the flow of lymph. In both cases a control check-up is required at least every 2 days.

Using the Y symbol is of outstanding importance in curing psychosomatic problems. The symbol is also able to neutralize the negative, harmful effect of imaginary or genuine ills and grudges. Further on, an entire chapter is devoted to discussing such a role of the Y symbol (see Chapter 11).

The Sine Curve

The third basic symbol in New Homeopathy is the sine curve. The following experiment shows its effect.

Experiment No. 1

Pick up an apple. If it is unflawed, the dowsing rod will swing horizontally. Take a large sheet of paper, draw a sine curve in the middle, and cut this shape out of the paper with a width of about 3 mm. Turn your desk lamp on and stand the cardboard with the 'sine-cut' on the table so that you let the lamp light shine through the cut, while holding an apple in the ray of light on the other side of the cardboard. Test the apple with the sine-shaped

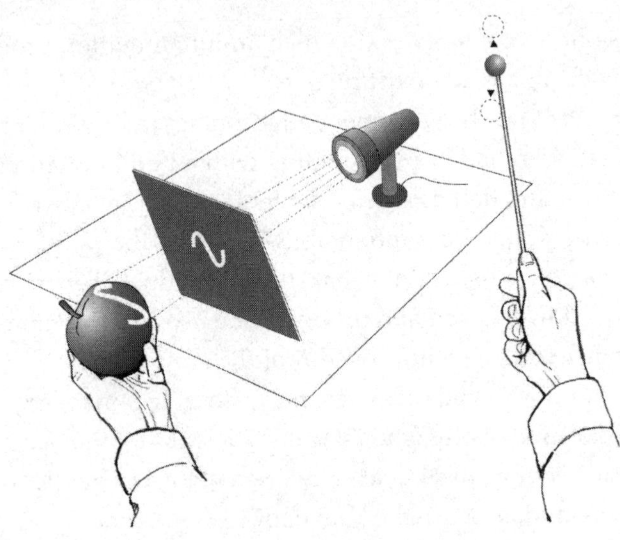

Figure 47. The effect of sine-shaped light on the subtle-energetic information of an apple

light on it as in *Figure 47.* You will find that as soon as the sine-cut appears on the apple, the direction of swinging will change to vertical *(Figure 47).*

Experiment No. 2

Take three new sheets of cardboard and draw a sine curve on each, following *Figures 48a, 48b and 48c.* In the first drawing we mark *the center of the sine curve* and name it **A**. On the second figure *the deepest point of the sine curve* will be **B**. In the third figure we name *the peak of the sine curve* **C**.

Touch point **A** – as compared to the starting point of the sine, at point **A** the direction of swinging changes, the dowsing rod swings in a vertical plane. At point **B** the dowsing rod starts moving in circles, clockwise. At point **C** – the circles will be reversed, anticlockwise. *(Figures 48a, 48b, 48c)*

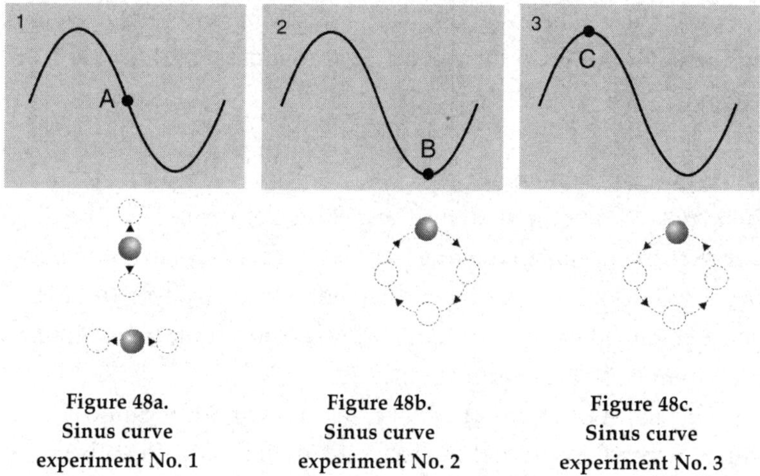

Figure 48a. Sinus curve experiment No. 1

Figure 48b. Sinus curve experiment No. 2

Figure 48c. Sinus curve experiment No. 3

Transferring information with the sine curve

The following information transmission experiment will allow you to test the effect of the sine curve. The vertical dowsing rod reveals how the sine curve reverses the electromagnetic information of a substance. The swing pattern of a substance affected by the sine curve will always be the reverse of the original swing pattern.

Experiment No. 3

Use a homeopathic remedy of dilution D23 and pour a part of it into a glass and some into a bottle. Draw some sine curves with a felt-tip pen on a strip of white paper and wrap the paper around the bottle. Hold the wrapped bottle in your left hand, and the glass in your right hand for four minutes. Now test both substances with the vertical dowsing rod. Surprisingly, the information of the homeopathic remedy will have been reversed in both the bottle and the glass.

Testing a homeopathic dilution D23 of greater celandine *(Chelidonium majus)* will result in 63 radial and 40 transversal swings. When wrapped around with the piece of paper bearing the sine curve, it shows the exact opposite – 40 radial and 63 transversal swings. Thus, the information of the substance has been reversed.

The sine curve in healing

In Körbler's vector system, the geometric symbol of the sine curve corresponds to the five parallel lines, that is the 5th vector *(see Figure 49)*. It causes the movement of the dowsing rod to become reversed compared to its original (horizontal) movement, i.e. it will switch to vertical.

This symbol is one that reverses 'information quality' of a substance: an unfavorable electromagnetic 'effect' can become favorable, and thus this is the most important symbol in healing. This is why it is the rapidest way of helping our patients. We know, however, that the sine curve will reverse every electromagnetic quality, which means that it will also turn favorable quality into unfavorable. Therefore its operation must be checked on at least once a week. The extended application of the sine curve can prevent the wound from healing, or reverse the process, and it can result in an oscillation of good and bad conditions. This may happen once a day or even every 5 minutes. As soon as the healing process starts, it is advisable to use a different symbol other than a sine curve.

A sine curve may be used for injuries and wounds if you draw this symbol next to the wound – the injured part will heal more quickly and pain will be reduced. It is applicable to backaches, problems of the knees, inflammation processes (e.g. sore throats) or bites, the method being to draw the sine curve on the affected body part. In the case of bronchitis we draw it on the left- and right-hand-side acupuncture point, which instantly soothes coughing. In the case of an irritable cough, we draw it over the thorax and the acupuncture points. It is extremely useful for overcoming infection in children. Körbler's daughter was never given medication, except for informed water made by the

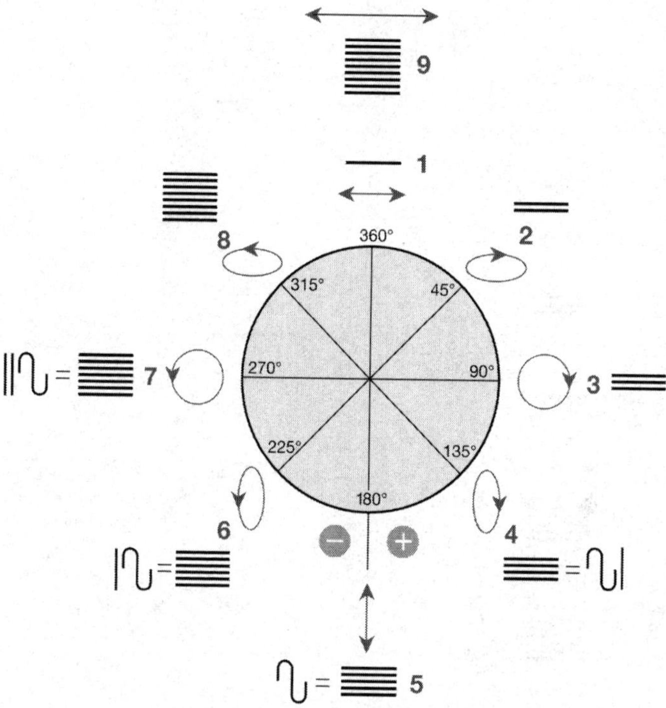

Figure 49. Körbler's vector system

daughter with the use of a sine curve. This proved sufficient to reduce the duration of the disease from 1 week to 1 hour. This can also help with toothaches. The sine curve may be used on several body parts at the same time, as long as you make sure that the effects of the various sine curves do not disturb each other.

Körbler's Vector System

Further basic symbols of New Homeopathy are introduced here as parts of Körbler's vector system consisting of parallel lines of varying numbers *(Figure 49).*

As we have already mentioned, in his article 'Die Neue Homöopathie VI',[5] Körbler offered a detailed analysis of the significance of the equal-armed cross and parallel lines found on Ötzi's body.

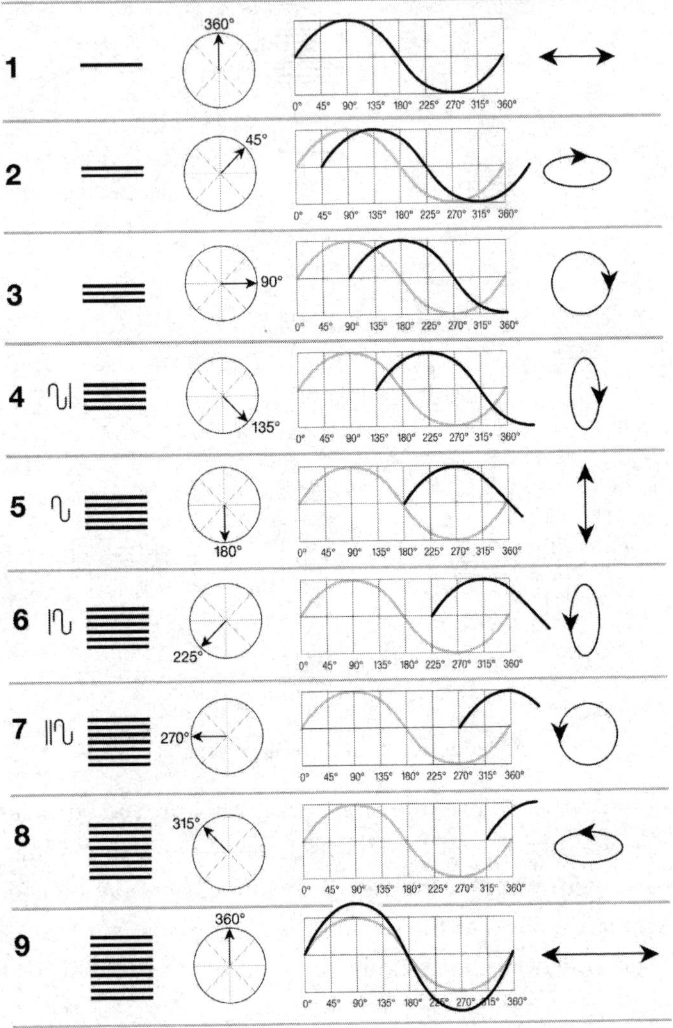

Figure 50. Wave representations of Körbler's vector system and the movement image of the dowsing rod

Körbler depicted the effect of parallel lines as geometric symbols in a vector system. These geometric symbols work as antennas as regards electromagnetic waves. If we depict a wave in a co-ordinate plane, the starting point of the wave will be at the origin of the coordinate plane, its apex at 180 degrees, and the end point at 360 degrees. When a certain amount of energy in the form of electromagnetic radiation reaches a line, it causes the line to become polarized, and since the line behaves like a 'conductor', or an 'antenna', the energy will propagate from the center. It will propagate until it reaches our body. *(Figure 50)*

Now let us examine one by one the vectors of Figure 50.

1.
First vector position:

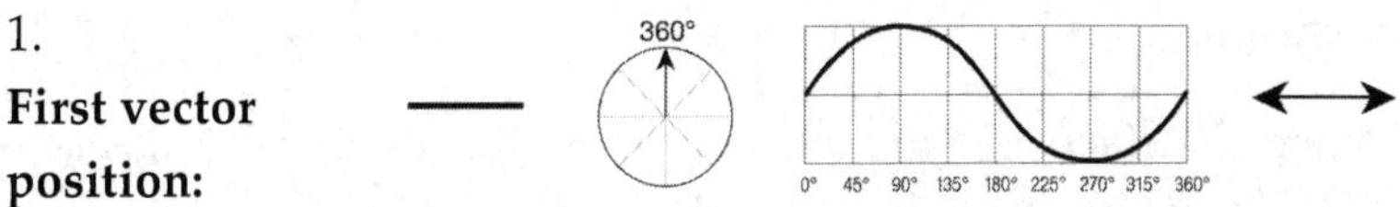

When the energy – in the form of electromagnetic waves – reaches *a geometric symbol consisting of one line,* the electromagnetic wave will start out at 0 degree; the dowsing rod moves horizontally.

Application: When we are fit and healthy, the dowsing rod shows horizontal movements both at top of the head and at the various meridian points. In healing, this geometric symbol is used to strengthen the function in question, e.g. an acupuncture point along a meridian. It is also suited for soothing established scars. Some scars may be soothed simply by drawing a vertical line across them.

2.
Second vector position:

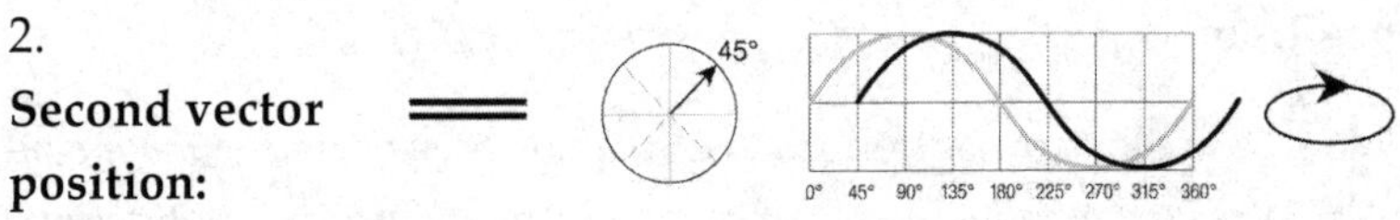

As soon as the electromagnetic wave reaches a *geometric symbol consisting of two parallel lines,* the phase of the electromagnetic wave will be shifted by an eighth of its cycle (45 degrees). As a result, the dowsing rod will move along a horizontal ellipse, clockwise.

Application: If there is a slight deviation from health (e.g. tiredness), the dowsing rod will move along a horizontal ellipse, clockwise, at the test areas, i.e. at the top of the head, or at the various meridian points. In order to restore healthy electromagnetic charge patterns, we apply two parallel horizontal lines either at the meridian points or on the body part concerned (e.g. in the last stage of recovery after an injury or blow).

3.
Third vector position:

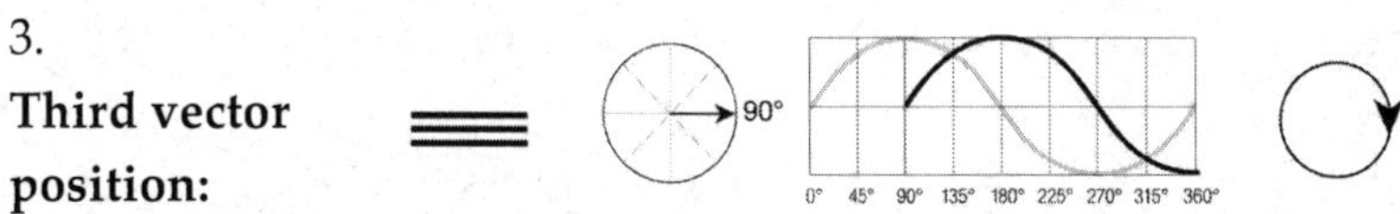

When the electromagnetic wave reaches a *geometric symbol consisting of three parallel lines,* the phase of the electromagnetic wave will be shifted by a quarter of its cycle (90 degrees). The dowsing rod moves in circles, clockwise.

Application: The same happens when there is a more pronounced diversion from a state of health (more drastic tiredness, air travel, electrosmog, extended work on the computer): the dowsing rod will move clockwise in a circle at the various meridian points or at the body parts we test. In order to restore healthy electromagnetic charge patterns, we use three parallel horizontal lines on the meridian points or the affected body parts.

4.
Fourth vector position:

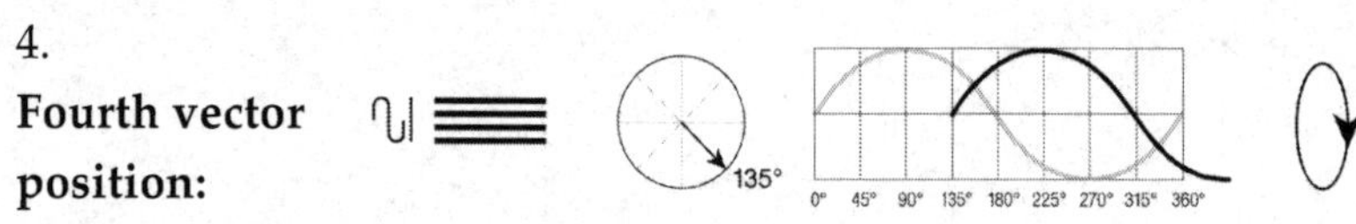

When the electromagnetic wave reaches a *geometric symbol consisting of four parallel lines,* the phase of the electromagnetic wave will be shifted by 135 degrees. As a result, the dowsing rod will move along a vertical ellipse, clockwise.

Application: If there is a painful diversion from health (in cases of a blow, inflammation or infection), the dowsing rod moves along a vertical ellipse, clockwise. In order to restore the healthy charge patterns of the affected area, we apply four parallel lines at the meridian points or the affected body parts, i.e.

at the inflammation spots (e.g. throat) or at the end-points of the various meridians (e.g. at point 1 of the large intestine meridian). If we draw four parallel lines at a right angle to the wound, bleeding will stop instantly and recovery soon begins.

If we test a body part and find a vertical ellipse going clockwise, and we draw four parallel lines on the disturbance zone, this will produce a far more intense electromagnetic activity in the affected area, and so the resonance in the disturbance zone will be restored to a near-healthy state from which full recovery will be brought about by the body's self-healing power.

In a condition that produces vertical ellipses going clockwise, the body part is under the influence of electromagnetic waves that are in a 135° phase shift, and we need to find the geometric symbol, or combination of symbols best suited to avert this electromagnetic effect (parallel lines, Y, equal-armed cross, a combination of Y's and crosses). In order to neutralize the 45° phase shifts, we use parallel lines. If this is not enough, a combination of parallel dotted lines, or other symbols may help us to get the desired result. We shall discuss the application in detail in Chapter 17.

5.
Fifth vector position:

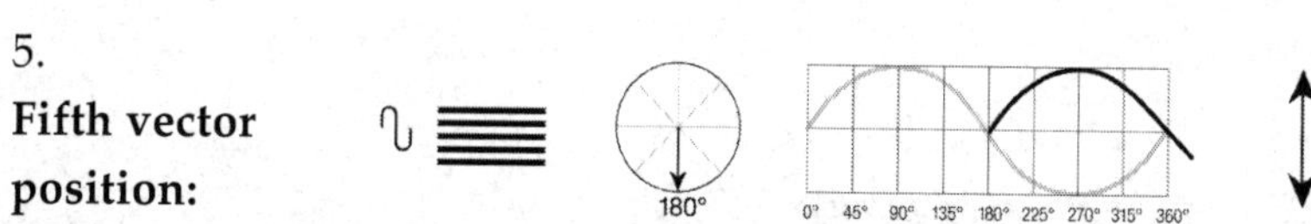

When the electromagnetic wave reaches a *geometric symbol consisting of five parallel lines,* the electromagnetic wave will be shifted in phase by 180 degrees (that is of one-half wavelength) compared to the original sine curve. Here, the crests of the waves line up with the trough of the other; it is a destructive interference *(Figure 51).* As a result, the movement of the dowsing rod will be reversed compared to the basic movement (horizontal); in other words, it will move vertically.

Application: In the case of painful diversions from a state of health (prolonged or deeper inflammation or infection possibly affecting more than one organ) when testing the meridian points and the various organs the dowsing rod will move vertically. This condition is the diagonal opposite of a state of health. In order to restore healthy charge patterns, we use the sine curve or five parallel lines at the meridian points or at the affected body parts. Up till now, each time we added a further parallel line, the energy intensified.

If we are using more than five parallel lines, the end of the dowsing rod will turn in an anti-clockwise direction.

Figure 51

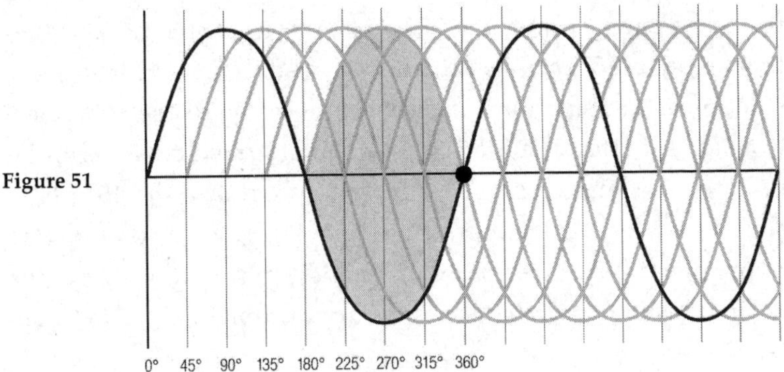

6.
Sixth vector position:

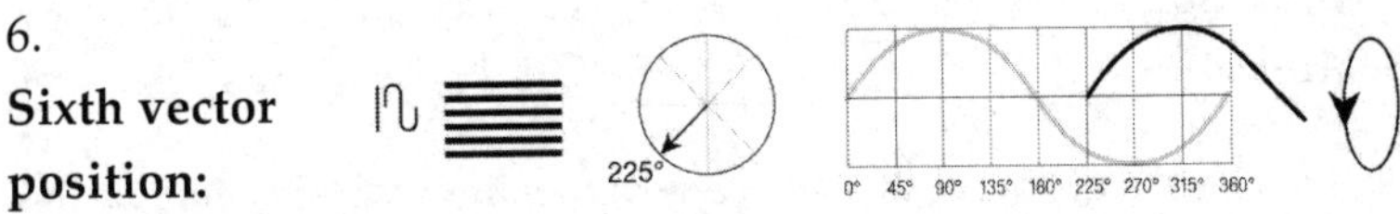

When the electromagnetic waves reach a *geometric symbol consisting of six parallel lines,* the electromagnetic wave will be shifted by 225 degrees. The dowsing rod shows this shift by moving along a vertical ellipse anticlockwise.

Application: In cases of a radical malfunction *(chronic inflammations, symptoms exhibited by a number of organs)* testing the usual points we find the same movement: the dowsing rod moves along a vertical ellipse, anticlockwise.

The dowsing rod will present the same movement when we are doing an allergy test by touching the allergy point right in front of the ear canal on the left side, and when *the body has an allergic reaction to the food we are testing*. In order to restore healthy charge patterns, we apply a vertical line and a sine curve, or six parallel horizontal lines at the meridian points or the affected body parts.

7.
Seventh vector position:

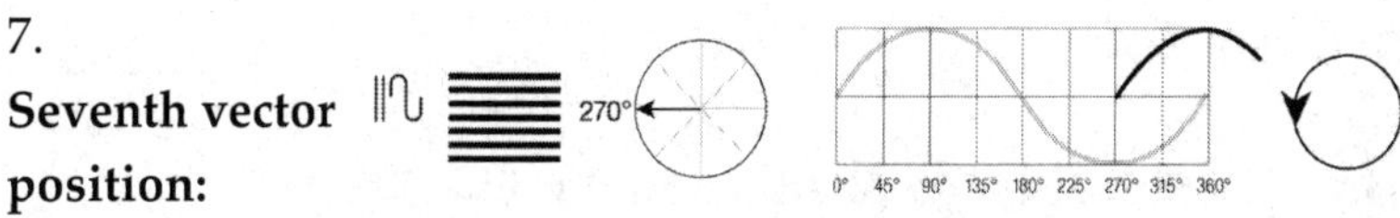

When the electromagnetic wave reaches a *geometric symbol consisting of seven parallel lines,* the electromagnetic wave will be shifted by 270 degrees. The dowsing rod shows this shift by moving in circles anticlockwise.

Application: In the case of serious, degenerative diseases (tumor, etc.) if we test the meridians or the body parts, the dowsing rod will circle to the left. In order to restore the healthy pattern of electromagnetic charges, we need to draw two vertical lines and a sine curve or seven parallel horizontal lines at the meridian points or on the affected body parts.

8.
Eighth vector position:

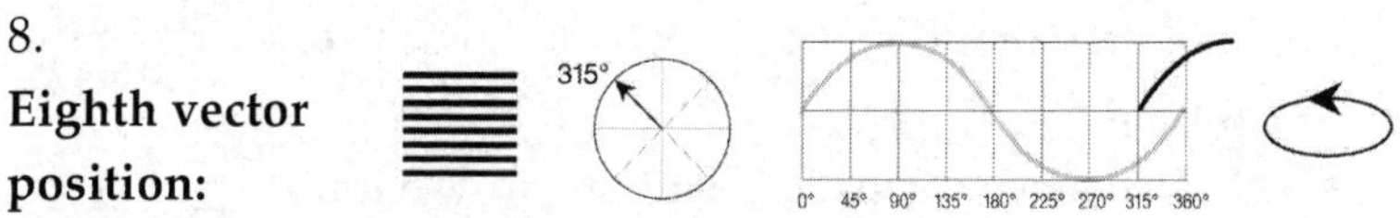

When the electromagnetic wave reaches a *geometric symbol consisting of eight parallel lines,* the electromagnetic wave will be shifted by 315 degrees. As a result, the dowsing rod will move along a horizontal ellipse, anticlockwise.

Application: In the case of terminal illnesses (e.g. in the last stage of cancer, that is, in the presence of metastases) the dowsing rod will move along a horizontal ellipse, anticlockwise. In order to improve the condition, we apply eight parallel lines at the meridian points or the affected body parts. Experience shows, however, that in many cases instead of eight parallel lines we need to apply only two.

The waves starting at the 6th, 7th and 8th vector positions constitute the negative side of Körbler's vector system. The energy of these positions is more forcible than the positive side of the cycle (vector positions one to four). These positions indicate that the biochemical state of the organism has shifted in the direction of disease.

The direction of the applied parallel lines

Parallel lines can be drawn in parallel or at a right angle to the affected area. If, for example, the need is *for improving venal circulation,* we first establish whether we need to apply two, three or four parallel lines, then we draw them *in parallel* to the vein.

Combinations of the basic symbols

Various combinations of sine curves and straight lines are often used. Experience shows that the effects of a combination of forms reach deeper strata than the effect of parallel lines alone, but their energy is somewhat reduced.

The most commonly used combinations are the following:

- A sine curve followed by a vertical line corresponds to the 4th vector.
- The sine curve corresponds to the 5th vector.
- A vertical line followed by a sine curve corresponds to the 6th vector.
- Two vertical lines followed by a sine curve corresponds to the 7th vector.
- Three vertical lines followed by a sine curve corresponds to the 8th vector.

Occasionally we position the lines above or below the sine curve because this ensures optimal healing at the given point.

Whether the lines are best positioned above or below the sine curve needs to be tested on every occasion.

The 9th vector

The 9th vector starts a new circle. From this point onwards the order of the numbering of vectors is reversed and becomes anti-clockwise. As regards healing, we need to focus on the 9th vector alone.

9.
Ninth vector position:

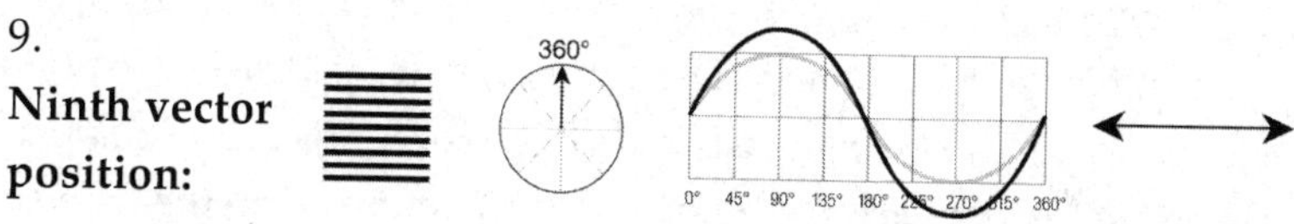

When the electromagnetic wave reaches a *geometric symbol consisting of nine parallel lines,* the electromagnetic wave will be shifted by a complete cycle, that is 360 degrees. This vector position is identical to the first one, except that a kind of 'miracle' happens here, which the dowsing rod shows by a very intense horizontal movement. This geometric symbol amplifies all electromagnetic energies regardless of the quality of the energy. Therefore it should only be applied as an amplifier at healthy points. The distance between the lines should be chosen so that altogether they constitute a square.

Application: If we wish to improve performance, e.g. for sportspeople, we draw nine parallel lines on healthy body parts (e.g. the kidney).

Körbler first tested the strengthening effect of the nine parallel lines on healthy individuals. He worked with a racing cyclist who decided that in the middle of winter, when the temperature was –5 °C, he would go training in his summer outfit. His outfit therefore consisted of shorts, a long-sleeved summer sports top and summer gloves. On his back Körbler placed a geometric symbol of nine parallel lines at the height of the kidneys. This is how the sportsman started out. During the training he felt pleasant, was not cold and in 45 minutes he covered the distance which normally took him 52 minutes.

On another occasion a cyclist with an injury asked for Körbler's help. The case was reported by Körbler himself in *Raum und Zeit:*[6]

> *Roland Königshofer, three times world champion cyclist in the amateur category (1989, 1990, 1992), was far from lucky at the World Championship held in Spain in 1992. Enfeebled after a sore throat, he was prevented from becoming world champion for a fourth time even though he was the fastest cyclist among amateurs. 'No problem,' he said to the journalists after his defeat, 'the world championship return race is coming up in November in the Vienna Cycling Stadium – there I will be the fastest again.' However, in November, when training a day before this great challenge (Saturday, November 28), he fell over and besides external injuries, he suffered a concussion of the brain.*
>
> *On the day of the return race he arrived in the stadium on time but was in a poor condition – so much so that an hour before the race he had to interrupt a conversation with his trainer and lie down in his rest-cabin.*
>
> *At this point, one of Königshofer's friends and well-wishers called my office phone and asked me what I could do for his friend in this situation. It was also clear from his voice that this was an occasion when New Homeopathy could gain considerable credit if the assistance proved successful. I traveled to the cycling stadium, was instantly given special permission and was admitted to Königshofer's cabin, five minutes before the warm-up training. Königshofer was lying down, as white as a sheet, and the loudspeakers were just beginning to explain that the local celebrity was probably not going to compete because of health problems.*
>
> *'I am poorly,' said Königshofer to me, then added, gesturing toward his wife, 'My wife is about to enter your seminar, so, as far as I am concerned, you can start your first class. I can only get better.'*

The first lesson was very brief. The dowsing rod signaled a disturbance zone at the side of the forehead. I drew four parallel lines and Königshofer instantly started to feel better. Next I went on to draw nine parallel lines on his back.

What came next was hailed as a miracle by the television commentator and 4500 exhilarated, jubilant fans. Königshofer won the race and declared to journalists that it was one of his best laps ever. He went in for several other races in the championship that evening and won every one of them.

Körbler gained a number of similar experiences with the nine parallel lines. These led him to connect the ways in which Western and Eastern cultures are thinking; he intended to connect the Western-style decimal system with the antient base-nine system of the East.

In Goethe's *Faust*[7] he found the sentence 'nine is one' in the 'Witches' one-by-one' that is a reference to using a numeral system of nines. I quote George Madison Priest's translation (http: / / www.levity.com / alchemy / faust07.html):

This you must ken!	*Du musst verstehn!*
From one make ten,	*Aus Eins mach Zehn,*
And two let be,	*Und Zwei lass gehn,*
Make even three,	*Und Drei mach gleich,*
Then rich you'll be.	*So bist du reich.*
Skip o'er the four!	*Verlier die Vier!*
From five and six,	*Aus Fünf und Sechs,*
The witch's tricks,	*So sagt die Hex,*
Make seven and eight,	*Mach Sieben und Acht,*
'Tis finished straight;	*So ist's vollbracht:*
And nine is one,	***Und neun ist eins,***
And ten is none,	*Und Zehn ist keins.*
That is the witch's one-time-one!	*Das ist das Hexen Einmaleins!*

The witches' 'one-by-one', in the most ancient Greek manuscript, the *Casselanus Codex,* found in Germany, was used by the English mathematician John Dee in his Latin text. This served as a model for Goethe.

Part II.

Using the System in Healing

Chapter 7

The Theory and Practice of Diagnosis and Therapy

Körbler offers the following introduction to the section on 'Diagnosis and Therapy' in one of his books:

> *My ideas follow the regularities of nature. Thus it is my purpose not only to demonstrate the disturbance zones of the living organism and outline them with the help of the principle (and practice) of the reversibility of systemic information, but also to change this disturbance, this information, with the help of symbols and replace them with new, stronger, 'positive' information. I call this process 'therapy with forms'. (Formentherapie).*[1]

Körbler repeatedly emphasized that healing with the help of geometric symbols (geometric codes) and optimizing the electromagnetic functions of the organism are processes in the terahertz band where the symbols optimize the paths which the organism requires for proper functioning. This re-launches the communication of body parts that had been electrically blocked. Despite the fact that the energy of the electromagnetic waves in the body is extremely low, the waves impact the living organism because their length is identical to that of our cells and therefore they produce resonance. Creating an effect on the body requires very little energy. These energy levels are so low that they cannot be measured by instruments. We can only establish their effect from the responses of the body. This is a type of energy measurable by the response alone, where influencing the human organism takes place through treatment using the geometric symbols of New Homeopathy. Each geometric symbol has an impact due to the fact that the symbol alters the radiation of light and particularly the UV segment of light.

Diagnosis

What is disease? From the perspective of New Homeopathy, disease occurs when electromagnetic factors come to affect, slow down or accelerate the biochemical processes of the organism that ensure healthy life-functions. This is true of both acute and chronic diseases. Körbler claims that the background of chronic diseases is a solidified 'charge pattern' which is not coherent with life functions.

An electric charge pattern is a specific and complex electromagnetic pattern characteristic of a particular state of health at a particular location. The dowsing rod demonstrates these conditions in different vector positions. For instance, in the case of an inflammation of the large intestines, by examining large intestine meridian point No. 1, the dowsing rod will show the 4th vector position, i.e. a vertical ellipse movement revolving to the right. Thus the function of diagnosis is to find those points and areas in the energy field of the organism where the charge patterns diverge from the healthy condition in a manner significant for the emergence and continuation of a disease. As we saw in Chapter 6, the vector system covers the possible energetic conditions of the body in steps of 45 degrees. The movement of the dowsing rod shows the extent to which the charge pattern at the tested point diverges from the optimal condition.

Körbler developed a special system for establishing the diagnosis. Essentially he is relying on the diagnostic approach taken in traditional Chinese medicine. His system incorporates certain meridian points of Chinese acupuncture, the meridians and testing points that he discovered, and certain points used in kinesiology and the testing of the organs, to mention just a few elements. Based on the examination of these diagnostic points we quickly get an idea about the condition of the patient and the cause sustaining the disturbance of biochemical functioning.

The diagnostic points discovered by Körbler are the following:

The inflammation point. Körbler found that examining wrinkles 2–4 on the inside of the wrists gives accurate information about inflammatory processes taking place in the body; therefore he named this area the 'inflammation point' *(Figure 52).*

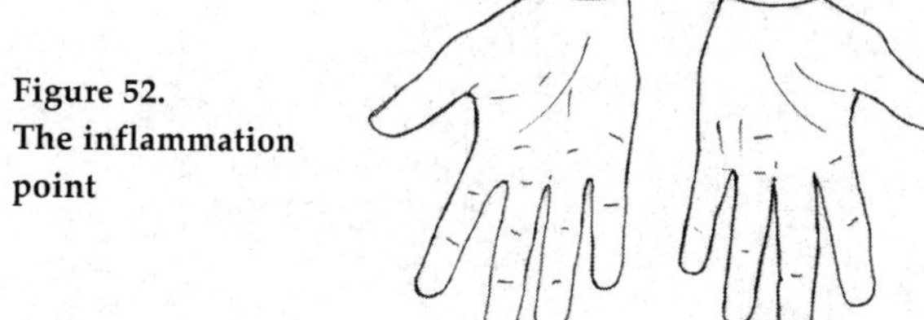

Figure 52.
The inflammation point

The mycosis point. Körbler discovered a point on the left-hand side of the chest, underneath the third rib, examination of which shows very clearly the fungus exposure of the body. He named this the 'mycosis point' *(Figure 53).*

The antibiotic point. Examination of this point in the center underneath the ninth rib under the shoulder blade serves to establish how heavily the organism has been exposed to antibiotics and whether it is permissible to give the patient an antibiotic treatment *(Figure 54).*

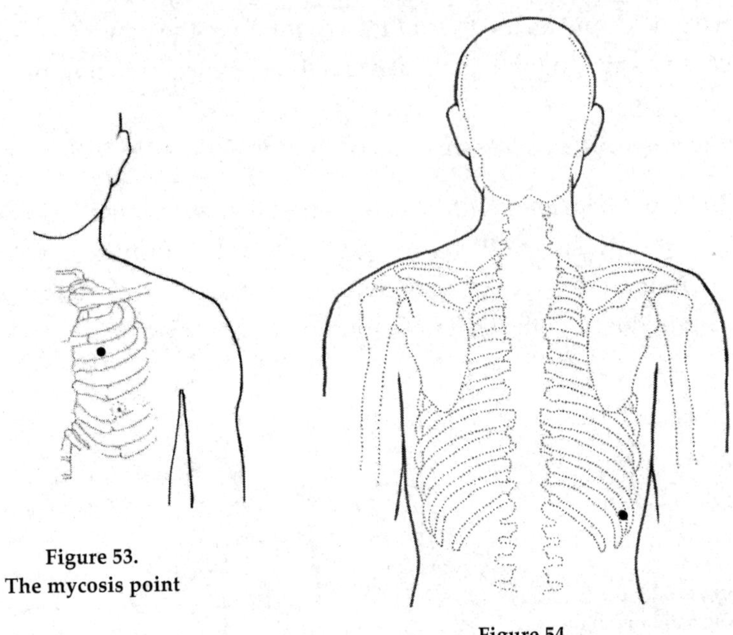

Figure 53.
The mycosis point

Figure 54.
The antibiotic point

Choosing the locus of the examination

It follows clearly from the complex system of electromagnetic effects that for carrying out these examinations we need to choose a spot which is neutral regarding intolerable radiations. The reason is that if you are standing amid unfavorable radiation, the movement of the dowsing rod will signal the unfavorable condition of your organism, i.e. the totality of radiations coming from the soil, from any kind of foundation you are exposed to, from heating radiators, electric equipment, or other persons. All of this affects our organism, and the condition of our organs is actually a response to these effects. If you shift your position by 1 or 2 meters, the condition of your organism will be different from what it was before. We get a new set of reactions, a new signal. We only get an accurate picture of the functioning of the body if we eradicate or screen unfavorable radiations. *This is why it is crucial to provide a neutral area for examining patients.* This is the only way to find out how much the condition of the patient has improved between one examination and the next.

The sequence of examination

Körbler proposed that in establishing our diagnosis we should first test the patient with the dowsing rod. The next step is to produce the *anamnesis,* questioning the patient about his or her complaint, and then comparing the results. If we start by questioning the patient about his or her complaint before the examination, then both the patient and the tester will be concentrating on the complaints and it might happen that imaginary complaints also manifest during the testing even though the source of the problem is elsewhere (since the electromagnetic functions of the organism are very sensitive to the quality of our mind and our emotions). In order for the examination to produce an accurate result, before the examination patients need to remove their glasses, jewelry, watch, mobile phones, and electric or metal objects. The tester draws a vertical line with his/her finger repeatedly along the back of the patient's neck along the *psycho-meridian,* moving down from the top of the head to the first neck vertebra *(Figure 55).* The aim of this is to render the organism free of its current psychological condition for 10–15 minutes and in this way ensure an authentic picture of the condition of the body during the examination. Next, the tester maps out the patient's bio-energetic field with the dowsing rod. The tester's left index finger, if directed at a certain point, will absorb the information both in the proximal examination of the patient's body and when testing the patient from a few meters' distance. We use our left index finger to test the meridian points and reflex zones, while the top of the head, the

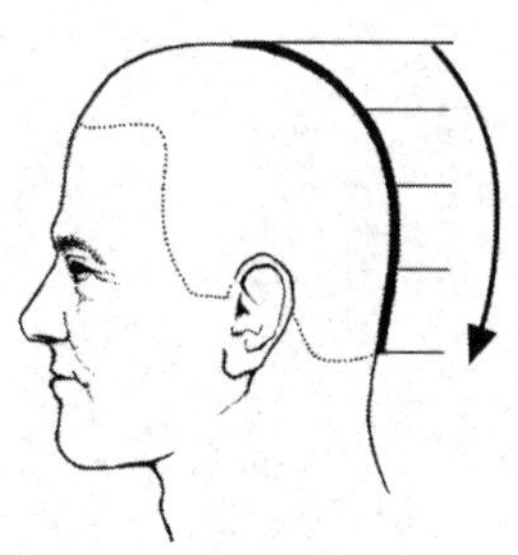

Figure 55

psychomeridian and the area of the organs are examined with our left palm. We note the vector position after testing each point.

The diagnostic points

Establishing the diagnosis consists of testing certain meridian points of Chinese medicine, as well as Körbler's diagnostic points, and the diagnostic areas he used. After Körbler's death we named these points *Körbler's diagnostic points.*

The diagnostic points identified by Körbler are the following:

- The top of the head *(Figures 56a and 56b)*
- Psychomeridian *(Figure 57)*
- Large intestines 1 *(Figure 58)*
- Small intestines 3 (Figure 59)
- Lungs 1 *(Figure 60)*
- Kidneys 3 *(Figure 61)*
- Spleen 6 *(Figure 62)*
- Stomach 36 *(Figure 63)*
- Gall 40 *(Figure 64)*
- Liver 3 *(Figure 65)*
- Circulation point *(Figure 66)*
- Thyroid area *(Figure 67)*
- Amalgam point *(Figure 68)*
- Körbler's mycosis point *(Figure 69)*
- Körbler's inflammation point *(Figure 70)*
- Solar plexus point *(Figure 71)*
- Heart 9 *(Figure 72)*
- Tooth meridian *(Figure 73)*

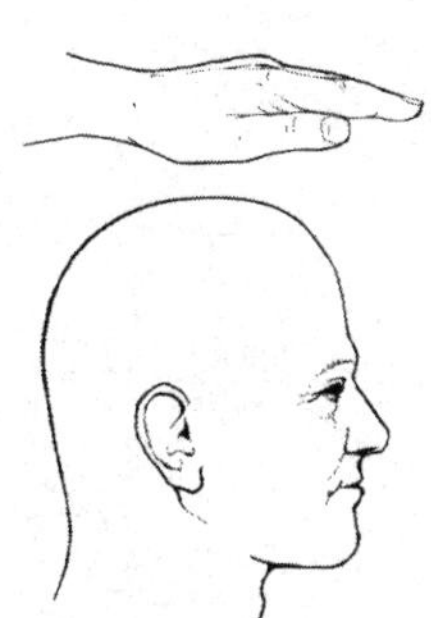

Figure 56a.
The top of the head

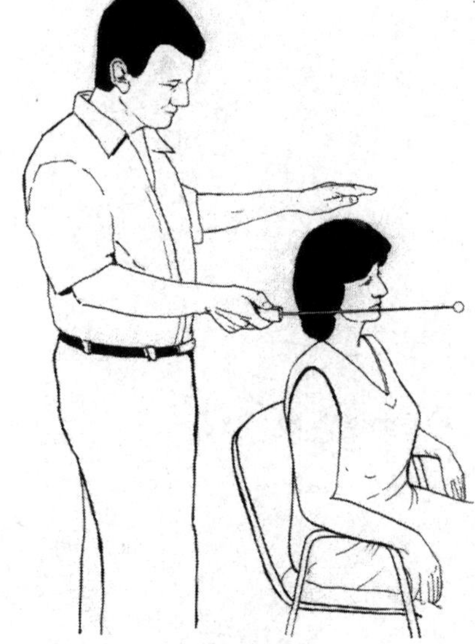

Figure 56b.
The top of the head

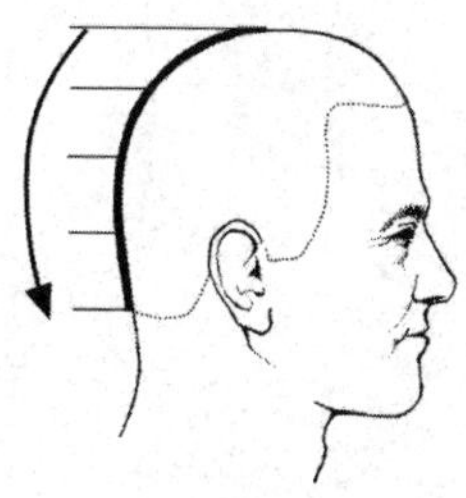

Figure 57.
The psychomeridian

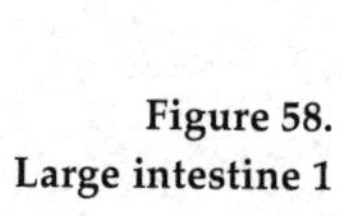

Figure 58.
Large intestine 1

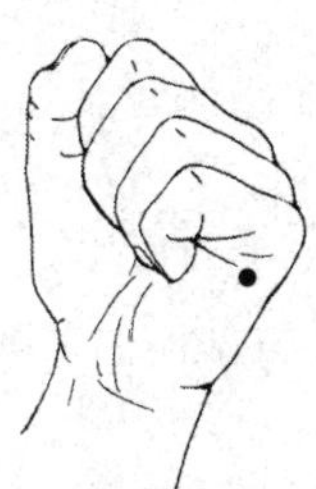

Figure 59.
Small intestine 3

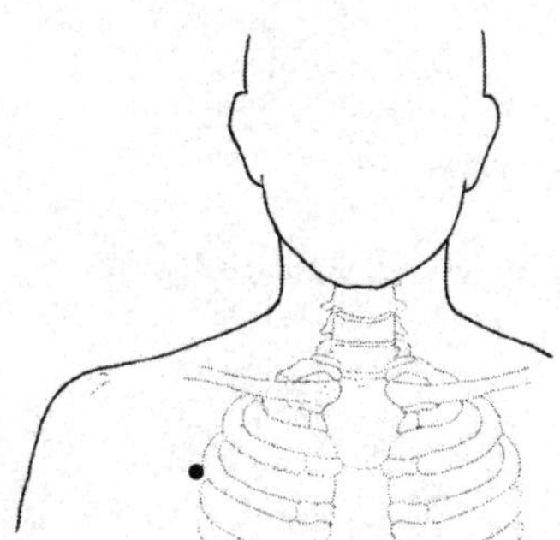

Figure 60. Lungs 1

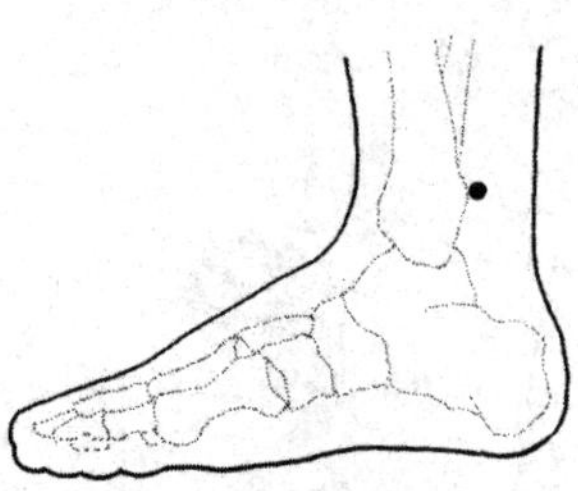

Figure 61. Kidney 3

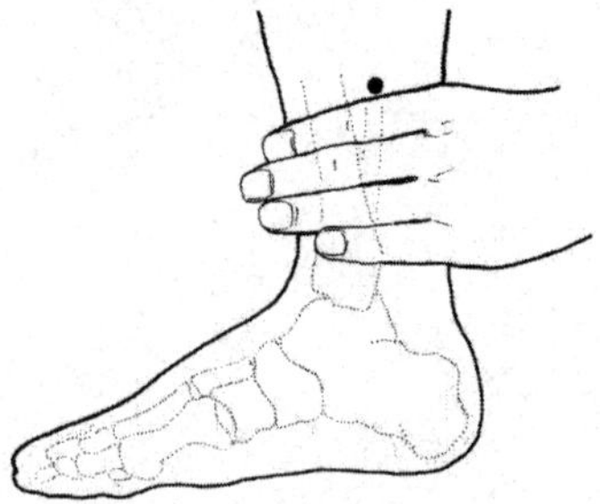

Figure 62. Spleen 6

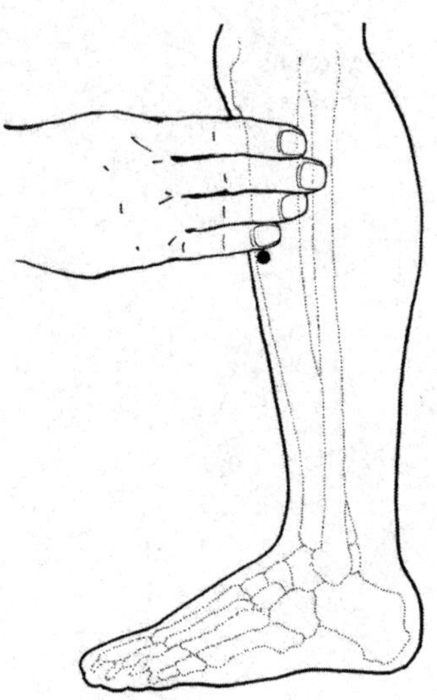

Figure 63. Stomach 36

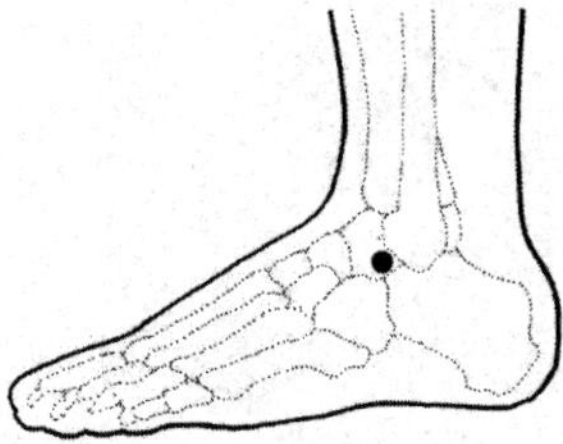

Figure 64. Gall 40

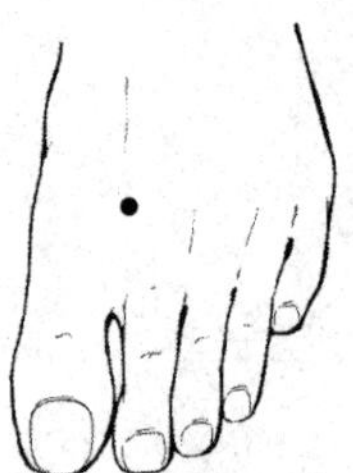

Figure 65. Liver 3

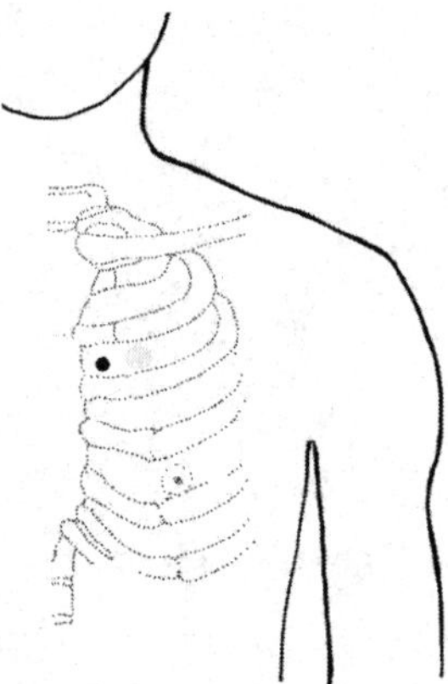

Figure 66.
Circulation point (third rib interspace on the left, next to the breastbone)

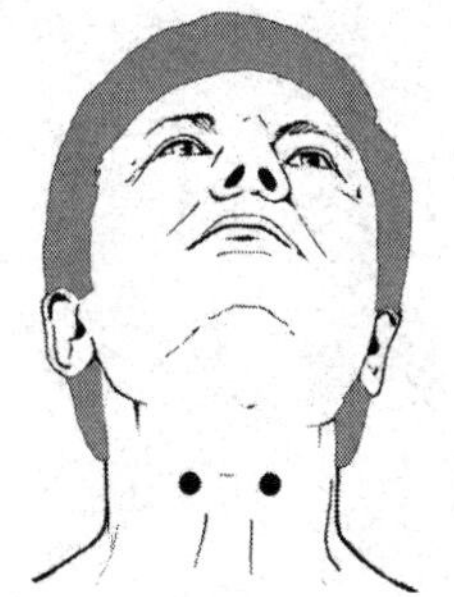

Figure 67.
Area of the thyroid gland

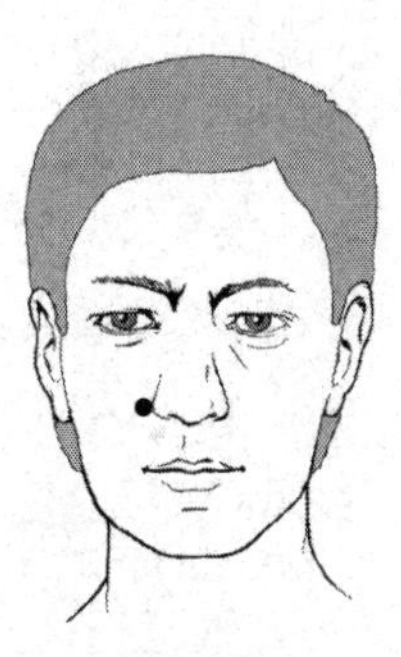

Figure 68.
The amalgam point

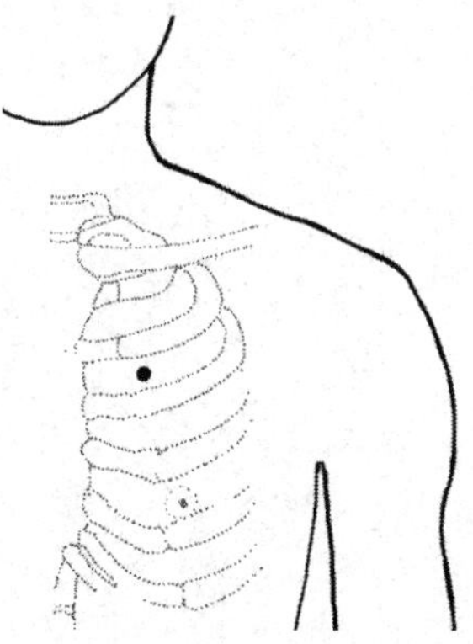

Figure 69.
Körbler's mycosis point (fungus point) on the left-hand side of the chest

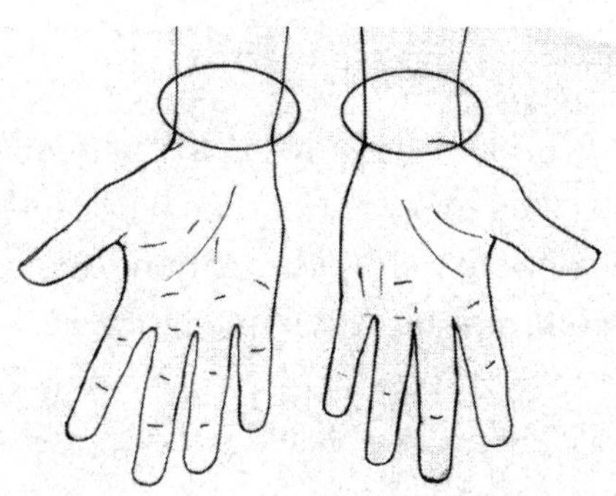

Figure 70.
Körbler's inflammation points – on the inside of both wrists

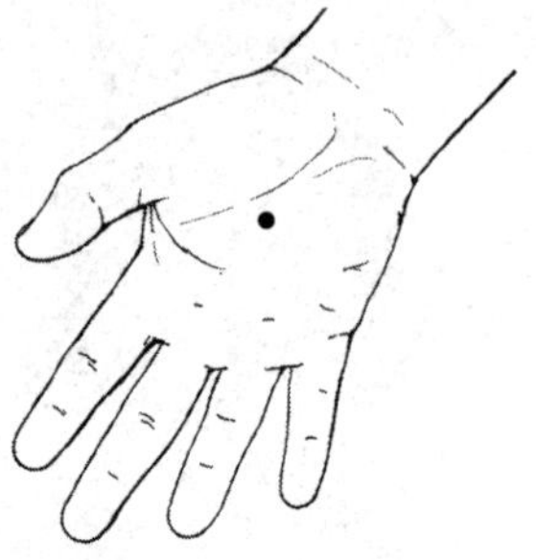

Figure 71.
The solar plexus point in the middle of the right palm

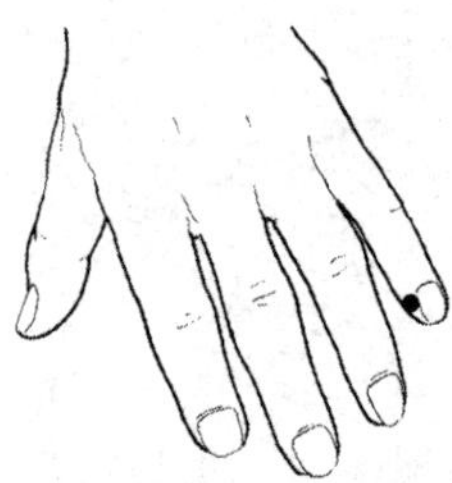

Figure 72. Heart 9

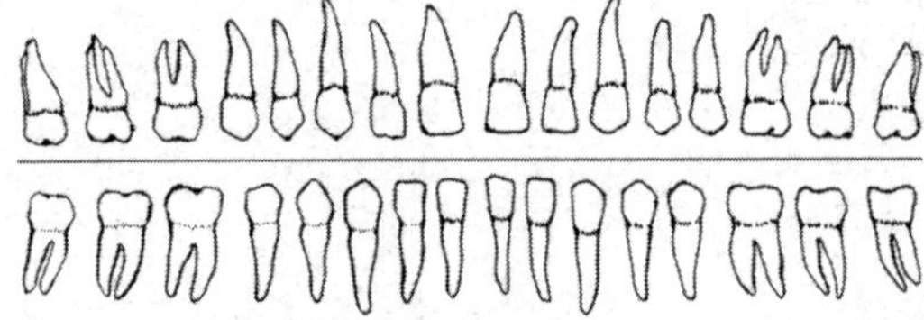

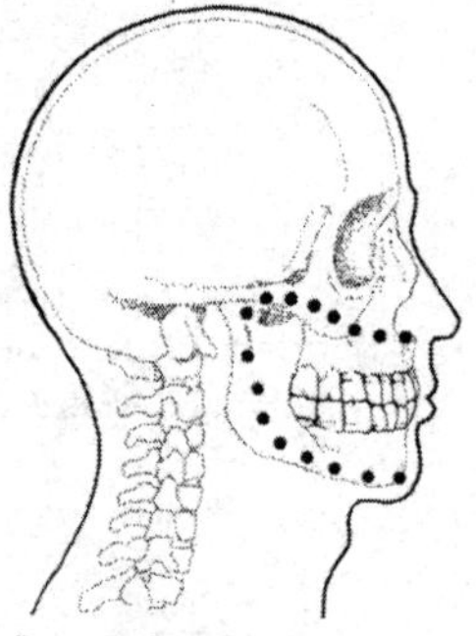

Figure 73.
The tooth meridian

Körbler often turned the patient's head left and right to see the extent of stiffness; then he would manipulate the muscles in the neck to reduce the tention. After establishing the therapy he would repeat the treatment, the neck stiffness disappeared.

In a case of allergy we examine the allergy point in front of the right ear, and test the foods, medicine allergies and allergies to chemicals, household substances and cosmetic substances.

(The diagnosis and therapy of allergies will be discussed in Chapter 15.) In order to grant full comfort for the organism it is important to test all objects such as glasses, dental braces, objects permanently worn on the body, etc.

Further diagnostic options

Körbler started examining his patient by testing the spine meridian *(Figure 74)*. The spine meridian running along the center line on the top of the head is the most neutral area for examination from the patient's point of view. From the tester's perspective it is important to work in a relaxed yet swift manner and only focus on the dowsing rod's movement at each point. This way the tester's attention will not wander and he or she will have no chance to conceive any preconceptions about the patient's diagnosis. It is also favorable for an accurate diagnosis to divert the patient's attention, for instance by asking to look at a picture on the wall. This way we can avoid the patient's emotional changes that can arise in the form of anxiety or euphoric anticipation of recovery.

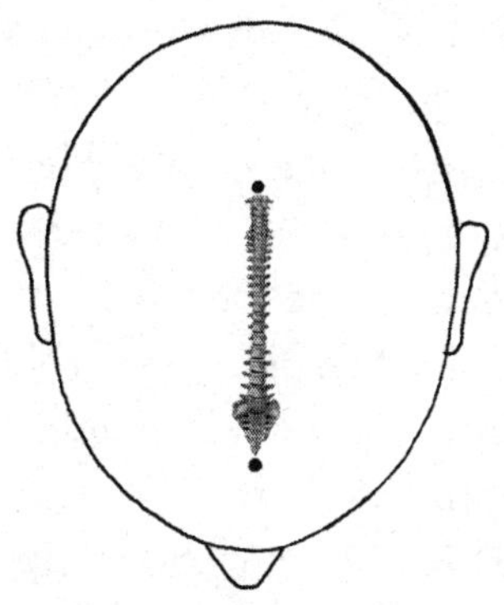

Figure 74.
The spine meridian

Once we have outlined the patient's condition, we can start elaborating the details. Based on the alterations we find on the spine meridian, we examine the vertebrae. Where the electromagnetic function diverges from healthy functioning, we manipulate the muscles to distinguish a momentary disturbance from a permanent one.

If we find vector positions 5 to 8, we examine Körbler's inflammation point on both wrists. Next comes the examination of the organs. When we wish to establish the depth of the disturbance in the body, we must use our entire palm. We hold the palm of our left hand over the disturbance zone at a distance of 1, 2, and then 3 cm from the skin while we observe the intensity of the swinging of the dowsing rod. We move on to a distance of 4 cm, 5 cm, and further. As we are moving away from the body, we see how the intensity decreases. The distance at which the dowsing rod moves most intensely refers to the depth at which the centre of the disturbance zone is to be found within the body. For example, if the intensity is the highest at 3 cm, then the centre of disturbance is 3 cm deep in the body. This way we can act like a 'tomographic' instrument and establish the depth of the disturbance point. Determining this depth is extremely important for the diagnosis.

If you are examining a very small area, instead of the left index finger you can use an acupuncture needle as an antenna. This will allow you to establish the depth of the focal point to the millimeter. This is extremely important because we are able to outline, even mark with a pen, the body part which requires intense examination with medical instruments.

An accurate diagnosis can also help to avoid unnecessary operations.

> *Körbler reported the case of a woman who went to him with severe pain in her knee. Her doctor had proposed an operation and even the date was set when the patient came to see Körbler. According to the latter's diagnosis the pain was related to a venal problem which he treated with a sine curve symbol ∿, and this rendered the operation unnecessary. The patient soon recovered.*

The importance of relationships between the disturbance zones

It is also possible to identify what kind of correlations are there between different malfunctions. This is done with the help of a coin. If the dowsing rod shows a disturbance rotating to the left somewhere in the body, the disturbance can be eradicated with a coin, because on testing the metal the dowsing rod will swing to the right. This indicates that the two opposing sets of information neutralize each other. If we have two points, point **A** and point **B**, showing malfunctions, and we wish to identify whether there is a correlation between the two, we place the coin on the disturbance point or reflex zone at **A** and then examine disturbance point **B**. If the disturbance at point **B** is gone, i.e. the dowsing rod is moving horizontally, then the disturbances at points **A** and **B** are related. If the disturbance at point **B** continues, then the disturbances at points **A** and **B** are of different origin.

Summary

It goes without saying, the manner of establishing the diagnosis is different in every case. Indeed, Körbler used to map out the patient's physical condition in a minute, discovering the correlations between the disturbance zones of the body. He never examined every diagnostic point, but proceeded according to the nature of the case. If faced with an acute condition, he formed a diagnosis by testing a few points only. In the case of chronic diseases he also explored the correlations between the causes creating the condition in a swift but thorough manner. Naturally, exploring the psychological causes took longer. In order to liberate the *psychological charge,* he examined the psychomeridian (see Chapter 12). He taught that with a sound knowledge of the diagnostic points we can proceed by using intuition and creativity in establishing the diagnosis.

Therapy

The greatest experience during our time with Körbler was the experience of healing itself. The most effective method he used was to heal the patient on the spot. He used admirably simple means to resolve blockages and put energy flow once again to the service of the body. He used each case as an occasion to introduce yet another new approach. He gave a great gift to anyone who ever took part as a healer at even a single lesson.

From the point of view of information medicine, he said, the job of therapy is to rectify the charge patterns that has changed as a result of flawed biochemical processes, and so they sustain disease.

The essence of therapy is to free up and, if necessary, rebuild the paths of electromagnetic communication. The goal, to use Körbler's analogy, is to secure a 'road map'. Building the road map is the purpose of the geometric symbols that rectify the charge pattern of the disease in line with its vector position. The next step of the therapy is to introduce the substances and information that can enable both electromagnetic and biochemical functioning. These include the necessary foods and the soft and allopathic substances needed for healing.

Körbler used the geometric symbols of New Homeopathy in healing sick body-parts, while also following the rules of Chinese acupuncture. He found that at the acupuncture points it is sufficient to introduce gentle non-coherent material information, such as the application of various geometric symbols in order to influence the stimulus–response processes of the organism. He also used natural substance, e.g. crystals, semi-precious stones, oils, flower essences, or the tree-blossom essences and Himalaya water, as well as a number of other treatments based on information transfer, which in the case of a correct selection positively influenced the information-based regulation system of the living organism, increased cell voltage, and supported self-healing mechanisms.

Therapy in practice

In order to propose a therapy we must identify which symptom or set of symptoms responds to which kind of therapy. Besides using geometric symbols, it is a good idea to try soft methods. These can prove effective even in the case of chronic problems existing in the case of dysfunctional malformations. Allopathic medication should only be used if we have run out of soft methods. Wave information that signals and maintains disease can best be changed by traditional and modern methods that influence the information systems regulating the biochemical processes and thus free up or reconstruct the communication paths of electromagnetic and other waves. Körbler's method is much easier to understand today, 20 years after its appearance, since studies in biophysics and quantum physics have gone through breathtaking development since then.

A number of different types of bio-resonance therapy prove that patients can recover under the effect of information that propagates the healthy resonances of the organism. The diseased organism can use this to transform the wave information that sustains the disease into healthy wave information that will normalize the relevant biochemical processes.

This is the purpose of both ancient traditional healing methods and soft healing methods of modern times, such as geometric symbols whether drawn on the body or worn as articles. These methods also include physical exercise of Chinese acupuncture and acupressure; the application of precious and semiprecious stones and crystals; the classic homeopathy of the modern period; Bach's flower therapy and other flower and aromatherapies; Körbler's blossom therapy; W. Reich's 'orgone energy' or the nearly 100-year-old method of radionic therapy, to mention but a few.

Treatment with Geometric Symbols

The use of geometric symbols in healing is of outstanding importance. Its efficiency can only be properly appreciated once it has been tested in practice. It is special in that it may be combined with any therapy but is able to produce near-miraculous results even when applied independently. I have used these symbols continually for 20 years in healing. Indeed, not a single day goes by without their application and they still amaze me with their efficacy. Below I offer a far-from-exhaustive list of the areas and types of illness where the role of geometric symbols in the healing process has been demonstrated:

- Treatment of small children with acute and chronic inflammations;
- Treatment of adults with acute and chronic inflammations;
- Treatment of injuries, blows, cuts, bites;
- Treatment of warts;
- Treatment of post-operative scars;
- Treatment of allergies;
- Treatment of pains and aches;
- Treatment of terminal patients;
- Treatment through remote healing.

It is worth noting that the use of geometric symbols is extremely useful also in curing animals. This rules out the possibility that the effect of geometric symbols is purely a placebo.

The use of geometric symbols in the treatment of small children

After April 1993, when our articles on New Homeopathy started to appear in *Természetgyógyász,* an increasing number of parents with small children began to contact us. Many of these children had been suffering from allergies for 1, 2 or even 3 years and found no relief through mainstream treatment methods. Observing their quick recovery with the Körbler method, these parents came to us for help even later when their child had any disease, and they chose information medicine over allopathic remedies. We always worked under simultaneous medical control. This way we gained a great deal of experience about how children's bodies react to the use of geometric symbols.

In the case of bronchitis, we test therapeutic points on the chest and back where we draw the symbols. If necessary, we also draw on point 1 of the lung meridian and the alarm points of the large intestines.

In the case of intestinal inflammations, we draw symbols on the large intestinal alarm points and, if necessary, also on the area of the small intestine.

In acute diseases such as sore throats, every day for 2–3 days,

1) we draw a sine curve ∿ on the throat area and

2) we draw one of the following three symbols on the large intestine area (the same symbol on both sides of the body), and one (probably another one of the three) on the small intestine area;

a) a sine curve ∿

b) a sine curve followed by a vertical line ∿|

c) four parallel lines ≣.

Balázs was about 6 years old when his mother called me and asked for help because the boy had a temperature of 39.6 °C for 3 days. Since they lived in a remote town, I treated Balázs through remote healing. Examination with the dowsing rod suggested only one type of therapy: two vertical lines followed by a sine curve ||∿. I had tried homeopathic remedies, allopathic medication, but applying the above symbols was the only way I could get a horizontal response. I applied the symbols for three hours, and Balázs's temperature descended and the little boy's condition improved. (Treatment by Mária Sági)

One of our training course members helped his 7-year-old son with the Körbler method he had only just learned. After he got home he used the dowsing rod to test a lump of unknown origin in the back of his son's left popliteal fossa. He drew the indicated symbols of two vertical lines followed by a sine curve ||∿ at the affected spot and redrew it every day. After 13 days the swelling disappeared without complications. (Treatment by István Sági) *(Figure 75)*

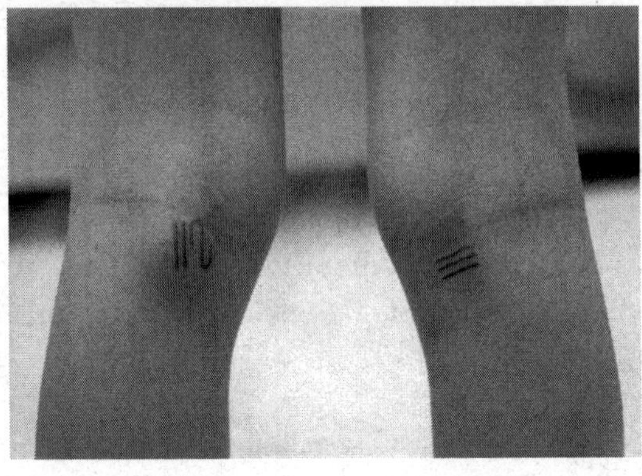

Figure 75

The use of geometric symbols in the treatment of adults
We follow a similar procedure as in the case of children.

Körbler told us a story about his own experience.

> *Three years before, he suddenly felt a sharp pain around his waist. Although he was extremely busy and had no time for sickness, he went to see his doctor to find out what was wrong with him. The doctor's diagnosis was shingles (herpes zoster) and he gave Körbler a heap of medication, tablets, and injections from his medicine cabinet. Seeing all these drugs Körbler answered that he only wanted a piece of paper. He drew a sine curve* ∿ *on the piece of paper and placed it under his shirt. Now he went back to his office and forgot all about his shingles. After a while he noticed that there was a piece of paper under his shirt and took it out. Ten minutes later he felt a very sharp pain again. Then he decided that he would put back the piece of paper with the sine curve on it and not take it out again. Three days later the shingles disappeared, never to return again.*

> *József was a man of 67 who had been suffering from asthma for 15 years. Early every morning, between 3 and 5 AM, he would wake up feeling bad. On my suggestion, following examination with the dowsing rod, he drew eight* ≣ *and seven parallel lines*

≣ underneath each other on his chest with a red felt-tip pen. He drew these symbols every day for 2 and a half months, and during the tenth week his complaints cleared up entirely. (Treatment by István Sági)

On one occasion a middle-aged man came to me with kidney complaints and pains, poor general condition, low mood and feebleness. I took out my anatomy atlas and asked the man to sit down next to me. I took out the dowsing rod, held it in my right hand, and with my left index finger I started tracing along the colored photograph of the right and then the left kidney in the atlas, while constantly keeping an eye on the movement of the dowsing rod. In both pictures (right and left kidney) when I reached the critical area the man hissed, indicating that he felt a burning pain in his kidney. Then we chose the appropriate symbol and applied it for a longer period of time (2–3 weeks); combined with a special diet and herb teas we reached a stage where he was free of complaints. (Treatment by István Sági)

Once I had a visit from a lady and her husband. She was in the fourth month of pregnancy. For several weeks she had felt a constant pain on both sides of her abdomen. She did not want to use medication; this is why she chose us. Testing with the dowsing rod I came to the following conclusion: on the left-hand side of the abdomen she needed four parallel lines ≣, on the right-hand side three parallel lines ≡ for a period of 4 days (strengthened by redrawing). A week later she came to me personally to thank me for the treatment – she was by this time complaint-free. (Treatment by István Sági)

Another patient was a man aged 32, working as a security guard. He complained of long-standing backache, particularly around the trapezoid muscles. He had been to a masseur, a doctor and a natural healer, but noticed no improvement. Testing with the dowsing rod gave the following result: heavy exposure at the mycosis point. Disharmony was established at the large intestines, small intestines, stomach, liver, gall and kidney meridian points; and he had problems with his stool. He stated that he reacted to stress with sensitivity of the stomach and the kidneys. The procedure of the treatment was the following: a large vertical (3–4 cm) line followed by a sine curve |∿ were drawn on both shoulder blades on his back for 7 days. He was also given Pianto Extra and some herbal syrup for his liver and gall, both chosen with the dowsing rod. On the eighth day the man came in person to tell me that he was feeling really well and in the gym he was able to do five times as many arm exercises as he had done before. His stool was now in order. (Treatment by István Sági)

A man of 40 was a watchmaker by profession, and an amateur football player who spent all of his free time playing. While he played, however, he suffered from a constant backache, particularly around the trapezoid muscle. He said his stool is in order. When I examined his liver, the dowsing rod showed a disharmony of the electromagnetic charge pattern. Therefore he was given Pianto Extra essence and a tea blend for protecting the liver. To remedy his backache I placed a large sine curve ∿ on both sides. He kept coming back for months asking me to redraw the symbols. After 4 months he became entirely free of complaints. (Treatment by István Sági)

On 28 September, 2012, I received the following letter:

Dear Mária Sági,
With reference to our telephone conversation I am sending you the case study I mentioned. I am Károly Kövesi (30/05/1954) retired army lieutenant colonel, by civilian qualifications an economist and commercial manager. With regard to traditional healing and medicine I profess Paracelsus' principles. I would like to describe my experience for

the reader's benefit, hoping that Körbler's method, which you are describing and developing further, will soon gain broad popularity.

In July 2012 I underwent a blood test where the laboratory found the level of c-reactive proteins to be at 92.18, which is some 8.5 times higher than the normal rate (0.00–5.00). I was shocked. This was the period when I came in contact with Erich Körbler's method which intuitively grasped my attention and I went on to perform one of the experiments on myself.

For 5 weeks I drew five parallel lines ≣ underneath each other at a distance of about 1 cm and a total width of 5 cm at the inflammation points on the inside of both wrists, using a skin-friendly green felt-tip pen. Once a day I redrew the lines because they got blurred. At this time I took no medication whatever of an anti-inflammatory nature and no antibiotics. After the 5 weeks I had a new blood-test done which produced astounding results – the value had gone back from 92.8 to 7.28 which is nearly within the normal range.

What I have described is a fact, and it begs the question – how can this be? Even if the excess is only 3 or 4 times, doctors start giving you huge doses of antibiotics, which is expensive and destroys beneficial bacteria in the intestinal system, while at the same time there exists another method based on ancient wisdom which heals people by placing the appropriate symbols on the appropriate meridians and harnessing quantum energy. I think what I am trying to say here speaks for itself and it should be clear for anyone which is the right path to follow.

I entrust to you the public use of my personal data; I have a large group of friends and contacts, I am a person of integrity, and I hope that all of this will contribute to expanding this core group.

The use of geometric symbols for injuries, blows, cuts and bites

In cases where we do not have a dowsing rod handy, we can be quite confident about using a sine curve ∿ or four parallel lines ≣. If there is a cut on the arms or legs it is best to draw a sine curve or four parallel lines at a right angle to the cut. The bleeding will stop and the pain will recede.

If we are faced with an injury or bruise from a fall, or with a bruise which has already turned purple, it is best to draw a sine curve.

> *A female acquaintance of mine fell down the stairs in her house and hurt her thigh and calf. We met about a week after the event and I saw huge blue bruises on her thigh and calf. I drew a sine curve ∿ on both, right in the middle of the spots. The pain decreased considerably and the recovery accelerated.* (Treatment by Mária Sági)

> *I was working in the garden when a large piece of ornamental rock rolled off a steep wall and fell onto my right shin-bone. In great pain I ran into the house and grabbed a ballpoint pen to draw four parallel lines ≣ on the injured area. The skin did not even turn purple and the pain disappeared straight away.* (Treatment by István Sági)

> *A group of friends were working together in the garden when one man drove the teeth of his saw into his right thumb. We rubbed salt into the open, bleeding wound, then drew a sine curve ∿ at a right angle to the cut. The recovery was pain-free and surprisingly quick.* (Treatment by István Sági)

> *Once I was in Tirol in February, in the middle of the skiing season. One afternoon my host came to me in despair, saying that one of his friends had injured both of his lower arms so badly dur-*

ing skiing that he had to be carried off and taken home by the rescue team. This young man was in so much pain that he wept silently as we began testing him with the dowsing rod. After the testing we placed four parallel lines ≣ on the outside of his left lower arm, on the wrist; and a larger sine curve ∿ about 10 cm higher up toward the elbow on the same arm. On the wrist of his right arm we drew a sine curve ∿, around 5 cm higher five parallel lines ≣, and another 5 cm up a sine curve ∿, and a further 5 cm up four parallel lines ≣. The pain stopped; he wore the symbols for another 3 days and made a full recovery. He told everyone the story of his fantastic recovery – this is how I was invited to the Basel conference of natural healers where he also attended and gave a personal account of the story of his recovery. (Treatment by István Sági)

This is the story of a hostess and her guests. One evening I was invited to dinner with some friends. I had only just arrived, and was still in the hallway when I heard a loud cry from the kitchen. The hostess had been trying to pour some hot cooking oil from one dish into another, but the dish slipped and she scolded the back of her left hand. Directly next to the burnt area I drew a large sine curve ∿ (3–4 cm) with a red felt-tip pen on her skin. The pain stopped instantly and the guests in the room did not even notice her injury – all they asked her as she served the dishes was why she had painted a red figure on her hand. (Treatment by István Sági)

The application of geometric symbols in cases of mosquito, wasp and tick bites

In cases like this we draw directly on the bite.

At the beach, in the grass I trod on a wasp which bit me at the base of my second toe. It swelled up and was very painful, so that I could hardly make the 5-minute walk home. At home I drew a symbol of a verticle line followed by a sine curve on it: |∿. The pain almost instantly abated and an hour or two later it stopped completely. (Treatment by Mária Sági)

After an outing I returned home carrying two ticks. After removing them I made a drawing on one bite and did nothing with the other bite. The place bearing a symbol made a quick and complete recovery; the other one left a small red mark at the center of the bite which only disappeared 4–5 weeks later. (Treatment by Mária Sági)

A lady medical doctor who attended our Körbler training course had the following experience directly on her return home from the course. She had hardly got home when her next-door neighbor rang her doorbell and asked for help – after working in the garden both her legs were covered in stinging-nettle bites and red rashes. On an impulse, the doctor took out her red lipstick from her handbag and, purely by intuition, drew five or six sine curves with the edge of the lipstick. This proved a huge success – the itch and the pain stopped straight away. She reported all of this in the training group the next day.

The application of geometric symbols in the case of warts

Sonja S., a woman living in Vienna, had been suffering for months from a wart on the sole of her foot. After testing her with the dowsing rod I drew an equal-armed cross of about 2 cm with a blue felt-tip pen. Sonja redrew the symbol every day and by day 24 this stubborn wart was gone without leaving a trace or any pain. (Treatment by István Sági)

The application of geometric symbols in the treatment of allergies

In chronic allergies, geometric symbols are used for re-programming the allergenic foods (see Chapter 15) and correcting the charge pattern of the organ in question.

For instance:

> *A 2-year-old boy (Gergő) had been suffering from milk allergy ever since he was born, with rashes covering his entire body. Method of treatment: testing and avoiding allergenic substances, all previous medication, previous formula, and foods, substituting all of this with a new diet (macrobiotics) and applying a sine curve ᔐ of about 1.5 cm around the liver for a month with testing repeated every day.* (Treatment by Mária Sági)

Alleviating pain through the application of geometric symbols

In the case of a headache, for instance, we draw three or four lines on point 1 of the gall meridian. Pain will abate or cease entirely in about 10 minutes. In the case of a toothache we place a symbol on the tooth meridian or the nape of the neck.

> *The father of one of the children we were treating was quite skeptical as he observed the process. Even though we had successfully treated his son's maladies for years with Körbler's method, he did not believe in New Homeopathy. On one occasion, however, this man had undergone some dentistry on a Friday evening and was in a lot of pain afterwards. He took painkillers but his complaints did not improve by the next day. It being a Saturday he could not go back to his dentist. So eventually he decided he would give these symbols a chance this time, so he contacted me for help. I drew three parallel ≡ red lines horizontally on the back of his neck over the first neck vertebra. His pain soon abated, so he now had first-hand experience of the effectiveness of the method.* (Treatment by Mária Sági)

The application of geometric symbols in terminal cases

> *One of our participants in a Körbler seminar for medical doctors in Budapest was a medical doctor living in the countryside. He used geometric symbols together with modern mainstream med-*

ical therapies in terminal cases where standard medical opinion held that the patient had only a few weeks to live. He used several symbols on a large area of the chest which brought improvement in these difficult cases.

The application of geometric symbols in remote healing

After Körbler's death I further elaborated his method and worked out the steps for using it in remote healing, as well as developing a new combined symbol system. [The method of remote healing will be discussed in Volume II. In preparation.] *Since that time, for 21 years now, I have been regularly treating patients living in other parts of Hungary or abroad by remote healing. If I am away for a longer period of time, this is the way in which I can continue to heal my family – first of all, my mother. The man with the toothache I described earlier contacted me again 10 years later. Now he complained about a severe pain above his heel at the Achilles muscle. I was abroad at the time, so I only learned about his problems through talking to my mother on the telephone, but she did not tell me which leg it was that was hurting. Using the dowsing rod I established that the pain was in the right leg above the Achilles muscle. So I chose the following combination of symbols: the* Y *symbol followed by a vertical line followed by a sine curve* Y|∿*, and I applied them for 44 hours. I also used a symbol consisting of two parallel vertical lines followed by a sine curve* ||∿ *for painful parts on the left leg, for a day and a half. My mother informed me that in 2 days the patient told her that he made a complete recovery.* (Treatment by Mária Sági)

Two friends, a couple living in Luxembourg, regularly received my help through remote healing. One night at 10 PM the husband phoned me to say that his wife had banged her head on the corner of the kitchen cupboard at 3 PM; she had a hard lump about the size of a largish coin and was in great pain. (I silently asked myself why they had not phoned me straight away instead of now, but did not ask the question.) Through remote healing I placed a Y symbol followed by a sine curve Y∿ on the affected spot. The next morning the wife phoned me to thank me. She woke at 3 AM, felt no pain at all, went into the bathroom, looked in the mirror and saw in amazement that the hard lump was entirely gone. (Treatment by Mária Sági)

Healing with Soft Methods

As the second part of therapy we identify and introduce into the diseased organism all the necessary material and information that normalizes both electromagnetic and biochemical functions. In the following section we describe the use of these soft methods.

Soft healing methods may be divided into two groups. One includes nutrients, medical herbs, minerals and trace elements. The necessity of these is common knowledge; therefore we simply note that in the case of disease it can be very helpful if we decide by testing which foods and natural supplements are needed. Introducing trace elements is extremely important, since they function as connecting elements in both electromagnetic and biochemical functions, so the lack of them can prevent the healthy operation of entire chains of functions. It is important to know that the necessary nutrients and trace elements cannot be replaced by information. For instance, in areas which are low in iodine, as in the greater part of Hungary, it is not enough to introduce the information of iodine – you also need the iodine itself.

The other group uses the geometric symbols regulating biochemical functions purely by information. These include information that occur in nature to which our body reacts either favorably or unfavorably. This explains the action mechanism of alternative cures such as high-potency homeopathic remedies, ancient symbols, physical exercises forming certain geometric symbols, yoga mudras, rune forces, sounds, mantras and reactions to colors.

Each treatment conveys a 'message' that our organism absorbs and thereby converts the malfunction into healthy functioning. How does all this happen and what is the role of the self-healing mechanisms? Today's science is not yet able to account fully for all these processes. However, Körbler's assumption about information transfer in the living organism is a milestone in trying to explore the action mechanisms of healing methods dating back millennia.

Information Transfer through the Body

Körbler discovered that in the body, a complex open system, information is transferred without modification. The information we absorb with the fingertips of our left hand is emitted again through the fingertips of our right hand. Körbler called this phenomenon the 'left–right meridian' of our body.

The left–right meridian is the most effective instrument for creating the medication you need. It enables you to use the radiation of the body to transfer the resonance pattern of any substance to water or to any substance (e.g. a crystal) that can conserve information.

Let us see how all this takes place in practice! You hold an object made of gold in your left hand, and some water in a glass in your right hand. Hold both for 4 minutes. Next you put the glass of water in your left hand and test it first with the hand-held dowsing rod, then with the vertical dowsing rod. Both will react as though you were holding the object of gold in your left hand. The vertical dowsing rod will produce the same movement.

If you now hold the glass of water with the information of gold in your left hand, and in your right hand you hold another glass of water for four minutes, testing the second glass of water will give the same result as the first. The experiment may be repeated any number of times – the result will always be the same.

If you place the index finger of your left hand on the electron microscope image of gold and in your right hand you hold water in another glass for a further four minutes, on testing the water you will get the same results as in the case of glasses of water. No matter what sort of object, crystal or herb you use, the process of information transfer always takes place in the same way. If, however, you place informed water into a water bath and heat it to 55–60 °C, the information will disappear. After it cools down, the water will absorb new information again. If you fix the information of a remedial substance onto a piece of jewelry or a dental crown, from that time on the jewelry or crown will emit the healing information for the organism.

Healing with Informed Water

Körbler also discovered a way in which the healing quality of geometric symbols can be increased. It is important how we introduce the charge pattern that helps restore healthy functions into the body. As we have seen, with the help of the left–right meridian the living organism transmits information to new information carriers: water, metals, crystals, precious stones, etc. If we choose water as the new information carrier, the informed water prepared by the given person will carry the kind of information characteristic of his or her resonance system and represent coherent information for his or her own organism.

As we saw in Chapter 3, Körbler worked extensively on the functional mechanisms of water molecules in the organism. We also noted that since Körbler's death, Del Giudice and colleagues have explored the relevant quantum electrodynamic processes as well.

These findings have allowed us to conclude that the healing effect of the informed water works through the quantum electrodynamic mechanisms of water molecules in the body. The water informed by the patient can retune the information that converts disease into health-sustaining information through quantum electrodynamic processes. This is the secret of the organism's capacity for quick recovery. There is no more effective way of producing a remedy. If the geometric symbol is well chosen, informed water made by the patient is the most effective soft remedy. Based on my 20 years' experience, I can affirm that it is effective for all patients and in all types of diseases.

Preparing informed water

If you have a sore throat, use the dowsing rod to test what sort of geometric symbol needs to be drawn on the throat *(Figure 76).*

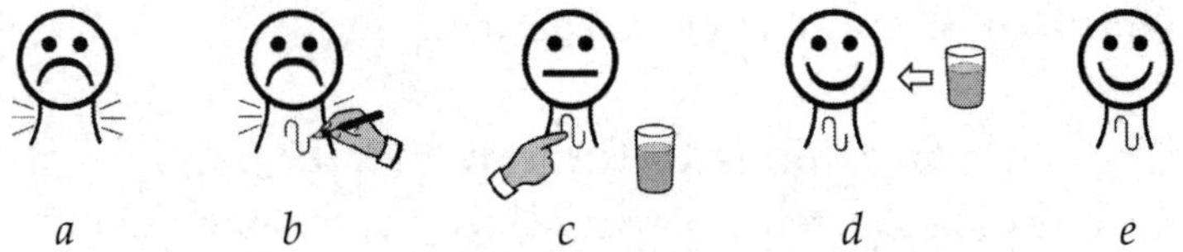

Figure 76. Making informed water

If the geometric symbol is appropriate, the dowsing rod moves horizontally.

Take a glass of water in your right hand. You hold the index finger of your left hand 1 cm in front of the symbol drawn on your throat and stay in that position for four minutes. Next you pick up the informed water with your left hand – in this case the dowsing rod moves horizontally in your hand. If it is not moving horizontally, this is due to an error, and you need to retest (b and c). When the informed water is produced, you drink it a mouthful at a time. Four hours later you repeat every step. After drinking three or four glasses of informed, water the complaint ceases in most cases *(Figure 76).* Adult patients usually produce their own informed water. For small children it is made by their mother.

Another way of producing informed water is to have the patient look at the correct information. In other words, instead of the left index finger, the information is absorbed here through the eyes. The procedure is the following. You take a sheet of white, unruled paper with no pattern on it; write on it the name of the patient, the name of the sick organ, and draw the geometric symbol required for the cure (e.g. 'Anna', *Figure 77*).

Anna is looking at the piece of paper, holding it in her left hand, while in her right hand she holds a glass of pure water for four minutes. Once that is done, she drinks the informed water that has been produced, one gulp at a time.

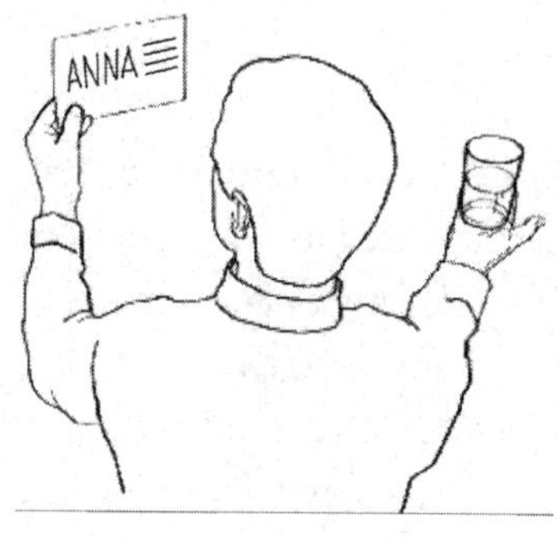

Figure 77

Using informed water is recommended in all cases where the malfunction is more serious than what the organism could rectify by correcting the electromagnetic pathways. Informed water needs to be used until health is restored and the healthy organism is able to produce the remedy by itself. This method is equally effective for children, and for adults.

The application of informed water in the treatment of small children

The informed water is prepared by the mother, having her baby on her lap. The amount of time required is again four minutes. If the symbol is in an easily accessible spot on the baby's body, the mother places her finger 1 cm over the symbol and holds the water in her right hand for four minutes. If this is uncomfortable, then with the baby on her lap, the mother holds the glass of water in her right hand while looking at the symbol for four minutes.

The application of informed water in treating older children

When they are somewhat older, children can make their own informed water. In acute processes (sore throat, flu) it acts really rapidly – in fact in most cases it is sufficient to drink the informed water once or twice to achieve recovery.

Körbler told us that at the age of eight his daughter would cure herself; indeed, she had even taught her friends how to do it. If at school she feels she has a sore throat, after getting home she draws a sine curve on her throat, holds her left index finger over it and at the same time holds a glass of water in her right hand for four minutes. Usually the sore throat goes away after consuming one glass of sine water.

The application of informed water in the treatment of adults

In the case of acute processes we produce informed water every 4 hours, usually using the same symbol. For instance, in the case of a high temperature and an inflamed throat we draw a sine curve over the throat and consume water informed with the same symbol about three to four times. This is usually sufficient for recovery. When treating diseased organs, we draw the selected symbol on the skin over the organ or follow the rules of Chinese acupuncture and draw on the relevant meridian point. Then this is used for creating the informed water.

> *I was teaching this method at a training course for doctors in Germany. One of the participants, filled with enthusiasm, told us the following story on the second day. The previous day he went home to find that his son aged 19, who had been healthy the same morning, had a temperature of 40 °C. He thought this was an occasion to try out the method he was learning, so he examined him with the dowsing rod, to find the appropriate symbol. The son was willing to experiment and prepared the informed water for himself. His temperature descended.*

Let us now offer an example of how Körbler once used water 'informed' with the Y symbol to cure István.

In spring 1991, János Déri, commentator on the television show Close Encounters of Type Zero, *presented Körbler's work. The program was to be shot in Vienna. One afternoon the crew set out in a minibus toward that city to get ready for the next day's shoot. My brother and I left separately by car, but before leaving Budapest we fulfilled a friend's kind invitation on our way and paid a flash visit. Istvan ate a fish sandwich and drank some mineral water and, after making a quick farewell which our friends received with understanding, we continued on our journey. Trouble began during the drive – Istvan began to feel increasing pain in both arms and both legs from the ankle all the way up to the hips. This was coupled with a headache and a general sense of indisposition. As we drove past Győr and approached the border (180 km), his condition worsened at such a rate that we had to stop – he could drive no longer. It was late at night when we finally arrived in Vienna (270 km from Budapest). His condition remained poor, and he developed a new symptom as well: both hands and feet swelled up. In the hotel we asked for a thermometer which showed 39 °C.*

After he woke up the next morning, Istvan identified a further symptom – on the inside of his right thigh there was a wide black stripe from the knee all the way up to the groin, surrounded by slight bruises and extremely painful. The film shoot itself was going to take place in the office of healer Thomas Steinmann. After we arrived we spoke to Thomas who, seeing Istvan's alarming condition, proposed instant diagnosis using the radionic device. For this, he took a colored photograph of the entire body with a Polaroid camera. This picture was then analyzed by the radionic device. In the meantime Körbler also arrived. Using the dowsing rod he identified that the required therapy was to draw a large red Y *lengthwise on the inside of the thigh (with the leg of the* Y *pointing toward the knee). He also said Istvan must make informed water using this body area and consume it three times a day. This took the following form. Istvan held the palm of his*

> *left hand 2–3 cm above the inside of the right thigh while in his right hand he held a glass of pure water for four minutes. Next he drank the informed water slowly, one gulp at a time, and repeated the same process three times a day. Whenever the red symbol* Y *faded, it had to be redrawn. The diagnosis of the radionic device revealed bad liver data, which indicated a case of poisoning.*
> *After we arrived home, Istvan was instantly given a referral by his GP to the Teaching Hospital of Vascular Surgery where they diagnosed thrombophlebitis, but the cause was not identified. At a Chinese clinic operating in Budapest it was established that the total set of symptoms pointed at poisoning and this can only have been caused by spoiled fish. This means that in all probability the fish sandwich contained some fish which had gone bad. Istvan followed Körbler's advice and regularly redrew the* Y*, as well as drinking informed water three times a day for 3 weeks. Using Körbler's method he completely recovered.*

The treatment of chronic processes requires thorough testing to determine how many times a day and for how many days you need to use informed water along with the appropriate symbol. Another examination will decide whether the use of a different symbol is required. Informed water is used in a wide range of arrangements from a few days to a period of several weeks, in treating almost any kind of disease.

> *Jasna, aged 55, is an ideal grandmother. She runs a big household in Croatia, on the isle of Brac, in a small holiday resort village. They live by tourism and producing olives and wine. Every time I go on holiday there I buy oil and wine from her, as well as anything else that might be growing in her biodynamic garden. She is a vigorous, sporty, open-hearted, jovial personality, positive and full of smiles, with a big heart. She is a joy to chat with under her huge vine arbor. Last summer, however, it was a pale, tired*

Jasna with sunken cheeks who met us. In response to my question she told me that she had been struggling for months with inflamed varicose veins on her left leg and the medical treatment was doing her no good, even though she had followed all the advice she had been given so far. Her doctor proposed an operation but she was reluctant. I offered my help; I explained to her that we would make informed water and that if she wished, I would examine her. She was more than willing, so the same day I returned with my dowsing rod and examined her. I suggested the use of informed water: the combination of a sine curve followed by a vertical line: ∿| *, three times a day for 5 days. A week later I visited her again. I was met by the 'old' Jasna – a lady with a happy face and ruddy cheeks. Her first question was whether she could have a course of treatment like this all the time or at least more often, say every month, because she had totally recovered. Her pain was gone; the swollen vein had retracted. Her daughter also encouraged her: 'Well, Mum, just keep drinking the informed water if it is so wonderfully effective.'*

The other day I met a representative of the Szeged University of Metaphysics. The Körbler dowsing rod was sticking out of my handbag so he approached me and asked where it came from. After we introduced ourselves he told me that he knew the stick well. He related that they had recently had a patient who had suffered from panic syndrome for years. He had tried many different kinds of medical treatment – to no avail. 'That was when we tried Körbler's method,' he went on to say. 'We tested to find out what kind of symbol she needed. We drew it on a piece of paper and, using the symbol, the patient made herself informed water every day for 2 weeks. Two weeks later she came to us to say that she was feeling much better. We examined her again, gave her a new symbol and then for 2 more weeks she prepared and drank informed water every day. Two weeks later she came back again and told us happily that her complaints were completely gone. Ever since then, every time she comes our way she pops in just to express her gratitude. She recovered from a really heavy burden of panic syndrome that she had carried for years.'

The application of informed water in alleviating pain

Informed water is an effective painkiller even in cases where we are unable to treat the root cause of the pain. In such cases we select a geometric symbol that matches the painful area, draw it on a piece of paper, and the patient prepares the informed water on this basis. It is surprisingly effective in soothing the pain.

An elderly female patient of ours suffered from intense pain around the ribs on her right-hand side, due to a mammary operation on the right and advanced osteoporosis. According to a diagnosis by Vietnamese medical professor Dr. Kiem Do Thanh, a specialist in spine function therapy, this was due to a pain of the rib nerve caused by scoliosis. Sadly we were unable to influence that condition. In order to help the patient rest and sleep at night we needed to soothe her intense pain. Medical treatment and allopathic remedies up till that time had proved ineffectual. The patient did not want to use morphine-based painkillers. Therefore we applied informed water which again proved so effective that the patient slept for 6–8 hours before being woken by pain in the affected area.

The application of informed water in remote healing

We use the water in the same way as in proximal healing. In my view the basic method of treatment in remote healing is the production of informed water. I send my patients the data required for informed water. The patient holds the sheet of paper in his/her left hand, looking at it, and makes the informed water in doing so. In most cases a one-time treatment is sufficient.

Informed water produced from natural substances

If we wish to use the information of a semi-precious stone or a crystal for a remedy, we can produce informed water by using a coin.

Körbler gave the following example.

> *A neurological patient was shivering with cold at the hottest time of summer. In cases like this the remedy was informed water using the information of silicon. This can be produced in a number of different ways. If you have access to silicon crystals, you need to hold the silicon in your left hand and a glass of water in your right hand. Hold it for four minutes, then drink it. If you do not have access to silicon crystals, you can do the same using the electron microscope image of the crystal. You can also produce homeopathic silicon using a solar powered calculator in the following manner. Place your left index finger on the solar cell of the calculator, while in your right hand you hold a copper coin for four minutes. Then take the 'informed' coin in your left hand, while in your right hand you hold a glass of water for four minutes. The primary characteristic of the informed water thus produced is that because it runs through the organism, the body will produce the homeopathic remedy at exactly the potency which is required. This is why it is crucial to make it over and over again, two or three times a day, as required.*

Testing the Effect of Allopathic Medicines

A novel consequence of Körbler's system is that it also demonstrates how the diseased organism reacts if allopathic medication must be used for its recovery. If the choice of allopathic medicine is not optimal, testing with the dowsing rod will show that despite the use of allopathic medication, the unhealthy charge pattern that sustains the disease in the energy field of the organism is still present. This strengthens the information of the disease or the harmful information of the adverse effects, strengthening negative influences rather than health. It also happens quite frequently that the allopathic medicine used to treat one organ has a bad influence on the condition of another organ or set of organs (i.e. the intestinal system in case of antibiotic treatment). Although we know that a strong organism will recover despite these medicines, this is not what happens in most cases. For the allopathic medicine to really serve the recovery of the patient, it is important to use the optimal substance. The optimal substance requires optimal dosage. Although we have long had the instruments for this (Voll, radionic, Nelson Scio and many other bioresonance instruments), an examination takes far longer this way than the time the public health service is willing to grant to their patients. The other factor is that these instruments are too costly for general, widespread practice. This means that they are only available to the private praxis of healers. As there is no instrument to measure the right dosage, most patients get a larger quantity than is required. If more than one allopathic medicine is used, there is no way to detect synergies and determine the optimal quantities of the various drugs with conventional methods. Since this procedure is highly time consuming, it is seldom employed.

Körbler was well acquainted with the available instruments. By developing his system and the dowsing rod, he was hoping to introduce a device which was accessible to all practitioners, and its use is rapid enough to cope with the pressure of time. Healers who were keen to learn the method were curious to compare the performance of the various instruments with the dowsing rod. It was common at the training courses for doctors in Austria to have so many instruments on the table that there was hardly any room for our notebooks.

On one occasion I asked Körbler, 'When I get a chance to buy an instrument, which one should I choose?' He answered, 'None of the above. The dowsing rod knows more than any of these. It knows just as much as a radionics device. If you have the means to buy just one, only the radionics device is worth acquiring.'

After Körbler's death it became clear to me how right he was. On one of the occasions when I was teaching in Germany I met Peter W. Köhne, head of the Pronova Energetik company, who, being a friend of Körbler's, had given him a radionic device. Peter invited me to try out the radionic system for reasons of comparison. We both examined the same patient and compared our therapies. The radionic device measures on a scale of 1–100 the quality of the suggested therapy. Optimal therapy would get 100 points, anything over 85 points is seen as really good and would bring quick help, while scores over 95 points are rare. In this case the therapy suggested by the radionic device was rated at 94 points by the device. Next we tested the therapy I suggested on the basis of the dowsing rod and the radionic device rated it at 96.7.

Choosing an allopathic medicine

When testing a medicine, the patient holds it in his or her left hand. The testing is done on the top of the head or over the right brain hemisphere by placing the palm of the left hand on the patient's head or holding it next to the head. If we are using more than one substance, we place all allopathic medications and all the soft medications in the patient's left hand. If the dowsing rod moves horizontally over the head, the choice of medication is optimal. The next step is choosing the appropriate geometric symbols. If we follow the reverse order, the geometric symbols could turn out to be wrong, since the allopathic drugs also change the energy field.

The application of allopathic medicines with geometric symbols

The unique feature of information medicine is that it is able to overcome the difficulties of allopathic medicine if we need to optimize the steps and paths of information levels. By using New Homeopathy we can easily ensure that allopathic remedies serve the recovery of the patient. For this we first need to identify the substances and then their required quantity. Next, of course, we need to apply the geometric symbols.

As a next step of the therapy, we apply the geometric symbols with the potential to harmonize the disturbed points and areas. We test the vectors of the diagnostic points one by one, then proceed to draw the geometric symbols. Vectors are helpful in letting us know which symbol we should start with when testing. If, for example, the point or an area shows vector position 3, it needs to be balanced by the symbol of three horizontal lines ≡, but it is also possible that two lines = will be sufficient. We might, however, need to use four horizontal lines ≣. In all cases we do the testing separately. The order of testing follows that of the diagnostic points: large intestine 1, small intestine 3, lungs 1, kidneys 3, spleen 6, stomach 36, gall 40, liver 3, circulation point (third rib interspace on the left next to the breastbone), Körbler's mycosis point on the left side of the chest, Körbler's inflammation point on both wrists, the reflex zones of the palm of the hand.

There is usually no need to correct all these points. For each patient we need to supply different combinations of points with the geometric symbols. This is why testing is recommended. It is important to make sure that the dowsing rod moves horizontally on testing every diagnostic point. By way of control we hold our left hand over the top of the head, and if the dowsing rod is still moving horizontally, we have chosen the right therapy. We have provided geometric information that has rectified the paths of electromagnetic communication.

Determining the dosage of the remedies

The last step of therapy is to establish the dosage of the medication. Once we have chosen the substances, we place the tablets and capsules in the patient's left hand and test on their head whether the dosage we had determined is appropriate. If it is, the dowsing rod will move horizontally. Once we have established the dosage of all the medicines, we place them all in the left hand of the patient and test once more. It is possible that when applied all together, some of the medicines will require a lower dosage. The total dosage of all of the medicines is only appropriate if at the final testing the dowsing rod moves horizontally when tested over the head.

Determining the duration of the treatment

Determining the duration of the treatment is likewise based on testing – we first test the medicines each on its own, then we test them all together.

Testing the medications one by one

We write down the name and dosage of the medication on a piece of paper and the duration recommended (e.g. acidophilus, 1 capsule before breakfast for 7 days), then put it in the patient's hand and ask him or her to look at it and read it silently. While they are doing this, we test over the top of their head. We keep changing the dosage until the dowsing rod starts moving horizontally.

Testing the ensemble of medications

Once we have established the dosage of all of the medicines one by one, on a fresh piece of paper we write the total list and again test on the top of the head. We may find once again that with the joint dosage we need to adjust the dosage of one or the other medicines. We carry on testing until we find that the dowsing rod moves vigorously in a horizontal direction. When that happens, we have reached the optimal therapy.

Chapter 8

Various Methods for Harmonizing the Flow of Energy and Information

If the electromagnetic condition of the organism is not satisfactory due to various blocks, this will sooner or later lead to a blockage, triggering harmful biochemical processes. These, in turn, lead to the appearance of disease. As we have already mentioned, despite the fact that their energy level is extremely low, electromagnetic waves have a substantial influence on humans, and other living organism. This is due to the fact that the wavelength of electromagnetic energy is the same as the wavelength of the building blocks of our cells and therefore they cause resonance in our cells. Optimal electromagnetic conditions are also extremely important in the process of healing.

If we provide the organism with the trace elements or other biochemical substances which are required for recovery, these can only make their beneficial impact if the electromagnetic condition of the body is suited to allow the biochemical substance to create its effect. In other cases the body is unable to make use of these substances and they produce more harmful side-effects than benefits.

In order to avoid this, it is vital to eliminate energy blocks in the body, to restore the flow of energy and information and optimize the electromagnetic condition.

Körbler developed several simple methods for this. He relied on the experience accumulated by ancient healing methods and studied their electromagnetic components. These methods are simple, quick, almost entirely cost-free; they are rapid to apply from the healer's point of view, are easy to handle even in the patient's home and, last but not least, are highly effective.

You can build energy and information flows with water, stone, color, sound, aroma, crystals, metal, geometric symbols, that is, symbols that carry balancing information according to the vector system, as well as with informed water carrying balancing information, and with a combination of these. The list is, of course, far from exhaustive. The essence of the above procedures is that the disharmonic information at the block is balanced by the information required for that spot, and thus the electromagnetic balance is rapidly restored. There is only one important criterion in applying and combining these methods, and this is accurate choice. No matter whether we are using one or several methods, we must test for the whole organism whether the effect is positive. We need to use the bio-indicator to guide the choice and application.

The Application of Precious Stones and Crystals

The use of precious stones and crystals as decoration, as jewelry and for healing has a tradition going back over two millennia in the Far East, in South America and in all places where the stones and crystals are found in nature. Using them as jewelry also aims to enhance the beauty, strength and radiation of the person who wears it. In traditional cultures people are still able to sense the different radiations of precious stones and use them appropriately for decoration and in the art of healing.

The literature regarding the effect of precious stones and crystals is enormous. For Western cultures this literature might be very helpful, even though the qualities it lists are not always sufficient to guide our choice for purposes of healing. Körbler demonstrated in his courses how to choose the right stone, whether for jewelry or for healing.

The application of precious stones and crystals as jewelry

If a precious stone is to be used as jewelry, we can use the top of the head for testing whether it is beneficial or not for the individual. It should only be worn if the bio-indicator is swinging horizontally. In all other cases the jewelry is not optimal in the condition tested. Jewels can have a different effect at different times, depending on the energetic condition of the individual. In most cases the wearer of the item can sense this and chooses different jewelry depending on what he or she senses.

The application of precious stones and crystals in healing

Using precious stones and crystals for healing is part of the art of medicine in traditional cultures and is seen as a highly effective method. It can be just as successfully applied in our culture if the stone is well chosen. Almost everyone is acquainted with the beneficial impact of well-chosen stones. The following story confirms this effect.

> *Last year's holiday took me back once more to my old friend Jasna. A year had gone by since we last met. Jasna is the same as she was – a beaming, good-humored, friendly grandmother serving an extended family and a farm. I surprised her with a tiny present – I gave her a piece of citrine the size of a walnut. When she saw it in my hand her face lit up and her eyes widened. She said she would wear it around her neck. We met again 2 weeks later to say goodbye. I had long forgotten about the citrine but she mentioned it. She said she had been wearing it ever since – over the solar plexus. She said she loved wearing it because she found that it helped her channel her sense of urgency from overwork in the summer season into a more normal rhythm. Under all the pressure, she had often experienced a bitter taste in her mouth – this unpleasant reaction had stopped completely since she had been wearing the citrine.*

In making the right choice of precious stones for treatment, we can rely on the help of the bio-indicator. People are different and every person's energy system differs too, as does their relation to precious stones and crystals. You can make the choice by testing the entire organism, but the precious stone which is appropriate today may not be so some time later, so the test needs to be repeated. You can also choose by finding the adequate balancing information for the disturbance zone. In this case the optimal precious stone is chosen for the particular disturbance zone and affixed to it, for instance, by adhesive tape. In cases like this you need to retest the entire body to make sure you find a positive energy flow. If an energy block or a new disturbance zone has emerged anywhere, you need to find a precious stone which will guarantee a positive energy flow in the entire organism.

It is an interesting experience that the optimal balancing information for a disturbance zone may come from a precious stone or crystal which is otherwise unfavorable for the person in question. It is also possible for a precious stone with a favorable general effect to impart too much energy for one organ or area and thus it can cause an inflammation or disturbance zone in areas with a poor energy supply. The size, the shape, and the structure of the precious stone also matter.

Small precious stones as conveyors of energy

Small precious stones can be used as mediators of energy. This is required if the functional disturbance has been around for a longer period of time and hence a longer time is required to restore the original functioning.

First we choose a beneficial precious stone for the patient and then we find the ideal geometric symbol that helps restore healthy functions in their organism. The healer draws the symbol on the left index finger of the patient, who then holds this finger at 0.5 cm from the disturbance zone while in his or her right hand he / she holds the selected precious stone or crystal for about 3–

4 minutes. The balancing information for the disturbance zone is now transferred to the precious stone. Now the healer puts the stone in his or her left hand and tests the patient with the bio-indicator while tracing the spinal column with the stone held in his/her left hand. If the body shows an optimal energy condition, the patient can proceed to make informed water with the help of the precious stone two or three times a day, as needed.

Neutralizing Unfavorable Sound Frequencies

In Chapter 10 we shall describe how various sound frequencies have an importance in the energy system of the organism. Sounds are the quickest way of making an energizing effect. You may also find, however, that certain sound frequencies are harmful. Long-lasting effects such as the noise of the workplace or machines which make an intense buzzing noise through the night can damage the immune system.

Körbler has demonstrated how you can neutralize harmful auditive effects with the use of stones. This is done in the following way.

Using a sound aggregator, Körbler sought out a frequency which had an unfavorable effect on the energy of the heart for the tested person. Under the effect of the sound, the bio-indicator moved vertically when testing the heart.

Körbler chose a small phial filled with little stones – if he held this close to the tested person, the bio-indicator began to move horizontally again, even if the sound continued. If he removed the phial, the movement once more became vertical. This shows that the stones in the phial are capable of correcting the negative effect of the sound frequency.

The key to this phenomenon is the difference of the 'antenna size', i.e. the difference in the wavelengths.

The small stones behave like a frequency converter, a medium that absorbs the sound wave, then emits it with a different frequency. This way the stones alter the effect of the sound reaching the body.

The application of varying grains of zeolite

The body's sensitivity to the various grain sizes of minerals is different in the same way as our sensitivity to various stones and precious stones. This is why they can be used in healing. Körbler kept zeolite of seven different grain sizes in seven small phials on his desk and tested them for healing. The smallest grain size was 0.06 mm; the largest grains were 10–14 mm.

If we select the optimal grain size of an optimal mineral, we obtain a very potent healing effect. Even an unpleasant case of tinnitus can be influenced and also stopped this way.

Körbler shared with us his most recent experience in this respect.

> *Professor König from Vienna, a famous ear, nose and throat specialist, had asked Körbler to look at one of his patients with tinnitus. The patient was an architect of 70 who had been suffering from severe tinnitus for 4 years. Various hospitals and private clinics had tried different medical approaches but had achieved nothing. The tinnitus did not abate. Körbler examined the patient with the bio-indicator, found the point on the face – right in front of the ear – at which he could test the zeolite, and then chose the appropriate grain size. Next he put the stones in the patient's hand and the tinnitus stopped. From this time on, the patient carried a phial containing zeolite of the optimal grain size, in his pocket so that it could touch his body through the fabric. The resonance of the zeolite neutralized the resonance of the tinnitus so the patient could no longer hear it.*

There was also a tinnitus sufferer at Körbler's Budapest training course who let himself be used to demonstrate the above method. Körbler chose that method to select the zeolite of the appropriate size. While he held the phials of various sizes to the testing points, the patient sometimes heard the tinnitus more loudly; with other phials he heard it softer. When the phial with the appropriate grain size was found, the patient indicated that the sound had again changed – this time it became deeper. This was the phial the patient had to wear close to the body. This grain size first neutralizes the higher frequencies, and then the lower frequencies. In the case of chronic illnesses the appropriate grain size may be incorporated in the wall of a person's home, for example, it is mired into the plaster (see Chapter 17), or hung on the wall. It is also possible to project the radiation of the precious stone on the wall; this way the wall of the room will emit a healing radiation.

Finally, it is a good idea to test the grain size which is unfavorable for the test person. Körbler used his own body to demonstrate that for him a grain size of 3 mm was unfavorable. If he were to lay a gravel path of this grain size in his garden and sit on the path, this would put a load on the energy supply of his heart. If this grain size was to cover the inside wall of a room, this would reduce healthy energies for him.

The Energy-Optimizing Effect of Sensory Information

Information arriving through the sensory organs always has a similar effect. Either the sensory organ absorbs electromagnetic waves in the first place or it transforms chemical information into electromagnetic waves. Optimal sound frequencies are the most potent means of building up energy. Our hearing perceives extremely low frequencies of slow resonances. Inside the inner ear, in the middle of the cochlea, these resonances become transformed into electromagnetic waves and this is the information which the brain receives. The process takes place near the speed of light, just like the reaction of the organs to sound. If the resonance of a sound (e.g. 400 Hz) is much lower than the organism's own frequency (10^{12}–10^{13} Hz), the sounds are perceived as a rhythmic effect.

Application of aromatherapy

In the case of aromatherapy, the aroma, i.e. the molecule which transmits the smell, penetrates right into the nasal cavity. In this case the information carried by the molecule is transformed by the receptors of the nasal cavity into electromagnetic waves and these make their way to the brain and the organs. If one of the organs reacts positively or negatively to this information, this also reaches the brain. This is the feedback of the immune system. If the feedback does not take place, this produces exaggerated or reduced functioning. This is what happens in allergic reactions.

Aromatherapy can help with allergic reactions. If the patient smells the scent, the bio-indicator will identify what kind of reaction the various aromas produce from the organism and from the individual organs. In the case of the optimal smell, the organ in question will instantly give a positive reaction; in other words its energy and information supply will be ideal. This needs to be tested in the same way as with precious stones. There is no general recipe; the required smell is always in harmony with the given condition. The bioindicator thest shows us when the aroma has fulfilled its role, and it becomes unnecessary.

Application of colors

Electromagnetic information arriving through vision is also decisive for the functioning of the organism. Colors provoke powerful reactions. These are different for each individual. It is known that colors do not exist as such; all we perceive is the reflection of light from molecules of different shapes and sizes.

What our eyes perceive as color, however, is also perceived by other organs. This is why it is possible to test which colors resolve the disturbance zones for each person, and which colors may generate disturbance zones. It is important to identify which colors act negatively or positively on malfunctioning organs.

By testing sheets of paper of different colors we may identify the beneficial or harmful effect of the color. Bright red has the most intense effect. We can also test which are the colors that help recovery in case of organic disease. If, for instance, the liver is showing a malfunction, the color white is most likely to aid recovery.

There is also such a thing as color allergy. Therefore it is advisable to test patients for 12–18 colors at the least, to ascertain their reaction to colors.

Application of the pyramid form

In terms of their effect, the geometric symbols we use can also be three-dimensional – the pyramid is one of these. The mysteries of pyramids have been intriguing mankind for millennia. Even today there are attempts to discover their effect.

Körbler was once invited by a group of architects from Los Angeles who asked for his urgent assistance with their problem. They were building pyramid houses and found that within a few months of moving in, some of the residents were hospitalized with serious psychological problems. One of these residents was Marlon Brando. The pyramid houses affected all residents negatively. In all probability, the reason was that the pyramid form massively densified and rarified the electric and magnetic fields inside the houses. Radiation coming from the outside, such as sunshine, cannot penetrate into the center of this geometric form. Thus, even sunlight in the 200 nm UV range fails to penetrate the pyramid. As a result, the organism inside cannot gain sufficient energy and this also shows in the reactions of the body. It is known that if a piece of meat is placed in the center of a pyramid it will not go bad; it will merely dry out. The reason for this is that the energy required for transformation does not penetrate as far as the meat. Also, the human organism has a constant need for energies from the outside to sustain its life.

We know that lots of explorers and researchers died at the exploration of the Cheops pyramids. The explorers spent days and even weeks inside the pyramids. It must have been as a result of the shortage of energy that they died abruptly. In cases like this, electric charge drops in all the cells at the same time.

Viewed from the outside, the form of the pyramid is favorable, since energy travels upward along its sides. This flow of energy touches all sides of the pyramid. The main point where energy exits is the peak. At the peak of the pyramid an 'energy wind' departs which strives upward and also affects the fields underneath. In churches there are very intense energy zones underneath the steeples. People feel wonderful there, but they must not spend too much time in that position, because they get too much energy. This is also true of pyramids we wear on our person as jewelry. For a short period they have a very good effect, but then all of a sudden their influence can turn very bad and unfavorable. As mentioned before, the overall effect of pieces of jewelry can be tested with the bio-indicator, with hands held over the top of the head.

Application of metals for storing information

Energy can also be built up by using metals, in that we can use them for storing information. As we saw in Chapter 5, we can transfer new information to metal objects with the help of the left–right meridian. This new information may come from any living substance (e.g. medical herbs), from lifeless objects (stones, other metals), or from thoughts and emotions. It can also come from the geometric symbols of Körbler's vector system, the balancing information of a disturbance zone, etc. The necessary balancing information can be transposed to a tooth filling, a metal bracelet, a wedding ring or a coin.

Körbler willingly and frequently used coins for storing information. Patients themselves can transpose balancing information to the coin, but the healer can also do this for the patient. In cases where there are several types of balancing information to aid recovery, coins are handy to use, since the patient can produce informed water for himself or herself at home, using the informed coin. Using the informed coin is also practical when the recovery of the organism requires the use of informed water through a prolonged period, possibly weeks. In the soft treatment of mycosis this is usually the case.

The metal will retain the information as long as it is not heated to more than a temperature of 55 °C or immersed in boiling water for more than 3 minutes. After such intervention the metal will again contain its own information. This is due to the fact that in the case of solid bodies during the process when molecules assume a clear structure, in other words the crystallization process, it becomes possible for electrons and atoms to assume new constellations and to modify. The reaction taking place in this stratum is similar to what happens inside the cell. In one sense we could even claim that metals are alive. But metals only allow for extremely intense reactions. This is why there can be no life inside metals, only single reactions. With the exception of noble metals, in their natural form metals represent unfavorable information for the human body. This is proven by the dowsing rod showing circular movement to the right when testing metals. The explanation is that the atoms of the human body and the atoms of metals are of different weight. The human body is built of lightweight atoms. The nucleus is surrounded by a small number of electrons. Our molecules are constituted of a great number of atoms like this, oxygen being just one. Those atoms, however, where the nucleus is surrounded by many electrons, are poison for our organism. The atom of lead, for instance, contains a hundred times more electrons than the atoms of the human body, and the nucleus of uranium is surrounded by even more electrons. These substances are poisonous for the body.

In the case of certain metals there is a great number of electrons around the nucleus. The information of these medium-weight metals is unfavorable.

The information proper to the metal itself may be used in establishing a diagnosis and in therapy. As we described in Chapter 7, if we want to establish the cause of the disturbance with our diagnosis, we can use a coin. We can test which disturbance zones are related to each other and which are independent. This is important information for identifying further therapy.

Using the coin as a therapeutic instrument takes the following form.

The dowsing rod indicates a disturbance by revolving to the left somewhere in the body; this can be eliminated with the use of a coin. This is a method that was tested in Austria by psychologists and neurologists in psychiatric wards. They attached a Schilling (the currency of Austria before the Euro) to the nape of the neck of their patients which caused their attacks to disappear. This came to be called *Körbler's Schilling method.*

The only metals which are favorable and indeed indispensable for the human organism are trace elements – these are crucial for the functioning of the 'chemical plant' of the body. Their name also indicates that they constitute important components of our cells in extremely small quantities, measured in micrograms. Each of the trace elements plays a crucial role. If there is a deficit in one of the trace elements it is not enough to introduce its information – the body requires the trace element itself. Thus it is known, for instance, that zinc is vital for the operation of the sensory organs (vision, hearing, taste), but what is less well known is the fact that in the absence of zinc the body is also unable to make appropriate use of the other trace elements.

Energy and Information Flow in Healthy Persons in Everyday Life

It is a natural part of life that the energy-condition of a healthy individual varies and changes over the day. After a good night's rest we tend to feel energized, which means that all points of the organism receive optimal energy and information supply. During the day's work the energy level drops, that, we try to normalize by eating, drinking, exercise or possibly a nap. Often, however, we neglect the commonly known signs of fatigue and carry on working, as if we were fully energized.

Körbler shared a few ideas to highlight what the fluctuation of the energy level means from the point of view of energy and information flow.

If the organism is properly energized, every cell gives information by its normal programming for its place and electric condition. This information travels to the brain via the nervous system, mediated by quantum electrodynamic processes. If a cell emits information showing that it is malfunctioning, the immune system will correct this based on signal of its location from the brain.

When electromagnetic conditions in the body worsen, regulation automatically becomes disturbed. In other words, if our energy level decreases, the information transfer which guarantees regulation will also be damaged and only takes place if there are extremely strong energy-flow processes in the body, e.g. in the case of fear, anxiety, or panic. In the case of a low energy level there are usually only 'high alert' programs at work and the normal balancing and regulating program of the body is missing, therefore the organism does not get a chance to rest up and restore the flawed functioning. Under the influence of what we call the 'alarm program' the impact of information coming through the sensory organs, primarily the eyes and ears, affects the tired and de-energized person as a high-energy impact, and the brain transmits this kind of information as a primary instruction.

The positive side of the 'alarm program'

The alarm program of our organism can be made use of. This is what happens in the Christian tradition when believers fold their hands together in prayer during a church ceremony. The same thing happens if they make a short visit to the church for a prayer. In the case of hands folded or palms pressed together, the energy circuit becomes closed and the normal program regulation of the energy flow is switched off. All we are left with is the alarm program, where information coming through the sensory organs is primary information for the brain, and so this kind of information will dominate the thinking and emotions of the individual. This is also the goal during a religious service, so the believers can be freed of all the personal problems troubling them. The priest, by contrast, conducts the ceremony with his arms opened wide in order to build up the energy and transmit as much as possible to the believers.

Disturbances in the Energy Flow

Disturbances in energy and information flow lead to grave consequences for any living organism and sooner or later lead to its demise. The organisms most exposed to this are plants that cannot move away to evade harmful external stimuli. Although plants give signals in case of danger threatening their lives, nevertheless there are parallels between the ways in which different species react. Körbler wanted to focus attention on the importance of the fact that injuries and scars in the human organism have the capacity to generate energy blocks and zones of disturbance. To demonstrate this he described the types of reactions common in the world of plants and drew a parallel between the consequences of disturbed energy and information flow in plants and in human organisms.

Today we face the unjustified destruction of trees and cultivated plants. The flora of the Earth suffers from the harmful effects of human civilization. The lessons Körbler drew from this illustrate this phenomenon and shows us the cause of the destruction.

> *A friend asked Körbler to examine the fir trees outside his house and try to find the reason why they show signs of perishing. There were three long-needled pines outside the house which had been healthy for 50 years but now something had changed. Körbler examined the polarization of the pines and found that, compared to some similar trees standing nearby, the needles of the sick trees showed reverse polarization. In fact, the total polarity of the three trees was reversed compared to the healthy trees standing further away. Körbler examined their environment and found that the harmful radiation was coming from an automated garage door. This iron gate was lined with plastic. If the garage door was opened, the polarity of the trees was normal; if it was locked, the polarity became reversed. Körbler drew six equal-armed crosses on the garage door, as a result of which the polarity of the three pines became normalized and they grew healthyly.*

It happens to humans, that due to an unfavorable influence or energy block the polarity of our fingers is reversed. In the normal case, the polarity of our fingers is the following as tested with the dowsing rod:

- In the case of the thumb the dowsing rod moves clockwise;
- For the index finger it moves anti-clockwise;
- For the middle finger it moves clockwise;
- For the second finger it moves anti-clockwise;
- For the little finger it moves clockwise.

If the biological environment has been badly damaged, the connection between plants and the soil changes and instead of growing in the direction of gravitational influence, the roots tend to grow upwards. As a consequence they perish. Körbler first saw this phenomenon during a visit to Arizona. He was the guest of a fruit farmer. In his orchards not one of the fruit trees had grown its roots properly. This was an area where the roots of fruit trees did not follow the physical structure characteristic of them – their form was modified and the trees died. Form and function are closely interrelated regarding the flow of energy and information.

Assisting energy flow in plants with the help of the dowsing rod

In the following section we describe a positive experience that has proven the use of the dowsing rod in horticulture. I first met Mr Egyed Világi in the 1990s after he read a series of articles we had written in *Természetgyógyász* and grew so intrigued by the subject that he visited our training courses. This was the beginning of a co-operation which has continued to this day and can be described as a series of success stories. As Mr Világi has repeatedly stated, he believes that the method can be applied successfully with plants the same as with humans. Originally trained as a horticultural engineer specialized in plant protection, Mr Világi had a consultancy career of several decades which rendered him one of the foremost experts in the field.

As a first step, we went on a tour of his extensive orchards planted on different soils and under different climatic characteristics. Most of our trips took us to the Danube Bend, the area between the rivers Danube and Tisza, the Nyírség region, the Buda Hills, and the Zsámbék Basin. Wherever we went we were exploring the same question – how can we optimize the nutrient supply of the orchard and eliminate shortages or, cases, resolve the dominance of certain nutrients in the soils, not only with the aim of increasing and improving the quantity and quality of the yield, but also with a view to enhancing the nutritional value, storability and preservability of the fruit after harvesting? To be sure, there are a number of factors which influence the flavor, aroma, color, consistency, value, fibrosity, vitamin and mineral content, attractiveness, tastiness and preservability of a fruit, primarily the weather and soil conditions of the area. Soil structure (packed, loose, etc.) powerfully influences whether plants are well nourished or not, combined, of course, with factors such as rain, the amount of sunshine, wind, etc.

Soil components (nitrogen, phosphorus, potassium, calcium, magnesium, manganese, copper, boron and zinc) represent a huge resource for plans. The proportion of macro and micro elements present in the soil is, however, a crucial factor. It is also known that plants absorb their nutrients in an ionized form and their circulation takes place via capillaries, therefore fluid supply is an indispensable part of their lives. The most important challenge is to influence the capacity of the soil to provide nutrients and determine the quantity of the nutrients present, as well as the order in which they need to be administered to enable the plant to take advantage of them. (In many cases, introducing substances in combination with spraying the leaves can be a quick first aid.) Boron, for instance, regulates the hormone system of plants, therefore it is enough to provide small quantities of it (3–4 ppm), but this small quantity is inevitable for the desired effect. By contrast, if sodium is present in the soil in large quantities (5–10%), this leads to salinification, which is harmful. Too much magnesium (30–50%) is downright toxic.

As regards the practical side of our collaboration, after soil analysis and leaf analysis in the laboratory, Mr Világi went on to make solutions (0.1%, 0.5%, 1% and 1.5%) of all the relevant elements and used this series of 18 steps in testing the trees with the dowsing rod. After choosing three to five elements, we also determined the desired sequence. His land is carefully tended from spring to fall and fall to spring each year, with Mr Világi indefatigably pursuing his job. Using the dowsing rod has proved to be a source of extraordinarily successful for more than 16 years.

The Role of Wounds and Scars in the Energy Flow

Wounds and scars play an important role in the energy testing of people. Detecting and eliminating energy blocks is a prime consideration for health preservation as part of securing optimal flow of energy and information and maximum energy supply. Based on the law of coherence, an acute energy shortage anywhere in the body will influence the workings of the entire organism.

Disturbances and blocks in energy flow cause malfunctions; prolonged conditions caused by constant blocks produce and sustain disease. Constant blocks are usually caused by internal damage to the organism: inflammations of the organs, tumors, internal and external scars after surgical operations.

All scars make information transfer difficult. In more fortunate cases the organism develops a supplementary channel in order to improve communication, but this will only work in a restricted fashion and to a limited extent. This is how scars can lead to serious diseases. According to research carried out in the United States, the anamnesis of multiple sclerosis sufferers showed more than three scars or injuries per case.

Internal and external scars do not always correspond to each other; in fact quite frequently they are in different locations. This is again an instance where the organism does not function in a linear fashion – a post-operative scar in an organ in one place can easily block the energy and information supply of another organ in a different location.

Körbler showed that disturbances in energy supply can reach a point, even without symptoms that is sufficient for a person to die. This cause of death is not included in any of the commonly known categories, even though these deaths are due directly to a chronic lack of energy.

Six months before the story was told, Körbler was requested by a noted physician to visit his dying wife who was also a doctor. In terms of classic medical knowledge they were at a loss; the patient and her family were waiting for death to ensue. She herself was prepared for death – she could not speak anymore and could only raise her arm to a height of 6–7 cm.

Körbler examined the patient's spine meridian from the top of the head to the front hairline and established that this was a case of total energy block. He launched the resolution of the blockage by a sound frequency treatment lasting for about 10 minutes. With a huge effort the lady raised her right arm, signaling that she could hear something. Now Körbler recorded the selected frequency on an audio tape. The patient listened to this sound every 3 hours for 3 minutes at a time. After 6 hours the relatives could see rapid improvement so they felt free to go home. The patient had an extraordinary reaction to the treatment – at 10 PM that day she asked for food, and ate for the first time in weeks. Three days later she traveled to the nearby mountains for some fresh summer air. A few weeks later she made a tour of Austria. Six weeks after the treatment she invited Körbler for dinner in a restaurant as a celebration. During their conversation it turned out that she could not remember having been sick at all. Körbler now pursued examining the patient in order to find the initial causes.

Twenty years before, the patient had had a gall operation, and 2 years before she had an intestinal operation. She had a post-operative scar on the right, not far from the esophagus. In organic terms this place seemed to play no part and be irrelevant. The combination of internal scars, however, could easily form an energy block which, instead of emerging abruptly, led to a slow energy shortage. This reached an extent where she could not believe in her strength to live.

The Treatment of Scars

If we wish to neutralize visible scars, we need to use a geometric symbol that will grant energy flow even across the scar by amplifying the flow blocked before. We use the dowsing rod for selecting the healing symbol: first we test a single line —, then two =, three ≡, and four parallel lines ≣, until eventually the positive response appears.

In order to help with internal scars we need to find the suitable skin surface. For this we must examine skin reactions at different spots of the patient's body. Körbler illustrated this with an example of his own. A scar visible on the outside of his body had an internal scar corresponding to it at a different place. Interestingly, however, there was a spot of discoloration on the skin between the two points. The geometric form of the discoloration caused by a skin reaction corresponds to the structure of the energy block or disturbance zone inside the body. Thus if we apply the appropriately chosen geometric symbol on the skin reaction on the surface, we also dissolve the energy block inside while simultaneously treating the internal disturbance zone. Thus it is a good idea to observe the skin reaction on the patient's body and find the internal disturbance zone that corresponds to them. All patients have more than one disturbance zones and these are related to skin reactions in different locations. By examining these we can find the optimal spot where we need to draw the geometric symbol. It is not necessary to treat every scar or every spot of skin reaction. Experience shows that treatment of a well-chosen skin surface can liberate a number of scars and disturbance zones.

As for the duration of treatment with the geometric symbol, we once again need to decide by testing. There are places where the geometric symbol only needs to be used for a short time, while at other places a longer use is required. Once we have identified the place for the longer use of the symbol, we can think of using a tattoo. If the spot is one where it would disturb the patient to wear the symbol, we need to find an alternative solution. For instance, we can sew a small pocket on the inside of a shirt and draw the symbol on the fabric of the pocket, on the inside. This way, the patient's body becomes released and the energy block is resolved. Naturally, this is just one of many possible ideas – the solution depends on the place where the patient needs to wear the symbol.

The next question is how the energy supply changes at the place or the scar. This is again something we need to test. It is possible that after a long-standing energy block the place receives too much energy from the parallel lines. This can also cause a problem. The patient might come back and complain that since the treatment he / she has found it difficult to sleep for more than 3–4 hours at a time. When this happens we need to replace the lines with a sine curve or a combination of sine curve and lines. We need to test which side of the sine to place the lines. We may place it on the left, the right, underneath or above the sine curve. In this case the symbol we apply provides the required energy flow.

Chapter 9

Körbler's Tree-Blossom Remedies

Körbler gave the title 'Information in Tree Blossoms' to the article he published on the subject in *Raum und Zeit*[1] (published in Hungarian as part of the previously mentioned series of articles[2]). By this choice he aimed to emphasize that humans are surrounded by the information system of the living reality of nature and are free to absorb information from this information system as necessary.

Knowledge and use of so-called biotopes (habitats) is an ancient form of knowledge. Everyone who has ever been on an outing with a group of people may have experienced how some people feel truly happy and refreshed if they get to spend a few minutes or even an hour resting under a shady tree, while for other members of the group a rest like that may mean nothing special, or they get similar feelings in a different kind of spot. The phenomenon is the same when we hear of people who spend their most restful or most creative hours under their favorite walnut tree or regularly visit their favorite weeping willow by the riverbank with a similar purpose.

The effect of biotopes is based on the fact that plants emit electromagnetic waves which are of a similar wavelength to human bio-resonance. These can be favorable, neutral or unfavorable for the human organism, just like, say, an apple or an orange. Certain plants contain higher-level energetic information compared to the hierarchy of the different energy levels in the human body. This is the quality of the 21 old, indigenous trees which Körbler selected for use in healing after testing several hundred plants. He transferred the information of the tree blossoms onto Himalaya water by electromagnetic means and fixed it. The energy content of the remedies thus produced and, accordingly, their influence on the body is significant.

The Effect of Tree-Blossom Remedies

Körbler claimed that the subtle-energetic regulation of all our organs happens in direct interaction with the neural paths along the individual vertebrae.

As a result, the central nervous system as a communicational hub acts as the immune and regulatory center of the organism. Thus if there is a center of disease in the organism, and if this reduces information and increases disorder, the entire regulating system will be affected and cause a reduced level of regulation in the entire system. Through the bridges of energy flow it can also disturb the functioning of previously healthy organs. Naturally, the disturbance of this system can also influence the psyche.

Tree-blossom remedies are suited to correct the information of places of a disturbed energetic condition. This means that a well-chosen tree-blossom remedy is an active ingredient which contains clusters of the balancing geometric symbol necessary for the disturbance zones of the organism and in this way frees up the path of energy flow. For therapy we choose two or three tree-blossom remedies. Most diseases can be covered this way, since introducing the information required by the body frees up the disturbed energy paths and as a result, the entire energetic system once more becomes functional or, to put it simply, physically and psychologically healthy.

Selection and Application of Tree-Blossom Remedies

Despite the fact that all tree-blossom remedies have their own unique sphere of effect, this is not what governs the act of choosing them. The flawed functions of the body are mere symptoms; their treatment is only effective if we can find the cause of the symptom. The movement of the dowsing rod can show us which tree-blossom remedies strengthen the bio-energetic field of the organism. The manner of testing is that the patient touches the jar containing the tree-blossom remedy with his or her left index finger, but it is also enough if they just look at the jar and the dowsing rod will reveal the strength of the attraction. Experience shows that the organism has a positive reaction to four or five tree-blossom remedies for each person. The required two remedies are chosen by testing specifically for the body parts whose energetic balance has been disturbed. If, for instance, someone has problems around the functioning of the lungs and the intestinal system, out of the most favorable four or five substances we choose the two which are able to optimize the energetic operation of the lungs and the intestines and in this way achieve the coherent operation of the entire organism. The remedies can also be chosen with the help of pictures taken of these blossoms. We use the same method as we did with jars containing tree-blossom remedies. The patient looks at the picture or touches it with his or her left index finger, and the dowsing rod will show the reaction of the organism.

The use of tree-blossom remedies is extremely simple. During the day we need to make a blossom drink every four hours using 2.5 dl of spring water and five drops of tree-blossom remedy each time. We drink the resulting drink slowly, one gulp at a time.

Even a 3-week treatment can bring surprising results. Whether the treatment needs to be continued is decided based on the condition of the organism. Experience shows, however, that it is more effective if we rub some of the diluted substance directly onto the sick body-part or if we also keep sniffing at the diluted remedy from time to time. Although tree-blossom remedies have no scent whatever, the sense of smell is still the quickest vehicle for electromagnetic information to travel to the nervous system. The effect of the information will be indicated by the most intense motions of the dowsing rod.

The ancient mammoth pine *(Sequoia giganteum)* is a 'living fossil'[3] towering to some 50 m which has hardly changed at all for millennia. It sheds its blue-green needles for winter. Its information is suited to activate the most ancient components of our organism.

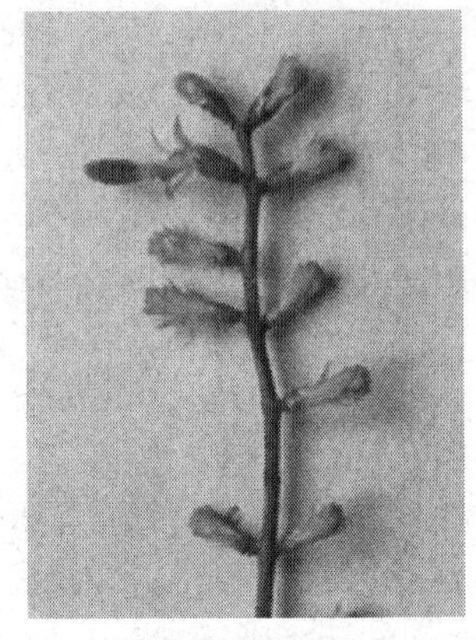

Figure 78. ***Sequoia giganteum***

The family of the ginkgo tree *(Ginkgo biloba)* existed as far back as 200 million years ago. Thus this plant is a miracle of a survivor. It is a deciduous tree which blossoms in May and sheds its spoon-shaped leaves in fall.

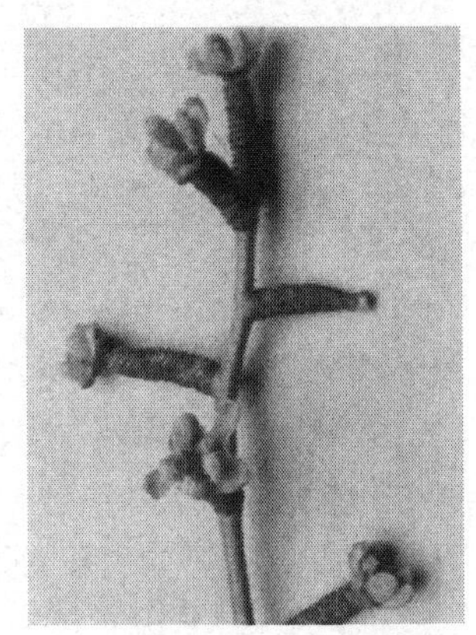

Figure 79. ***Ginkgo biloba***

Witch hazel *(Corylus colurna)* has 'only' been around in our forests for 60 million years. It blossoms in February. North American Indians thought of it as an important medical herb. It granted them the strength for major efforts.

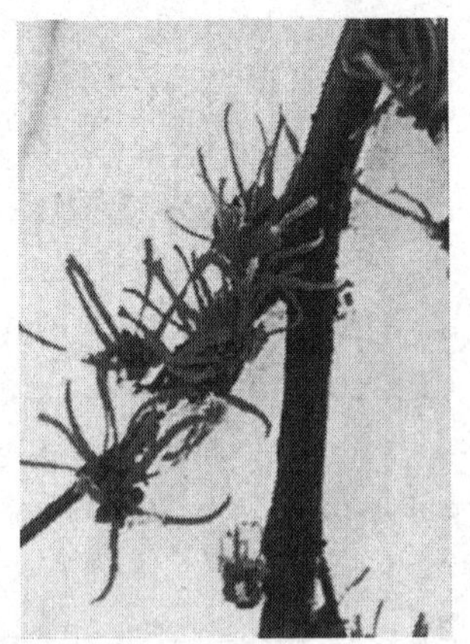

Figure 80. ***Corylus colurna***

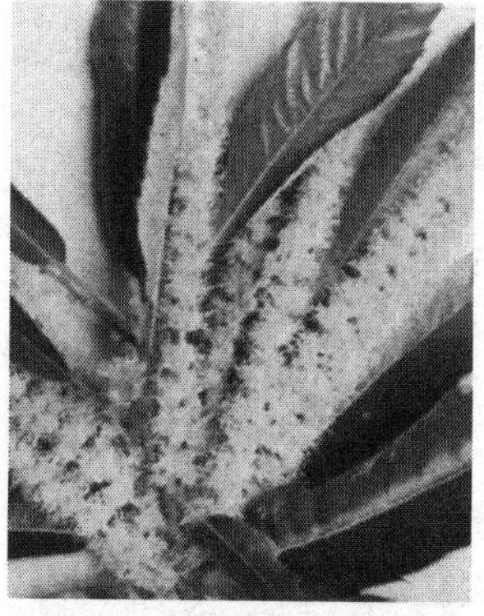

Chestnut trees *(Castanea sativa),* as archaeological diggings in Northern Italy have proved, have been cultivated ever since the Bronze Age. Everyone knows its catkins and the spiny cupules of its fruit. It is a remedy for the stomach and the intestines.

Figure 81. ***Castanea sativa***

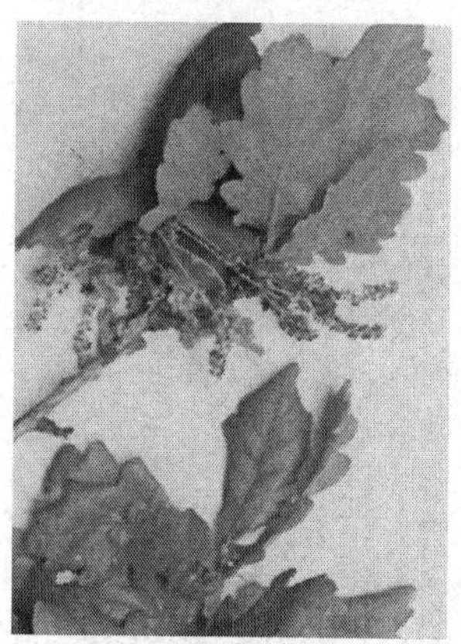

The English oak *(Quercus robur)* is the most important subspecies of oak in Europe. Sadly, it is so sensitive to environmental pollution that it is becoming an ever shrinking component of our natural world. Tinctures made out of its bark have been used for healing since the most ancient times. Its blossom information is most welcomed by the skin and the fatty tissues.

Figure 82. ***Quercus robur***

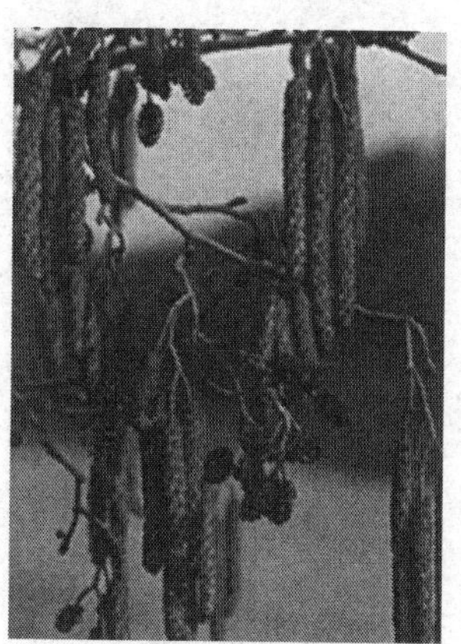

Green alder *(Alnus viridis)* is a particularly resilient tree. It strengthens people's psychological resilience. It is occasionally found in the forests of Bavaria; its knotted, twisted branches do not respect forest boundaries.

Figure 83. ***Alnus viridis***

Turkish hazel *(Corylus colurna)* comes from Asia. It is indigenous over vast expanses of the Balkan Peninsula and is known for its large, egg-shaped leaves and small, hard nutshell. Its information has a positive influence on disturbances in practically all organs.

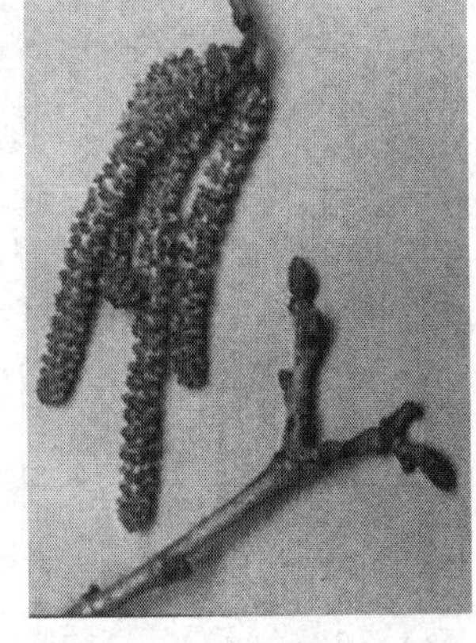

Figure 84. ***Corylus colurna***

The wood of the hop hornbeam *(Ostrya carpinifolia)* is particularly hard and tough. It was used in the past for making the cogwheels of mills. Its fruit resembles hops, hence its name. Its information gives strength.

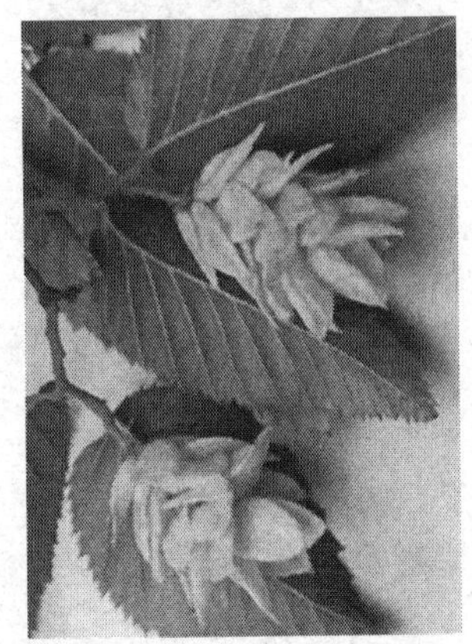

Figure 85. ***Ostrya carpinifolia***

Walnut trees *(Juglans regia)* go right back to the Cretaceous period. Glaciers of the Ice Age gradually squeezed it out of Northern Europe. Its leaves, fruit and wood are all remedial. Its information is received most favorably by the energy flows of the neck area.

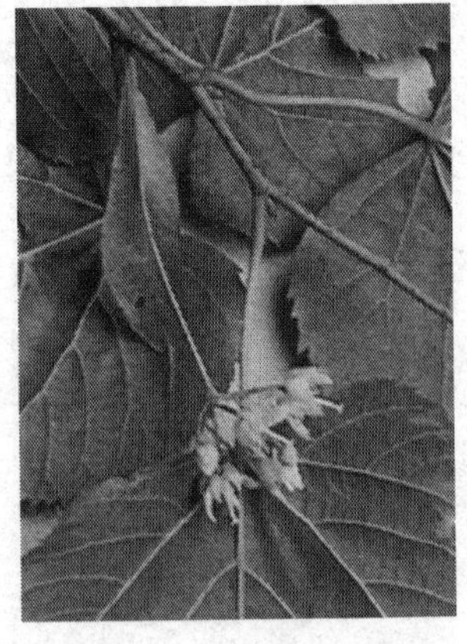

Figure 86. ***Juglans regia***

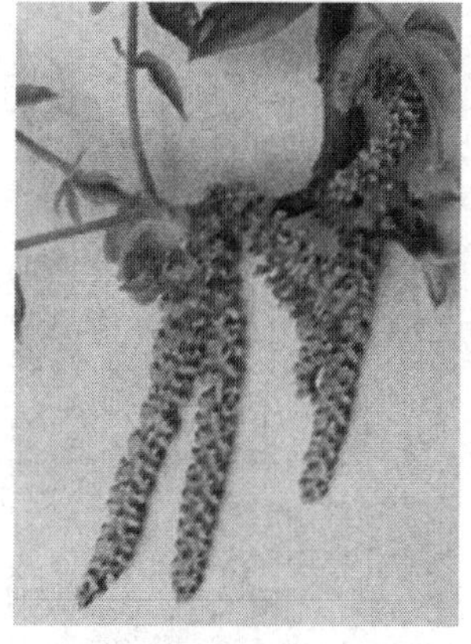

St. John's Wort *(Hypericum perforatum)* and its subtypes are very tough plants. They migrated from the subtropical area and the Mediterranean region. Its evergreen leaves remind us of its origin. It helps with psychosomatic disorders.

Figure 87. ***Hypericum perforatum***

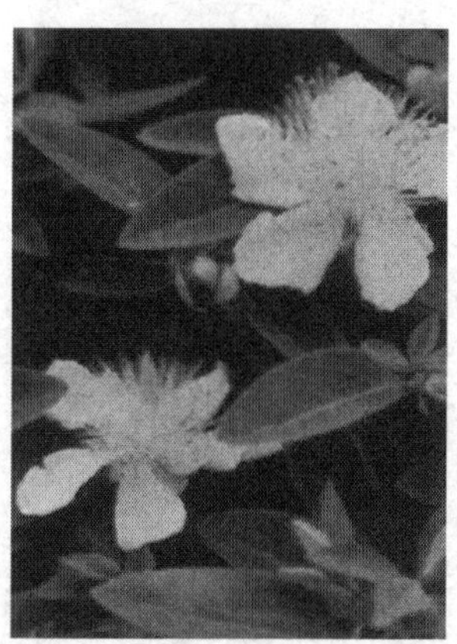

American linden *(Tilia americana)* has leaves 20 cm across. The tree grows to a height of up to 40 m. It is usually seen in giant parks and avenues. Its information secures free energy flow around the forehead and nose area.

Figure 88. ***Tilia americana***

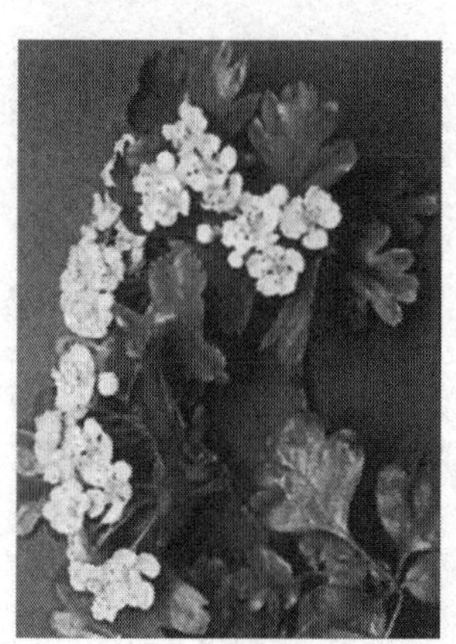

The common medlar *(Mespilus germanica)* was grown in cloister gardens in medieval Germany. In actual fact it comes from ancient Greece. It grows to about 5 m tall. Its information strengthens the energy of the gall, liver and kidneys.

Figure 89. ***Mespilus germanica***

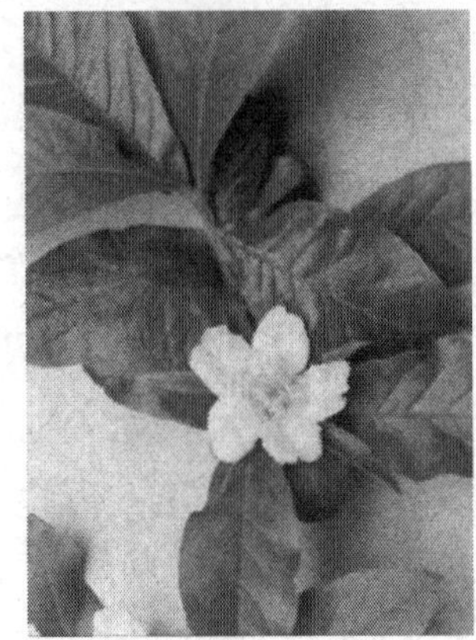

With their intertwined branches, hawthorn bushes *(Crataegus)* are a characteristic sight of forest clearings. Their branches spread wide and form an impenetrable mass. It is a medical plant with a long-standing and broad tradition. It improves circulation.

Figure 90. ***Crataegus***

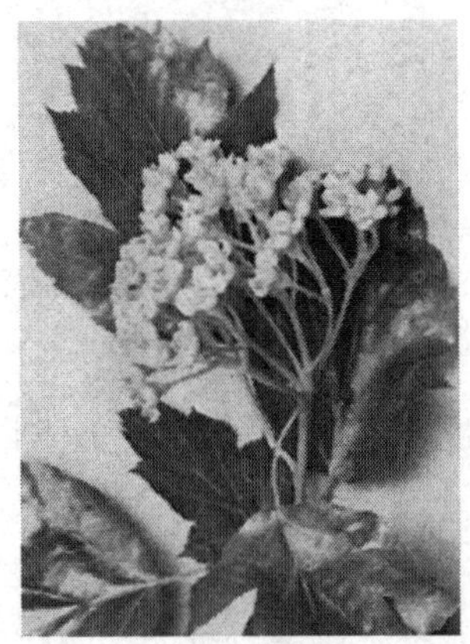

Checker trees *(Sorbus torminalis)* like a warm climate. In such places they will grow to 25 m. The fruit is small and sharp. The information of this tree supports the energy of the bladder.

Figure 91. ***Sorbus torminalis***

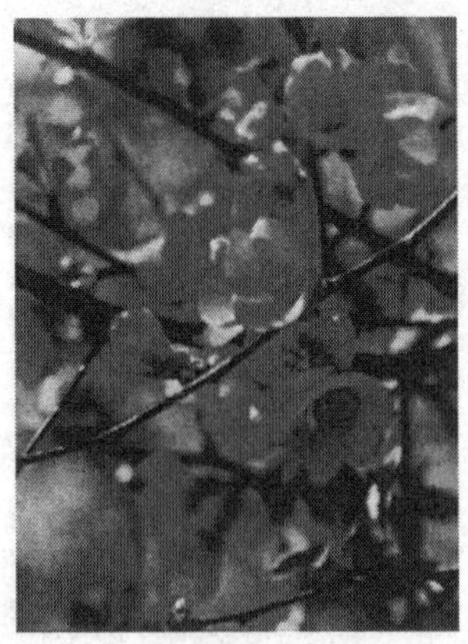

The fruit of the Japanese quince *(Chaenomeles japonica)* was for a long time a subject of debate – the question being whether it should be called an apple or a pear. It was only introduced to Europe 200 years ago. Its information supplies the spleen with energy.

Figure 92. ***Chaenomeles japonica***

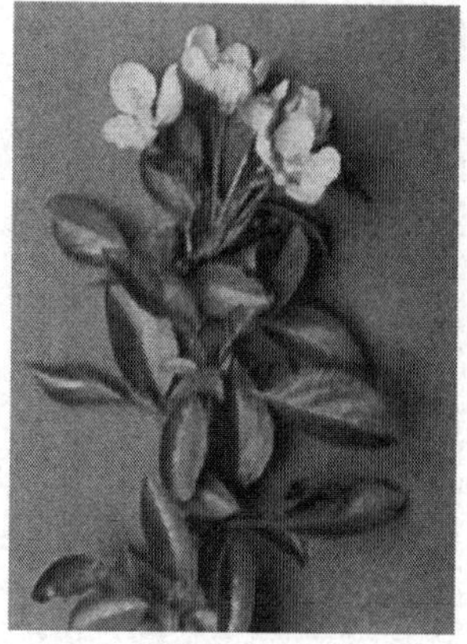

With crab apples *(Malus silvestris)* it is hard to tell whether they are wild or just run wild. At any rate, crab apples were found even in Stone Age 'gardens'. It energizes the gall.

Figure 93. *Malus silvestris*

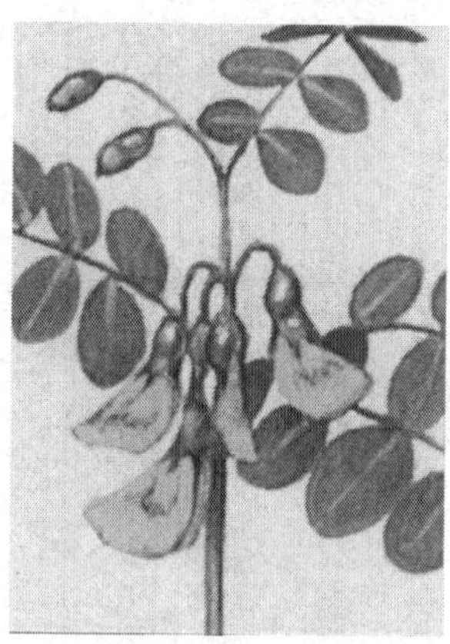

Common bladder senna *(Colutea arborescens)* grows to a height of 4 m and is extremely hardy. This is why it is often planted along railway tracks. In the winter the bushes freeze, but they always regenerate. The kidneys and the small intestines are perceptive to the information carried by this plant.

Figure 94. *Colutea arborescens*

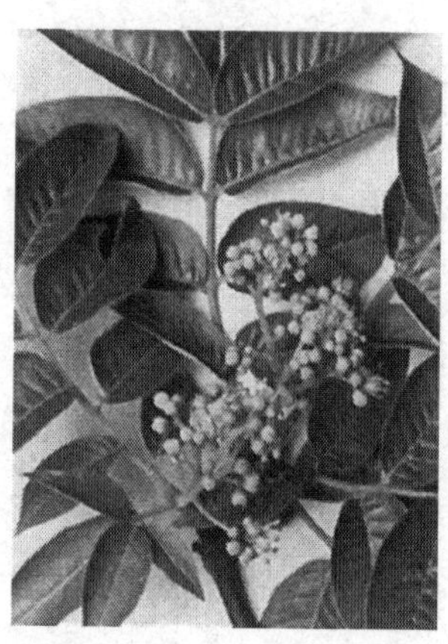

As its name indicates, the Amur cork tree *(Phellodendron amurense)* comes from the region of the Amur. It breeds well in deep damp soil. A popular tree for gardens, it grows to a height of 15 m. It lends effervescent energy to the region of the stomach.

Figure 95. *Phellodendron amurense*

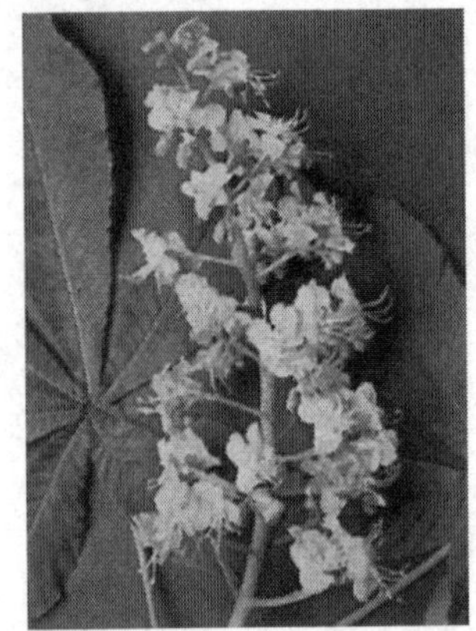

The common horse chestnut *(Aesculus hippocastanum)* was introduced into Europe from Turkey. Its lovely candlestick blossom and attractive leaves inspired people to plant entire avenues of these gorgeous trees. Its radiation improves the lymph circulation.

Figure 96. ***Aesculus hippocastanum***

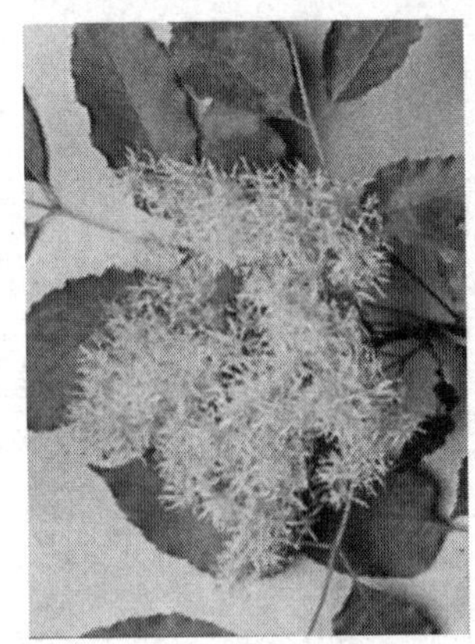

The holly tree *(Ilex aquifolium)* is an ancient medical herb. Its tough evergreen leaves cover a tree growing to a height of 15 m. It lends energy for extended, strenuous effort.

Figure 97. ***Ilex aquifolium***

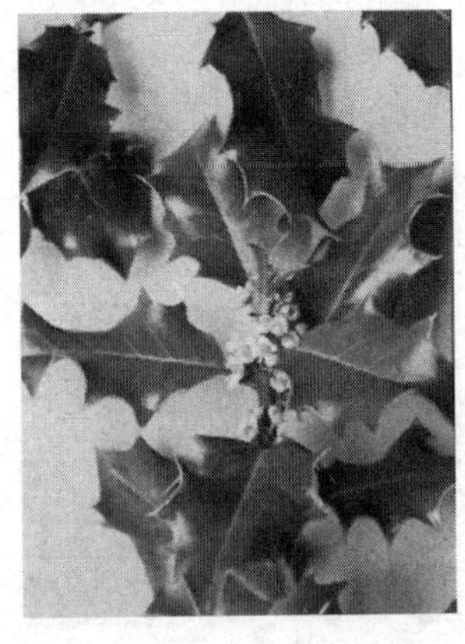

The flowering ash *(Fraxinus ornus)* is an insignificant-looking tree with panicles of simple flowers of four petals. It reaches a height of 16–20 m. In the Mediterranean area it has been used for medical purposes for millennia. Its information assists the heart and the circulation.

Figure 98. ***Fraxinus ornus***

To sum up, the action mechanism of tree-blossom therapy is based on the electromagnetic information of these substances provoking the same reaction in the organism as it would give to an intact biotope. This kind of information is active on the level of the integrated bio-energetic field regulating the biochemical processes of the organism.

Since in most cases we do not have the chance to live close to the kind of biotope most favorable to our body, we supplant this radiation by using the tree-blossom remedy.

Chapter 10

Sound and Music as Healing Information[1]

Sounds mediate the most crucial information in the living world, both for animals and humans. For animals, making sounds is the means of communication – the more highly developed the species, the more differentiated its sounds. The sounds are different if an animal is calling its mate, if a mother animal is calling to its young, or if the animal is alerting others to danger or indicating fear.

Sounds used by humans also have their signaling function. Sounds inform us, call our attention to danger, and inform us about its distance and quality. Humans have also created other communication systems beyond the use of sound for signaling: we have speech and we have music. Perceiving and interpreting sounds takes place in the right hemisphere, while that of speech and language use happens in the left hemisphere.

But what is music? One encyclopedia claims that:

> *Music is constituted when regularly repeated sounds which cause a pleasant audial sensation are connected together by means of melody, rhythm and harmony into compositions of varying length; or the sound of such a work when performed. A melody is a sequence of musical sounds of different height shaped into a rhythmical whole. Rhythm is regular alternation manifesting in temporal phenomena such as regular alternation of long and short sounds. Harmony means balance or accord between things.*

As we can see, capturing this phenomenon in words is far from easy. It is even more difficult to account for the experience of perceiving and emotionally attuning to music or understanding it as a form of communication – all of which takes place in the right hemisphere. The complex effect of music can only be sensed through its impact or effect. Its scientific measurement has not been possible in any way until the last 10–20 years.

The effect of music is most easily captured in its two extreme forms: one is when it has a harmonizing and healing effect; the other is when it impacts us as tiring, destructive and sickening. Recognizing and harnessing the harmonizing and healing effect of music has been around as long as mankind has existed. Producing healing sounds has two possible avenues – one is the sound produced by humans; the other is that of instruments. North American Indians and certain African tribes still preserve traditions which successfully use vocal music or rhythms for healing. The various meditation techniques of the Far East are still in use today, including those where in order to produce the desired effect we can create the required sound ourselves by sounding either single vowels or combining them with consonants. The sound spiral thus produced permeates the entire body; it harmonizes and balances the person.

Let us look at a few examples. In one meditation technique used in India, various vowels are sounded at a long held-out pace, at an even volume, and while we do this we observe our body parts to discover where one or other of these vowels is creating a resonance. The vowels are sung in the following order: 'i'; 'e'; 'a'; 'o'; 'u'; and are accompanied by hand gestures where we connect our fingertips with the tips of our thumbs in a determined sequence, shaping separate little circles with both the left and the right hand.

First we sound the vowel **'iii'** and touch our little finger against our thumb. The sound **'iii'** creates heightened resonance in the head.

The next vowel is **'eee'**, accompanied by the touching of the second finger and the thumb; the body part which resonates is the throat.

The vowel **'aaa'** corresponds to the chest and requires the touching of the middle finger and the thumb.

The body part that goes with **'ooo'** is the abdomen; the thumb touches the index finger.

The sound **'uuu'** produces heightened consonance in the groin and the body part beneath, while our hands lie relaxed one on top of the other on our lap. This exercise needs to be repeated until a complete state of relaxation sets in. We will find that our body spontaneously crouches forward, our head bends down, and our breathing becomes superficial and barely noticeable.

According to an ancient Japanese method the vowels are sounded in varying sequences and in combination with different consonants in altogether 50 forms *(Figure 99)*.

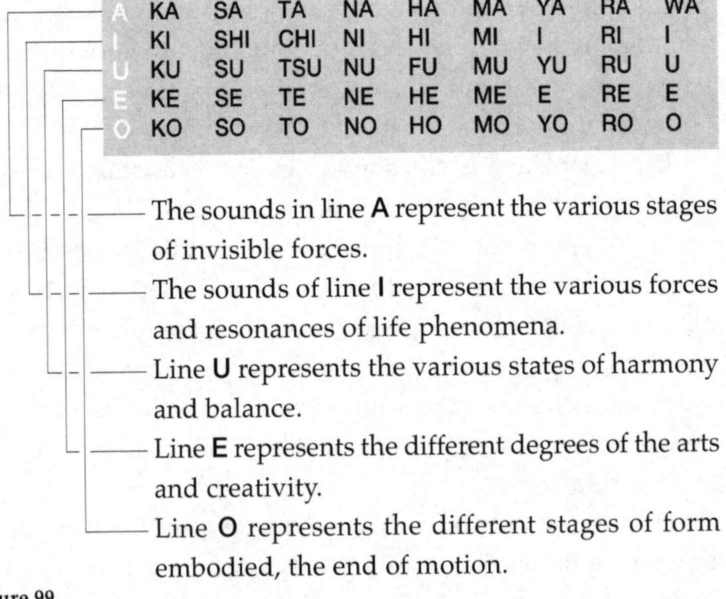

A	KA	SA	TA	NA	HA	MA	YA	RA	WA
I	KI	SHI	CHI	NI	HI	MI	I	RI	I
U	KU	SU	TSU	NU	FU	MU	YU	RU	U
E	KE	SE	TE	NE	HE	ME	E	RE	E
O	KO	SO	TO	NO	HO	MO	YO	RO	O

Figure 99

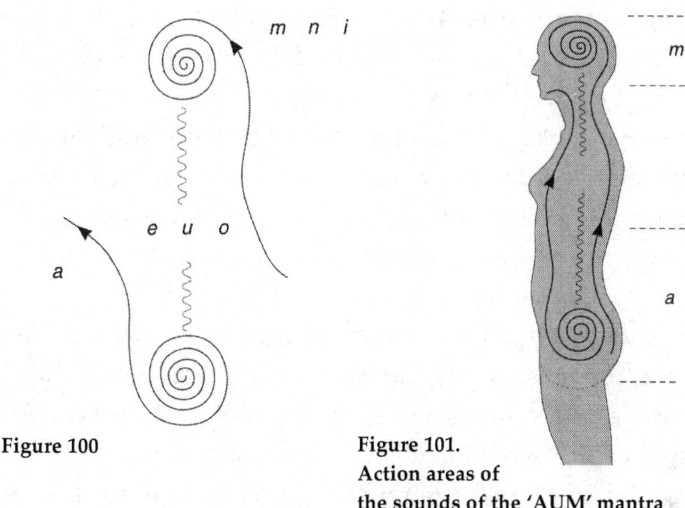

Figure 100

Figure 101.
Action areas of
the sounds of the 'AUM' mantra

Figures 100 and *101* show how people used to imagine the effect of sound spirals. Figure 100 shows the projection of the human body into a spiral form, including the sounds which correspond to the main parts of the human body.

In ancient China several hundred years before the start of the Christian calendar, during the Han dynasty, a bronze plate was rubbed so that it produced a sound and this was used for healing. Due to its unique qualities this plate was once used by the Chinese emperors, the 'Sons of Heaven', as it helped them live longer and healthier lives than ordinary mortals. The characteristics of this interesting, old green dish is of noble simplicity; a simple form ornamented inside by four embossed fish or dragons, while the handles were made of bright, glittering brass. When it is used, they pour water into it and rub the bright handles with wet hands sliding in opposing directions at an even pace. After a while this causes an odd, near-magical apparition – the water comes to life. At first we note mere ripples on the surface, and then it begins to make a low whispering noise, almost starting to dance, and produces four regular whirlpools on the four sides. Eventually it breaks into myriad tiny drops and spurts high up in the air like a fountain. It looks as if the water was bursting forth from the mouths of the four fish or dragons, while the dish itself makes a sound like a musical instrument. The tone and timbre of the sound depends on how full the dish is with water and on the strength and direction of the rubbing. The better the quality of the dish, the higher the water spurts. This resonance therapy was used to help individuals attain a higher state of inner harmony and health.

In the mid-19th century, scientists began to explore the effect of sounds, foremost among them being Helmholz[2] and Stumpf[3]. In the early 20th century Géza Révész[4] provided an excellent summary of the psychology and problematic of sounds, and a bibliography of its contemporary literature. To this very day one of the important fields of exploration is the sensation of sounds and its impact.

What is most exciting for us here is what science has achieved in terms of measuring the impact of sounds.

Mapping out in an exact manner the physiological effect of sounds by gentle means and applying this knowledge in appropriate ways are among Körbler's noted achievements. The way in which people react to sounds and different kinds of music is totally unique to the individual. One man's meat is another man's poison. Sounds and noises we are exposed to over a long period (e.g. the buzz of pipes or machines) can make people sick. In cases like this it is a good idea to examine what sort of bodily reactions are produced by the noise in question and, if this reaction is not favorable, it is best to avoid it.

Körbler discovered that extremely low frequencies of sounds are perceived as vibration (as wave) not only through our hearing organ but also through every cell of the body. The cell receives the information through the pressure of the sound wave. This process is independent of the volume of the sound. This is how it is possible for us to measure the blissful or harmful effect of sounds outside of the audible range. The dowsing rod also enables us to establish the effect of individual frequencies.

Sounds are extremely low frequencies when compared to the resonances of the human body. It is easy to imagine that if the body reacts positively to a sound of 300 Hz (= 300 vibrations/sec), then the body's own vibration of 10^{15} Hz will perceive this vibration of 300 Hz as a rhythmic pulsation. Naturally, changes in frequency of the 20–10,000 Hz range are not suitable for direct intervention in the communication between the organs and the immune system, since these are at a frequency discrepancy of approximately 100 000 000 000 000 (10^{14}) Hz from each other. If, however, we find the rhythm which creates new patterns of chaos, similarly to the Sterpinsky reaction, this will instantly affect the structures in the cell.[5]

Körbler's Sound Frequency Test

Körbler spent years experimenting with the effect of sounds. His experience was that sounds and rhythms have the most potent healing effect. However, the sounds which are healing for any individual need to be found separately in each case, since it is different from person to person and even from time to time. For identifying these sounds we can use any instrument or Körbler's computerized sound program. The program consists of a self-regulating scale where the intervals are different from those in the commonly known musical scale. The advantage of sounds produced in this way is that we can work with even resonances and can also experiment in the non-audible domains of sound.

The first surprise in this respect comes when, proceeding from low frequencies upward, we reach the sound of 50 Hz. This is the network frequency of the household energy supply which we are exposed to always and everywhere and which is present around various electric machinery as 'network noise'. Certain parts of our body react to this as 'incompatible'. Which part this is varies from person to person.

If we go on experimenting we will find the frequencies which are healing for the individual. This is done in the following manner: we choose an area on the tested person where we sense a disturbance zone with the dowsing rod. At times like this the rod swings vertically. (For measuring we hold our left index finger in front of the examined area.) Now we switch on the automatic sound programmer or if we are using an instrument we start moving up half a note at a time, starting from the deepest sound and at the same time constantly testing the body part in question. The dowsing rod continues to swing vertically, i.e. it indicates the disturbance zone.

At a certain height the movement of the dowsing rod suddenly changes and becomes horizontal. At the next sound the amplitude of the horizontal oscillation will be far greater and for the next one possibly even greater. We record the musical note or the frequency shown on the computer screen and continue testing. With the next musical note the horizontal swinging of the dowsing rod will slow down and then with the next sound it will again turn vertical.

The automatic sound program continues in the domain of inaudible frequencies but we can stop experimenting once we have found the three favorable frequency hubs, i.e. musical notes. We continue testing with these sounds, set the computer to produce held-out notes, or keep sounding the note on our instrument. At the same time, we perform the counter-test; in other words we explore whether there is an organ or body part which produces a disturbance under the influence of the sound, where the dowsing rod moves vertically. If there is no such response, we record the selected sound at rhythmical intervals.

It is sufficient for the patient to listen to the recording two or three times a day for 3 minutes at a time – this will eliminate the disturbance of the affected area and the process of self-healing will be set in motion. Used in the treatment of chronic disease the effect of the audio recording needs to be tested weekly.

We take a similar approach when selecting rhythms. The various rhythms (e.g. Viennese waltz, tango, samba) need to be played at their original tempo. If we compose melodies consisting of sounds and rhythms which are positive, i.e. increase cell voltage, the patient will react intensely and fast to the healing effect. We can record the 'work of art' thus produced and use it as healing music.

This new healing method, combined with the usual approaches, accelerates the regeneration process considerably, while it also reduces the amount of medication required.

What is man's subjective experience of music? A multitude of works in the psychology of music and art are seeking to answer this question with a whole series of interesting experiments. The first thing we need to bear in mind is that a piece of music can only be interpreted within its own cultural context and only there will it produce the emotions it was designed to awaken and only there can it harmonize the personality in the required manner. Western cultures live with different kinds of music than those of the Far East or Africa. What is similar all over the world, however, is the way in which music makes its impact. It offers a mirror to our emotional world and wherever the harmony of the personality is flawed or deficient, the sound of music will smooth out, recharge or harmonize our emotional world. It leads to the unfolding of an all-pervasive sense of love and assuages sorrow, pain or anger. This discovery is far from new – any reflection on music going back over the millennia remarks upon these impressions. In *The Republic,* Plato[6] talks about the effect of musical tonality on our emotions. He believes that in an ideal State the Dorian or Phrygian harmonies *'only are to be used in'…'songs and melodies'*[6] because he wants *'to have one warlike to sound the note or accent which a brave man utters in the hour of danger and stern resolve, or when his cause is failing…' 'and another to be used by him in times of peace and freedom of action'*[6]. And Lydian and Ionian harmonies *'must be banished'*[6], for they *'are the soft or drinking harmonies'* and *'drunkenness and softness and indolence are utterly unbecoming the character of our guardians.'*[6] We could go on to quote many authors where each applies a philosophical or psychological approach to describe how listening to music brings our energies to the surface, while also reinforcing and mobilizing them.

They speak of the sense of *'becoming a whole person'*; Schopenhauer calls music *'a special reification of the cosmic will'*.[7] In Hungary, studies exploring the physiology and psychology of music were summarized by two authors: Tibor Halm[8] and Iván Vitányi[9].

Emotional and affective changes which occur under the effect of listening to music were examined by Mária Sági using a whole series of experiments in music psychology. She applied projective personality tests (free associations, color pyramid, Rorschach test, etc.) in order to trace how drawings and paintings made by the subjects – children, university students, students of the Music Academy and young artists (painters) – exhibited the effect of music. The results showed that the content and form of the cathartic process experienced under the effect of the parallel creative processes always manifested through the filter of the personality and the structure of the personality. Description of the experiments and the results may be read in Mária Sági's book Esztétikum és személyiség [Aesthetics and Personality].[10]

Haffelder's Music Therapy

Is it possible to measure the effect of music on humans as regards brain research?

Brain researcher Günter Haffelder, head of the Stuttgart Institute of Brain Research, developed a special method for measuring the electric activity of the brain. The project began in the 1970s and his experimental measurements continued for more than 10 years. The method he developed has been used successfully in curing his patients for almost 30 years. In his methodology, electrodes are placed at points of measurement other than in EEG testing. This allows for registering the activity of the limbic system – the area which connects the cerebrum with the sensory centers. Separate graphic representations of the left and the right hemisphere render it possible to image the differences in the rational and the associative activities. Results are processed by computer according to a pre-determined mathematical algorithm, analyzing the resonances into their components. As a result, vibration components can be represented in a three-dimensional image, in the form of a temporal sequence. The method opened the way to measuring and representing components of the modern EEG curve in the domain between delta and beta waves, thus allowing for an even more accurate diagnosis.

With these developments Haffelder opened up new vistas in treatment. He discovered that certain peaks of the brain-wave diagrams are in conjunction with certain neurotransmitters – namely dopamine and serotonin. If these waves are introduced into the brain, the related neurotransmitters are produced in increased quantities in the central nervous system. At such times an exact analysis of the brain waves allows us to identify the neurotransmitters that the patient needs and what kind of waves could be used in their treatment.

Haffelder's experiments have proved that the optimal medium for introducing the healing audial waves into the brain is music. He found that while listening to works by Mozart, if played at a slower tempo than is customary today, the synchronization of the two brain hemispheres becomes optimal.

There is, however, another audial effect which is healing for the brain – and this comes from a mixture of dolphin sounds. This sample includes, for instance, some of the dialogue between a mother and her calves, but communication among grown individuals is also present. Remedial music is thus composed of dolphin sounds added to Mozart's music. Each music CD consists of five different music sections, each of them 6–10 minutes long. The total length of the CD is usually 35–45 minutes. The first part is a composition of dolphin sounds combined with Mozart's music, which is specific for each patient based on the analytic measurement of the EEG spectrum. Subsequent musical segments are chosen in a similar manner but consisting uniquely of Mozart's music. The CD has to be heard through headphones, at a low volume (preferably choosing headphones with a frequency spectrum going up to 20,000 Hz). An extra remedial effect arises due to lateralization while listening to the music – in this case the audial effect takes place from the left and the right as well as through the lower dorsal lobes, with different phase discrepancies and frequency settings. Therapeutic music travels from one ear to the other in different ways for all individuals, while the volume also changes from place to place. The feeling it produces is as if the music was truly coming through only at certain spots of the brain, sometimes on the right, at other times on the right back, now on the back left or on the left, and so on.

The effect of the CD with therapeutic music is manifested on several planes. Sound effects at around 18,000 Hz – that is very high frequency for the human ear – can rebalance the brain. As a result of the effect of the CD, the level of acetylcholine increases in the brain, which allows for the emergence of new learning neural paths. This happens in order to improve synchronization between the two hemispheres through the corpus callosum. This serves the co-ordinated and synchronized operation of the two hemispheres, broadens the possibility for learning, thinking and other mental activity, and thus creates new learning processes. If EEG measurements show a discrepancy in phases between the two hemispheres, this is taken into account and corrected when compiling the CD.

At first, the CD must be used twice a day for 10 minutes at a time. In every case, regardless of the duration, listening must take place during some kind of physical or mental activity, such as exercise, walking, housework, needlework, studying or reading.

After about 1 week the patient can start listening to the full length of the CD several times a day. Listening during meals or when sleeping is, however, prohibited. The therapeutic CD can be applied in all situations aimed to improve intellectual skills, and in the period of rehabilitation, in the service of restoring the optimal physical functioning of the body. Schoolchildren can listen to it while solving math problems or studying, while adults can apply it in order to improve their desired activity such as language learning, improving computer skills, composing, visualization, etc. Sick or injured people can listen to it while they practice their missing motoric skills, first in passive ways (with a helper) and then in active ways. Use of the therapeutic CD and practice jointly result in the emergence of new neural paths for learning.

Let us look at an example.

> *A physician took her son, aged 8 years, to be examined, the complaint being that while the boy was doing excellently in all subjects, he was close to a failing grade in mathematics. They had experimented with a number of different methods, but to no avail. The mother said that she did not actually believe in music therapy but she had decided to give it a try, just in case. After the CD was made, the boy listened to it all the time while doing his math homework every day. After a month there was a test paper coming up at school in math. The family were very curious how he would do. The boy did well in his test. The mother was very happy and phoned the Brain Research Institute to tell them about his success. Mr. Haffelder invited the boy to the Institute in order to find out about the exact circumstances. It is true that the CD method can do wonders, but it usually takes months of practice for the new neural pathways to develop, and 1 month is not enough.*

The boy told him in happy tones that the way he was able to do the test was by imagining that he was still listening to the CD.

As a healer, I have been participating in the research activities of the Institute for years. We are exploring the ways in which healing impulses and subtle-energetic effects can be transferred from person to person in experiments with proximal and remote healing.[11]

Chapter 11

The Informational Aspect of Psychosomatic Problems

Although there is a vast literature on the effect of psychological functions (such as belief, thoughts, emotions) on the condition of the body, on health and sickness, it is still hard to comprehend how and why this influence takes place. This is no surprise, since in the modern period the healing of the body and the mind took separate paths after the Newtonian mechanistic view of the world became predominant. Observation and therapy of the physical body became limited to the field of the natural sciences, while functions of the soul were relegated to the field of religion. Cartesian dualism, which claims that the human body is made of matter, while the mind is immaterial, the manifestation of some unknown power, has laid the philosophical foundations for centuries for the practice of Western medicine and biology based on materialism, and the separation of body and mind. The influence of belief and other psychological functions on the body has become questioned, as a scientific explanation of these phenomena was not directly forthcoming. In fact, psychological functions such as harboring belief, promoting positive thinking and anticipations of recovery played a huge part in curing the body right up to the modern period.

What is the current state of scientific thinking?

The picture is complex and colorful. Modern medicine uses the concepts of psychosomatics, placebo and nocebo to account for the influence of various psychological functions on the condition of the body.

The practice of *psychosomatics* examines physical symptoms and disease and their psychological background in a context of causal connections.

The concept of *placebo* takes account of the healing effect of belief.

The concept of *nocebo* refers to the harmful, pathogenic effect of belief.

Although the exact action mechanism of these phenomena is not yet fully known to science, an increasing number of exploratory experiments prove the reality of the unity between the body, the soul and the spirit; there are more and more biochemical and biomolecular research projects hoping to shed light on the deeper regularities of the processes which finally lead to perceptible symptoms. In the 20 years that have gone by since Körbler's death, more and more scientists are looking for and offering explanations regarding the action mechanisms of these phenomena and exploring ideas about how they could be influenced.

Körbler also worked on the frontiers of the new science. He did in-depth studies on the psychosomatic processes which appear as a result of the interaction between the human psyche and the human organism. He studied the information mechanisms of both recovery and disease happening under the influence of the mind. He believed that 'placebo effect' and 'psychosomatics' were names for two sides of the same coin. The placebo effect is a positive outcome; psychosomatic disease is a negative outcome. The placebo effect is a psychological regulating factor originating in the cortex, a positive, healthy outcome of communication between the immune system and the organs. Psychosomatic disease is the opposite – it is the negative outcome which sustains disease. Körbler studied the electromagnetic information components of these phenomena and the possibilities of information programming in the service of recovery. He published several articles on the subject in *Raum und Zeit*.[1]

Since the time of his death, several medical disciplines and trends have indeed emerged which look at the human being in the holistic fashion as a unified system. They take into account the body, the soul (emotions) and the intellect (thinking); in other words the unity of matter, energy and information. This is the approach taken by psycho-neuro-endocrinology or the complex method developed by the GUNA corporation operating in Milan, called 'physiological regulating medicine'.

The Informational Background of Psychosomatic Processes According to Körbler

Although there is now almost universal agreement about the fact that nearly all diseases have a psychological origin, the true reason causing symptoms is still difficult to find. This is partly due to the fact that all people react differently to various impacts, i.e. there is no regularity in the connection between psychological processes and objective physiological processes. A thing that makes one person sick will be unnoticed by another.

Environmental stress and the physical reactions of the organism can produce a whole range of diseases, while the effect of lasting environmental stress can cause or sustain chronic or frequently recurring diseases (such as high blood pressure, heart attack, rheumatoid arthritis, chronic diseases of the respiratory tracts or the intestinal system, etc.). Everyone knows the kind of stress resulting from emotional frictions and misunderstandings in everyday life. This happens in the closest emotional bonds inside the family, but also within the looser ties we have with colleagues and friends. Even a slight misunderstanding, a misinterpreted remark or an opinion which was actually meant to sting will leave us with profound traces of stress. Real and imaginary ills weigh heavily on the balance of our emotional life. This acts as a burden on our physical well-being, our stamina and health. We also know the kind of tiredness which goes hand in hand with a disheartened condition, or the physical disease which can come from grudges people have carried for a long time.

As for the causes, on the one side we find the environment as a source of independent events; on the other side is the human organism as a source of conditions which developed as a result of the personal history of the individual.

Körbler emphasized that the organism reacts to events both from the inside and the outside and is unable to separate these various impulses. Intellectual or emotional information coming from the inside is as likely to affect the degree of organization inside the human organism and its immune system as the disturbances of the immune system caused by information from the outside. Over the long term either can cause disease focuses. A disease focus creates a locus of reduced information which gives the entire system a reduced rate of organization.

The cause of psychosomatic problems is to do with the content of the information flow taking place in the individual. If the content is harmful for the individual, this will appear as an acute psychological and physical interaction; in other words the emotionally disturbing information will appear as a physical symptom. Psychosomatic symptoms are easy to recognize, because of the typical way in which they keep reappearing in spite of treatment. Information about old, long-forgotten traumas is stored away in the subconscious, but they continue to act as influencing agents in organizing the current set of symptoms or even just the way in which current bodily functions are organized. They form parts of not only the personality but also the physical function.

The human organism is a complex network system in which the operation of the parts is determined by the coherent macroscopic operation of the whole. It consists of a great number of hierarchically organized subsystems (organs, cells, molecules, atoms, particles, sub-particles) which are themselves also constituted of a multitude of parallel systems. It is obvious that not one of the partial functions can change without influencing the operation of the whole.

If we explore the information processes of the various parts, we find that information travels more rapidly between particles than could be expected from the normal physiological functioning of the cells or organs. On the macroscopic level this calls for larger spatial structures and time constants but lower energy values. In other words, the organism is ruled by spatial, temporal and energetic hierarchies. The highest level of the energetic hierarchy is the mind.

The information content of the functions of the mind, such as thoughts or emotions, affects the organs through the existing structures, no matter whether they are conscious or unconscious. They function not immediately, not directly, but step by step, strictly in line with the hierarchic structure. Körbler claimed that within the subtle-energy system of the organism, the functioning of the mind also manifests in the form of electromagnetic waves just like any other communication.

In the brain, every impact, whether consciously or unconsciously absorbed, is evaluated as information and becomes integrated with a marker of favorable or unfavorable. Every cell constantly informs the brain, i.e. the information storage unit, about its own condition and the external impulses and internal processes through the natural information channels using electromagnetic waves in the bio-resonance domain. Every brain cell transmits information inside the web of the synaptic network of several hundred thousand connections, with a capacity of approximately 10^{30}.

Evaluating this information content happens not through the co-ordinate switches but in a non-linear fashion, according to whether the information is 'system-friendly' or 'system-harmful'. The corresponding feedback may become consciously perceived (e.g. as pain) or it may manifest through the immune system and regulation. Its aim is to grant ideal living conditions for the cell among the given circumstances.

The life processes of the organism are determined by the interaction of the structures and the electromagnetic information. If a conscious or unconscious effect is stored in a symbolic form, e.g. it is linked to a word or a sound, the information which is stored can be accessed at any time. If the experience is linked to an abstract word or phrase which carries the affective content of the experience, the latter may be accessed instantly by pronouncing the word or phrase. The electromagnetic information content of the word is in charge of communication in the organism. If this information content is positive, the electromagnetic communication of the organism will also be ruled by a positive trend; the message will be positive for all cells. If this information content is negative, the electromagnetic communication of the cell will also show a negative trend and the message will be negative for all cells. This is a resonance chain which functions automatically through the information system of the regulatory and the immune system.

This theory by Körbler is in line with the theory of Nobel Laureate brain researcher Roger Sperry. Sperry demonstrated that the condition of the mind influences the functioning of all brain cells. He claimed that human consciousness (the neocortex) is actually the manifestation of the functioning of the entire cerebrum. Consciousness is more than the sum total of the properties of the parts constituting the hemispheres. Consciousness as the mirror of the total functioning of the brain influences the functioning of neuron networks. In other words the positive or negative contents of consciousness affect all the cells of the body through the central nervous system.[2]

Informational Aspects of Positive Thinking and the Placebo Effect

Körbler attributed special importance to positive thinking and the possibility of the placebo effect both as regards health preservation and healing/recovery. The fact of the placebo effect also shows what holistic medicine keeps emphasizing, namely that the organism has self-healing processes at work. The job of the therapist is to free up these processes, to resolve blocks and to trigger and support self-healing processes. When these are at work, the organism is capable of even miraculous recoveries. This is the reason why we must give this topic some attention without aiming for an exhaustive treatment. All we are going to cover in this chapter are the aspects which bring us closer to understanding Körbler's information-based therapies. We do, however, suggest a full review of the literature.

Contemporary medicine uses the term 'placebo' when a patient recovers under the effect of medication containing no active agent or a fake medical intervention or operation, purely because they believe in the effectiveness of the 'medicine' or 'treatment'. Although medical science recognizes the reality of this phenomenon, Bánki[3] (1994) explains the reasons why doctors are negatively disposed regarding the placebo effect:

1. The phenomenon is nonsensical from the point of view of modern natural sciences; although the most recent scientific exploration provides considerable certainty, these results are not yet widely accessible.
2. In our methodologically trained way of thinking, the placebo effect appears to be just a 'disturbing factor'.
3. It questions the validity of several 'standard' procedures.
4. Finally, it blurs the boundaries between the professional working with scientifically based methods and the lay healer operating with the placebo effect.

Thus, the daily practice of official medicine is left with a duality. On the one hand there is no room for acknowledging the healing effect of the psyche, of belief and of thinking, in other words of the placebo effect; while on the other hand every good doctor instinctively makes use of this effect. They use it in the treatment of their patients by the sheer fact of believing in the effectiveness of the treatment and thus they raise and confirm the patient's belief that with the help of medical treatment they are capable of recovery.

The subject is rarely treated in contemporary literature. Up until the turn of the millennium there were only two books published in English about the placebo effect – A. K. Shapiro and E. Shapiro's work[4] (1997), which is a historical review, and Spiro's[5] (1986) more philosophically inspired monograph. The situation is quite different as regards reports about placebo. Over 20 books and 50–100 articles have been published in the field. The effect of placebo on the various organ systems was described mostly in the 1950s and 60s. The discovery of endorphins[6] (1977), substances produced by our brain which act similarly to morphines, have steered placebo research in a new direction. The role played by endogenous opiate peptides in the placebo effect has remained a vast research area to this day.

An important contribution in Hungary has been a stream of research activities carried out by György Bárdos[7] and the PlaceBio research group at ELTE (Eötvös Loránd University, Budapest) over the past decades. These in-depth studies have covered the concept, history and applications of placebo, the connections between psychosomatic disorders and the placebo effect, the explanatory theories concerning placebo, the ethical issues around application in therapy,[8] interactions between placebo and the personality, the evolutionary background to placebo,[9] and the phenomenon of nocebo.[10] They offer very circumspect analyses of the various aspects of the placebo phenomenon from the point of view of both international and Hungarian literature and have introduced a new model for the explanation of the placebo phenomenon.

Scientific research takes a multidimensional approach to the phenomenon of placebo. Hungarian scholar Zsuzsa Kulcsár devotes a number of articles to presenting research findings on the psychological background of positive thinking and the placebo effect.[11] M. Csaba Bánki summarizes the technologies of molecular research used in contemporary medical science which enable us to observe the brain processes which accompany this phenomenon. They also allow us to describe the brain metabolic components of the biological changes which take place as a result of the placebo effect, including the different types of endogenous molecules which affect the central nervous system; as well as to explore the way in which the endogenous opiates become activated in the course of analgesics by placebo.[12]

There exists no theory to date which could adequately explain the placebo effect. Researchers approach its analysis and explanation from multiple angles. In the literature we find around 20 explanatory theories, which may be classified into six major groups (Cziboly, Bárdos, 2003):[13]

1. biological theories (endogenous opiates, peptide functioning, classical and operant conditioning, etc.);
2. theories related to the 'total medicinal effect' (the anthropological approach, the doctor as placebo, etc.);
3. social-psychological explanations (attribution, reducing cognitive dissonance, self-fulfilling prophecies, etc.);
4. further psychological explanations (psychodynamics, hemispheric lateralization, etc.);
5. theories related to suggestions;
6. the personality trait approach.

Cziboly and Bárdos propose a complex bio-psycho-social model which deals with biological, psychological and social factors in one combined system. Its essential new element is that it distinguishes the type of placebo effect based on conditioning from another type based on expectation. While the former can easily be explained by what we know about conditioning in general, the action mechanism of the placebo effect based on expectation is practically unknown to this very day. The model retraces expectation-based placebo effect to psychophysiological causes. They propose the existence of two 'gateways' (neural blocks) which developed under evolutionary influence – one filters the information which is to be processed after it arrives from the vegetative nervous system (bottom-up); the other filters the instructions arriving from the consciousness toward the vegetative nervous system (top-down). The expectation-based placebo effect is probably due to a temporary opening of the second gateway when the mind contents make their way 'down' into the vegetative system. The opening is supposed to take place under the influence of social interactions and suggestions. Besides, a genetic tendency for opening can also be imagined and this would explain a receptiveness to placebo which many scholars assume to exist within populations.

Over the past decades, research into the psychological and biological/biochemical mechanisms of the placebo effect has become intensified and continues so even today. Volumes summarizing the current stage of research are appearing almost annually.

A few examples

In the medical sciences, placebo is mostly used in double-blind testing of potential medication. Examinations of blind tests have repeatedly shown that placebo has proved as effective as the active drug (Bitter,[14] 1994). The analgesic effect of placebo was first discovered during the first blind-test experiment carried out in 1916, when, as a control to morphine, patients were given physiological salt solution. Some of the patients experienced the same

relief from pain as those given morphine. Since that time there have been innumerable experiments to demonstrate the analgesic effect of placebo. We only describe one of them here.
In an experiment, two types of injections were used to treat the chronic pain of an oncological post-operative wound: 15 mg morphine or placebo. Morphine reduced the pain in 60% of cases, the placebo injection in 43% of cases (Fürst,[15] 1997).

Experiments have also shown that the placebo effect can appear not only in analgesics, but in other therapeutic situations also. Körbler quotes the following experiment, carried out in the USA and published by *Yale Medicine* at Yale University. The test covered over 2000 patients after a heart attack. One group were given beta-blockers; the other group were given a placebo. The result was surprising – survival rates were the same in both groups.

The placebo effect can be provoked not only by drugs, but also by any intervention which appears as medical treatment to the patient. In the following case study a counterfeit operation was used as placebo.

The July 2002 issue of the *New England Journal of Medicine* published a report on a medical experiment[16] discussing the recovery of patients suffering from inflammation of the knee joint. Surgeon Dr. Bruce Moseley and his team of eight carried out a series of experiments overarching more than a year at the Baylor School of Medicine. The main question in the experiment was which component of the knee-joint operation was most effective. In order to answer this, they carried out three types of operations. There were 180 participants in the experiment, divided into three groups. The first group included 59 patients where the deformed, crumbled parts of a damaged vertebral disc were removed by arthroscopy and the joint itself was rinsed. In the second group of 61 patients the affected joint was rinsed with at least 10 liters of fluid. In the third group a counterfeit operation made an incision of 1 cm depth in the skin and stitched up the cut 40 minutes later, just as in the case of the other operations. During the operation a similar noise was caused by circulating some fluid as in the other two groups where the lavage of the knee joint genuinely took place. After the operation all three groups were treated in the same way in all respects. They all received physiotherapy and exercise. According to records, all three groups of patients took the same amount of painkillers. After the operation their condition was tracked for 2 more years. During that time the placebo group did not find out that they had not undergone a genuine intervention.

The experiment led to shocking results. Members of the placebo group made the same recovery as patients in the other two groups. Moseley stated, 'The only benefit of the intervention for these osteoarthritis patients was the placebo effect.' American television also reported on the series of experiments. One elderly man from the placebo group, Tim Perez, used to walk with a stick, but now he was playing basketball with his grandchildren. In an interview he gave to Discovery Health Channel he declared, 'Everything in this world is possible, if only your determination is strong enough. Now I know that the mind can perform miracles.'

Placebo can considerably improve psychological conditions by improving general mood and resolving anxieties and depression. According to clinical testing in America, 80% of the effect of antidepressants may be attributed to the placebo effect[17] (Kirsch et al., 2002). According to tests exploring the effect of leading antidepressants, in more than half of the cases the effect of these drugs did not exceed that of the sugar tablets used as placebo.

The broad range of placebo experiments shows that placebo can influence any bodily functioning which is under the regulation of the nervous system, including all systems innerved by the vegetative nervous system, such as the endocrine and the immune system.

Cziboly and Bárdos arranged systematically the result of placebo experiments[18] (2003) and found that placebo mostly affects the following organ systems:

- the central nervous system and the vegetative nervous system (e.g. in schizophrenia, stress, analgesics, as tranquilizer, sleeping pill, against migraines or in EEG, etc.);
- the cardiovascular system (e.g. angina pectoris, cardiomyopathy, arrhythmia, blood pressure problems, pulse, ECG, blood count, etc.);
- the gastro-intestinal tract (e.g. intestinal motility, secretion of gastric fluids, peptic ulcers, etc.);
- the immune system (e.g. tumors, temperature reduction, rheumatoid and degenerative arthritis, hay fever, coughs, SLE, etc.);
- to some extent, the respiratory system, the reproductive system, the secretory system and the endocrine system.

Körbler on the Placebo Effect

Körbler claims that the placebo effect emerges because the content of the negative stimulus reaction taking place in the organism is transformed into a positive content by positive thinking, by hope and joy, as energy types which are higher in the hierarchy of different energy levels. This causes an energy surplus and results in a chain reaction in the positive direction. On each occasion when a patient is given a placebo tablet or any treatment leading to a placebo effect, the positive effect is multiplied and this gives substantial support to the body's self-healing mechanism. Placebo manifests its effect through belief. It is an extremely important and useful tool for anyone who requires positive thinking, optimism and belief in success for their recovery. In the absence of positive belief the doctor or healer can give this to the patient with the help of the placebo. The healer supplements the use of the placebo by positive belief. This way, each time patients take their placebo, they strengthen their belief in their own recovery and this generates the chain reaction required for an energy surplus in their organism which in turn triggers the self-healing mechanisms and leads to recovery.

Placebo tablets work even if the patients simply hold them in their hands with the knowledge and conviction that the effect exists – the recovery will take place. The tablet may be replaced by any image of the object, too, as long as the patient knows that every time he or she looks at the object, the disease keeps on getting better. If this positive response comes to be associated with any word or object and the patient believes in this, the placebo will be effective beyond any doubt.

Positive thinking and various self-suggestion techniques (e.g. Coué's method[19]); anticipations of recovery; imagining the organ as recovered; or active expectations of recovery serve the same purpose. Any kind of complaint and pain can be remedied in this way as long as the cells involved in the symptom are capable of functioning.

Energy Surplus

The regulation of open dissipative organisms is a complex and complicated system which, instead of giving single answers one by one to individual stimuli, makes a coherent decision on the systemic level whether the stimulus in question is positive for it or not. Looking at it from this point of view, our organism distinguishes favorable and unfavorable effects both as regards external stimuli and higher-level energies coming from the organism itself. Accordingly, there are positive and negative response reactions within the body. Positive and favorable effects bring an energy surplus to the organism, while harmful and negative effects mean a drop in energy.

As we saw earlier, Körbler deduces the energy surplus from the consequences of the electromagnetic effects affecting the cell. In the presence of a favorable electromagnetic effect the cell voltage builds up and reaches –60 mV or even more. The molecular structure of the cell might develop preferences which enable new chemical connections. As a result of coherent regulation this process will spread over the entire organism. In consequence where the voltage is too low (–15 to –30 mV) cells are no longer able to influence healthy cells, and they become isolated and perish. As we have already mentioned, it is indifferent for the reaction of the cells where the higher-level energetic information is coming from; the bodily cells will respond in the same way whether the stimulus comes from the brain or from the outside world. In fact, the information from the brain is capable of overwriting the information from the environment. But positive thinking is only potent during waking hours. During sleep, this cortical function is not active. In that period, information from the body takes the leading role. The psychological domain of the unconscious is mostly determined by the information content of cells and organs. If an organ is under constant load or an overstimulated condition due to some unfavorable influence, the cells react in a negative way and this information (an identical, repeated, unfavorable and harmful information content) is transmitted to the brain. In cases like this, according to Körbler, the cortical functioning is determined by the negative information content arriving from the cells. Due to the feedback from the cortical function, a vicious circle develops with the vegetative system where the negative information content will become the dominant influence. In parallel with the disharmonic functioning of the physical body, the psyche also comes into a disharmonic condition. In order to prevent this, Körbler proposes that the functioning of the organ must be reconstructed, starting with eliminating the pain. Next comes the treatment of the psychological cause. Once the patient's pain has stopped, they will be trusting and open to the therapist. In the opposite case, if the patient is resistant, this conscious resistance will appear in the system as a decisive, higher energy. This will prevent the treatment of the psychological cause. In fact the presence of a higher-level positive energy in the patient's consciousness is crucial for recovery.

Sperry claims that positive consciousness promotes the coherent functioning of the cells. The essence of co-operation is that every cell should function in optimal harmony with every other cell. This is the condition of optimal functioning for the body, in other words the highest possible level of coherence. Körbler came to the same conclusion. Any stimulus, whether external or internal, which proves positive according to Körbler's testing will enhance coherence and promote harmonized functioning of the cells.

Sperry's discovery was confirmed by Bruce Lipton's laboratory experiments on endothelial cells. Lipton succeeded in demonstrating on the cell level that instructions arriving from the mind can overwrite instructions from the organism. Bruce Lipton's experiments in cell biology are extremely interesting. He studied cloned endothelial cells – the cells which line the inside of our blood vessels. The endothelial cells in the tissue culture change their behavior actively in line with the signals from the environment. If the environment is rich in food, they move rapidly toward the source of nourishment. In a toxic environment, however, these cells distance themselves from the toxins which represent a harmful stimulus. Lipton did not stop exploring at this point. He was curious what kind of sensations on the cell membrane were triggering the above behavioral change. He discovered a receptor protein which responds to the presence of histamine. This molecule plays an important part in the local alert system of the body. He found that the same histamine signal could provoke two possible responses, H1 and H2. If receptor protein H1 becomes activated, this produces a defense reaction, just like the one shown by endothelial cells in a toxic tissue culture. If receptor H2 becomes activated, the presence of histamine leads to growth in the cell, just like when the endothelial cells are given nourishment.

In his further experiments Lipton introduced adrenaline into the cell culture. Again, there were two types of receptors sensitive to adrenaline, called alpha and beta. These alpha and beta receptors provoked precisely the same cell behavior as receptors H1 and H2 in the case of histamine. When alpha receptors of integral membrane proteins[20] became activated, in the presence of adrenaline this launched a defense reaction. When the same adrenaline sign provoked a reaction in the beta receptors, the cell began to grow.

The most interesting result of this series of experiments happened, however, when Lipton introduced both histamine and adrenaline into the cell culture at the same time. He found that the adrenaline signals issued by the central nervous system had priority over the local effect of histamine. Cells mostly function based on the signals of the central nervous system even if these conflict with the local stimuli (Lipton et al., 1992).[21]

Körbler's Experiments

It is undecided whether Körbler was acquainted with Lipton's research. He did not refer to it in his teaching or his writings. His own approach led him to the same results as Lipton's cell biological research. In his experiments Körbler also demonstrated that the dominant role is played by the higher-level information coming from the mind. Participants at his training courses at both Budapest and Mönichkirchen were able to witness how the dowsing rod indicates the psychological factors present in the physical system.

We tested these effects in two series of experiments – one set was related to the transfer of ideas and information, while the other aimed to demonstrate manifestations of emotional effects in the energetic system of the body.

Körbler's Experiments on the Transfer of Emotionally Changed Information

These experiments demonstrate that the subject of the experiment transfers emotionally changed information through the left–right meridian. Mental information may be demonstrated on the object which the subject holds in his/her hands during the testing. These experiments require three pieces of metal and several glasses of water. The course of the experiment is as follows:

1. Test the pieces of metal with the dowsing rod – in all three cases you will experience a circular motion.
2. Lay the dowsing rod on the table. Pick up one of the three pieces of metal in which you had held the dowsing rod. Now spend 3 minutes thinking positively. This is easiest if you think of a word which carries a positive meaning for you, such as 'perfect' or 'peace' or 'love', and carry on repeating it continually. After the end of the 3 minutes lay the piece of metal on the table, touch it with the index finger of your free hand and test it. Instead of a circular movement the dowsing rod will now move horizontally. The positive idea has been transferred onto the piece of metal. This piece of metal will retain the information until some other information is transferred onto it or until you extinguish the current one. (Over a heat of 55 °C the previously transferred information becomes deleted.)
3. As a counter-test you can do the experiment with the help of a negative thought, e.g. 'war'. Take another piece of metal in your hand and keep repeating the negative word. If you retest after 3 minutes, instead of a circular movement the dowsing rod will swing vertically. This means that the negative thought has been transferred to the piece of metal.

4. Put the three pieces of metal on the table in front of you – the one that has been treated with the negative idea, the other one which had the positive idea transferred onto it earlier, and the third, untreated one. Test them one by one. You will get the following result – the untreated piece will generate circular movements, the one treated with the positive idea will provoke horizontal and the one treated with negative ideas will produce vertical motions.

5. If you transfer the information of each of the three pieces of metal in the already described fashion onto a glass of water, the result will be the same as when you test the pieces of metal.

Experiments Demonstrating the Manifestations of Emotional Effects in the Energetic System of the Body

The dowsing rod reacts sensitively to changes in psychological condition just as it does to information from the environment. It indicates how far an emotion is tolerable or intolerable for a person. It will also show how psychological changes influence the physical state of the body. The effect of negative, destructive or harmful events will appear on the physical level and affect our bodily functioning even if the event affects someone else or we merely see it on television, on a screen, or witness something going on in the street. Even though we are all aware of this effect and are horrified at the sight of harmful events, it is still interesting that these changes even manifest on the physical, bodily level.

The following series of experiments is one we repeated at every training course and always came to the same results.

1. In order to test the initial state, students tested each other at the following meridian points: large intestine 1; kidney 3; spleen 6; stomach 36.

2. After looking at some pictures of the horrors of war they retested each other at the same points. The value at the tested meridian points had changed drastically in all cases. The energy at large intestine 1 and kidney 3 meridian points had shifted in the direction of disharmony between vectors 4 and 7. If it was vector position No. 1 before the test, it became vector position 4 or 5 after looking at the pictures of war. This means that the dowsing rod showed an elliptic circular movement to the right, or a vertical movement, and the points of the stomach or the heart meridian, depending on the individual's weakest point, also signaled in a similar fashion. At points where the dowsing rod showed vector position 4 or 5 before the test, after looking at the pictures of war they changed to vector positions 6 or 7; in other words they indicated the changes in energy condition by a revolving movement to the left. The counter-test will also produce observable change – if you think of a much loved person or repeat the word 'love, love', the dowsing rod will move horizontally.

Applying Körbler's Method to Modify Information

The experiments described above show clearly that higher-level information coming from consciousness or our psyche in general is determining for the informational functioning of our physical being. These findings resonate with the results of Sperry's and Lipton's research; in other words the functioning of the cells is determined by the signals of the central nervous system, even if they conflict with local stimuli.

Körbler studied in depth the possibility that unfavorable energetic information of mental origin, which occupies a higher level in the hierarchy of energies, could be transformed by simple informational means into high-level energetic information favorable for the organism, and therefore promote health.

In his experiments, in order to modify the information content of the mind he used the Y symbol, the sine curve and the symbols of the vector system that have the capacity to influence physical processes. Experience shows that these offer extremely quick help in the already known areas of healing. In the following section we present experiments where unfavorable information mediated by the mind and the psyche is transformed into positive, favorable information.

Transforming Information with the Y symbol

The experiments in Chapter 6 have shown us that electromagnetic information which is unfavorable for the body becomes positive under the effect of the Y symbol. The positive significance of the Y symbol for the living organism is self-evident, as the defenses of the immune system are themselves based on the use of a geometric symbol – that of the antibody – against the undesirable influences coming from the outside.

During his experiments Körbler found that the use of the Y also played a prominent part in treating psychological problems of an affective nature. The Y symbol is able to neutralize and rectify the information of emotionally painful input.

The technique for using the Y symbol may seem strange at first sight, but it is very simple and experience has shown it to be very effective.

In treating ourselves we follow the following procedure. We use the Y symbol through our own body. We cross the middle and index fingers of the left hand, which produces a Y symbol. We lay our right palm over our right hemisphere and in the meantime keep repeating for 3–4 minutes the name of the thing or person giving us a disharmonious relationship. If you now go on to test the problem or the person in question on the right hemisphere, the dowsing rod will move in a horizontal direction. Körbler says that the effect clearly takes place through the left-right meridian, as a result of which the effect mediated by the central nervous system changes under the influence of the Y symbol. The method can be used equally well for children and adults.

Applying the method to children

Körbler tells a number of stories about the capacity of 5–10-year-old children for reception and reaction, relying on his experience with his daughter and her classmates. His daughter and her friends used nothing other than Körbler's method whenever some kind of sickness made treatment necessary. Körbler frequently used the Y method for curing the various emotional and health problems that used to occur in the children's lives. He taught them how to form a Y using the index and middle finger of their left hand, and how to then lay their palm over their right hemisphere and repeat for a few minutes the name of the person or object causing the difficulty. Should they quarrel with a classmate, the tension can be instantly assuaged with the distribution of the 'Y-treatment'. Should some ice cream consumed the previous day cause digestion problems, repeat the name of the ice cream and apply the method. Also he taught them how to draw the relevant symbol on point 1 of the large intestine meridian and explained the treatment by applying informed water.

Applying the method to adults

Körbler used the same approach with adults. He did his best to find solutions to personally painful problems whether in our close or more distant emotional relationships. We used to do exercises in Mönichkirchen where we listed our colleagues and friends and then tested them on our right hemisphere. The testing was done in pairs in the following manner: the subject would list and repeat the names of the persons to be tested. We evaluated the movements of the dowsing rod according to vectors just as in the case of any other testing. Wherever the movement of the dowsing rod diverged from the horizontal at the mention of a person, we applied the Y-method. Experience showed in the course of time that this always helped. To be sure, one could claim that this was all placebo effect. As we have seen, however, Lipton has shown that it had physiological reasons (Lipton at al., 1992).[22]

> *It is interesting that animals are also sensitive to the* Y *symbol. On one occasion we led a training course at Gut Schlickenried. We usually spent our afternoon break walking or hiking around the fields near to the building. One evening, in the early twilight of December, Istvan and I went for a walk. We suddenly noticed that a herd of cattle were rushing in our direction. As they approached I was overcome by an increasingly fearful and sinister feeling, while we made haste to return to the building. There were still some 200–300 meters to cover. I kept entreating Istvan to try and think of something, but I got no reply. Suddenly I thought of the* Y*-method. With my left hand I shaped a* Y *and with my right arm outstretched I pointed my right index finger at the herd of cattle. To our great wonderment, the thundering herd of cattle suddenly halted and turned backwards.*

Applying the method in the treatment of allergies

Körbler looked on allergies as a type of psychosomatic disease. He used the Y-method to re-program the information of the allergenic substance causing the symptom.

In order to identify the information of the allergenic substance we proceed in the following manner. We test a list of foodstuffs in order to identify which foods are allergenic for the subject. The subject keeps repeating the names of the foods out loud, while the tester carries on testing by holding the left palm near the right hemisphere of the subject. When the latter reaches the allergenic food and is repeating its name, the dowsing rod will circle to the left in vector positions 6 or 7. All allergy testing proceeds in the same manner in establishing the allergenic substance.

Körbler proposed the following technique in order to re-program and correct the information of the allergen.

The subject keeps on repeating the name of the allergen while they cross their left middle and index finger. During this time the therapist lays his or her right hand over the right hemisphere of the patient's head, placing the fingertips in the middle of the top of the head. They both stay in this position for 4 minutes. During this time the subject may be overcome by various bodily sensations. After the treatment is over, the patient names the allergen once more and if they find that the dowsing rod is moving in a horizontal direction upon testing the right hemisphere, the information of the allergen is favorable at that moment.

The Role of Visually Perceived Körbler Symbols in Modifying Information

In Chapters 6 and 7 we described the capacity of the sine curve and of parallel lines of varying numbers in changing information. We saw the broad applicability of these symbols when drawn over injured body parts or dysfunctional meridian points or organs.

Körbler emphasized during all his teaching at Budapest and Mönichkirchen that cortical absorption of the Körbler symbols through the iris was extremely potent.

At Mönichkirchen we carried out experiments to rewrite allergy programs in the following manner. In the case of a milk allergy we would first establish which symbol was suitable to correct the information of milk as an allergen.

The subject would be sitting at a table. On the table in front of them would be a glass of milk. The subject would gaze at the glass of milk with the symbol for 3–4 minutes. If the dowsing rod still failed to produce a horizontal movement, the subject would carry on looking at the glass of milk with the symbol until the movement of the dowsing rod became clearly horizontal during testing. In order to secure the long-term effect of treatment, we use a combination of gentle treatments to influence the disharmonious functions of the intestinal system.

Visual information programming for babies and small children

In Hungary after our article on 'Diagnosis and Therapy of Allergies' was published in January 1994, we were contacted many parents with small children who suffered from allergies. Since you cannot use the adult method with small children, as they do not use abstract concepts about their food, we developed a method for testing and information transformation which is suitable for use with small children.

For testing, we hold the food, drug, etc. which is to be tested close to the sleeping baby's head.

In order to change allergenic information the procedure is the following. As we have already discussed in the Preface, a small piece of the allergen (formula milk, cheese, medicine, etc.) is placed in a sealed phial and a Y is drawn on the outside of the phial. Next, the children were given the phial to play with, along with their other toys. At the same time, we eliminated allergenic foods and drugs from the children's diet. We established an optimal diet and started treating the malfunctioning organs with the Körbler method. The children spent 1–2 weeks looking at and handling the phials containing the allergenic food or drug, and then we retested, on their head, their relation to the allergen in question. If the dowsing rod showed a horizontal movement upon testing the former allergen, the unfavorable information had changed. As a result of combined treatment, skin symptoms changed at a remarkable rate – urticaria which had been in evidence for a year or two vanished within a matter of 5–7 days.

Chapter 12

The Psychomeridian

Remedying Psychosomatic Problems with the Help of the Psychomeridian

Psychosomatic problems are usually extremely difficult to treat by conventional methods. Bringing them into conscious awareness or using medication does not help over the long term, because previous conflicts may be re-activated either consciously or unconsciously and start causing problems through their interaction with various organs. In the case of psychosomatic disturbances several functions become disharmonic at the same time. Patients usually come to us with a number of complaints. For instance they may have digestion problems, frequent stomachaches and unhealthy intestinal functioning. In cases like this, Körbler's testing will also reveal several dysfunctions. It is important to identify, however, which dysfunction is in a primary connection with the psychological cause. In the present example, is it the dysfunction of the intestines or the stomach complaint? Once we have found the primary connection we also need to find the psychological reason which goes with it – i.e. the information which has provoked the injury. This is the information that needs to be changed, since the central nervous system stores the effect of the events experienced. Things undergone in the past influence the operation of the cells in the present. If we wish to eliminate the effect of an internal conflict which affects the body negatively, we need to disconnect the negative interaction between body and mind and transform the negative information content. This information may overwrite the current local information, as we saw in the experiments discussed in the previous chapter (including those by Lipton, 2005[1]).

As regards the exploration of information from the past, a number of different methods exist within psychiatry, psychology and several Far Eastern healing methods. The approaches used in Western culture are all lengthy, tiring and costly. Körbler, in turn, discovered a very simple method of diagnosis and therapy that helps us find the traumas experienced at different ages, the pieces of information that disturb functioning. As part of his therapeutic method, the Körbler-symbols also proved useful in transforming disturbing electromagnetic information from the past. Once the disturbing electromagnetic information has been transformed, the central nervous system works with the new information and this information constitutes the basis of recovery.

In *Raum und Zeit,* in his article 'Die Neue Homöopathie XIII',[2,3] Körbler reported that he had discovered what he called the 'soul meridian' *(Seelischer Meridian).* In this essay he presented for the first time the method for identifying the psychological components of psychosomatic problems. In subsequent writings he useed the term 'psychomeridian', therefore we are going to use the same appellation.

In the following section we offer a technical description of psychomeridian therapy and its functioning.

The Psychomeridian

By finding the psychomeridian, Körbler identified a self-repeating function of the body which enabled him to test the life events of his subjects. This testing was able to show the favorable or unfavorable effect of the life events undergone in the past. During the testing of favorable life events the dowsing rod moves horizontally. During unfavorable life events the dowsing rod produces a vertical or a circular motion. The latter testifies to the traumatic nature of the event the subject had experienced, as well as the degree of the trauma.

The psychomeridian is a vertical line at the back in the middle of the head, starting from the Atlas and running to the top of the head. At this spot of self-repetition, the body is capable of manifesting the information of the life events of the individual, whether they were favorable or unfavorable, difficult or even traumatic. *(Figure 102)*

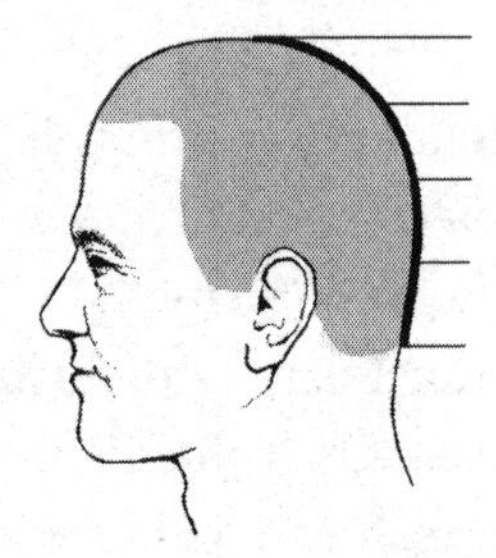

Figure. 102

At the Atlas we can test the birth point of the individual, and on the top of the head their present age. No matter how old the person is, the line can be divided in chronological order. If we are testing a child who is 1 year old, this stretch allows us to test the information between 0 and 1 year. If we are testing a person of 80 years, the stretch allows us to test the information of the past 80 years, starting from birth. In this case, the units indicating the years or months are obviously smaller.

Testing the psychomeridian serves the purpose of therapy. It allows us to find critical life events and the point in time when they took place. We may identify the unfavorable information of the critical life events which had decisively influenced the current psychosomatic functioning of the individual and played a decisive role in the possible emergence of psychosomatic conditions.

The significance of Körbler's discovery was proved by therapeutic practice, since the psychomeridian contributes considerably to the holistic recovery of the subject. Körbler showed us during his courses both at Budapest and at Mönichkirchen how to test for subconscious representations of emotional relations, but the systematic methodology for examination and therapy using the psychomeridian was developed by the present authors.

In testing the psychomeridian we use practically the same procedure as with all the other diagnostic points, with the exception that this time our examination is on a different level. You must bear in mind that these examinations take you to 'deep waters', in that you touch upon the profound layers of the personality.

When we test the meridian points of the physical stratum, we establish the harmonious and disharmonious degrees of the body functions. When people come to us with physical symptoms, they are eager to see whether we can find the disharmonious area, and especially the causes of the functional disharmony with the dowsing rod. If the signals of the rod supports their statement, this usually satisfies them. When we test the psychomeridian, the situation is very different. With the help of the dowsing rod we can refer to points in time when a trauma has happened. It happens often that the tested person cannot recall any traumatic event of that time. If he or she does, this can revive unpleasant or painful memories of the event. In this case the person re-experiences the event. The aim of the therapy is to transform the information that is unfavorable for the person according to the signals of the dowsing rod into something that is tolerable.

The test procedure

We use our left index finger to scan the consecutive points of the psychomeridian starting from the Atlas and pause if the dowsing rod produces a vertical movement or circles to the left. We establish the approximate time when the information was generated, i.e. how old the person is likely to have been when the event happened. *(Figure 103)*

If, for instance, the relevant event took place when the person was about 5, we carry on testing in order to find the exact time of the event, which the dowsing rod will indicate by circling to the left. The procedure is the following. We ask the subject to keep repeating the statement 'I am 5 years and 1 month old', a few times over, then move on to 'I am 5 years and 2 months old'

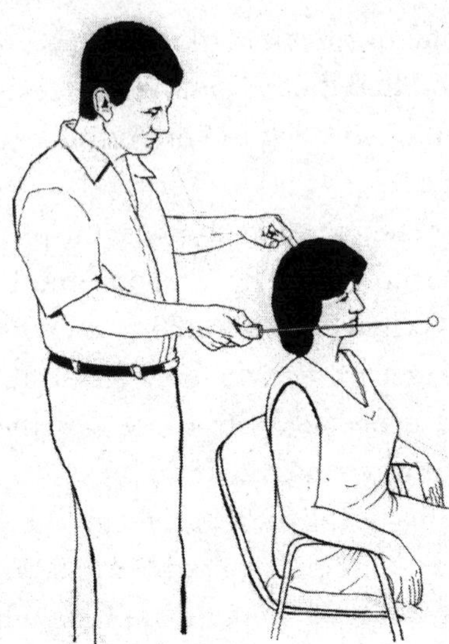

Figure 103

or 'I am 4 years and 11 months old', 'I am 4 years and 10 months old', 'I am 4 years and 9 months old'. When we have found the critical month, we can move over to establishing the critical week and the critical day. This way we can identify the exact time of critical life events and map out the course of the person's life. We record the points in time at which the dowsing rod circles to the left according to vector positions 6, 7 and 8. The effect of the events that happened at these times has contributed to the present physiological structure of the subject, the functional unity of their organism, including the existing psychosomatic problems.

We may find several critical moments or periods in a person's lifetime. The recollection of the traumatic event and the impact of this recollection are reflected in the leftward circling movement of the dowsing rod. Often the subject cannot personally remember the critical event, but their organism reacts to the recollection in the same way as it did when the event happened. It is possible for one of these points, free of personal memories, to produce the same kind of emotional shock as the recollection of a traumatic event. The subject might cry or feel physically sick. In an elderly male patient, the testing and recollection of a critical point in his babyhood resulted in bitter crying just like that of a baby, accompanied by spasmodic movements of the arms and legs. Should we be faced with such a reaction, we instantly move on to therapy.

Therapy

We start the therapy at the point in time that produced the intense emotional reaction. We choose a symbol that calms the patient. In the case of intense emotional reactions, this is a sine curve. The patient holds the symbol in his or her left hand and looks at it while we are testing his or her right hemisphere and the top of the head. If the movement of the bio-indicator changes while the patient looks at the symbol but the movement is not yet horizontal, we ask the patient to hold a vertical line followed by a sine curve |∿ instead, and we retest. If the movement of the dowsing rod is still not horizontal, we add another line to the symbol, that is two vertical lines followed by a sine curve ||∿, and we test again. Once we have the appropriate symbol, we ask the patient to hold it in his or her left hand and look at it for a few minutes. Three or four minutes are usually enough to restore emotional balance. Once the subject is fully composed again in body and soul, the dowsing rod will reflect this by powerful horizontal motion. This means that we have chosen the right symbol for altering the information of the trauma. This requires a lot of practice.

During the therapy, the subject reinforces the connection between the selected symbol and the traumatic information by *looking at a paper with his or her name, the exact date of the traumatic event, and the choosen symbol on it.* When the information is producing favorable response, we consolidate it by applying the Y symbol. In order to attain this, the therapy proceeds in the following manner.

If the traumatic event is known (e.g. the person had suffered a car accident), we prepare a sheet of paper in the manner described below for the individual to keep looking at over and over for several days at home. We use a blank A4 sheet of paper in a horizontal position. On it we write the first name of the subject, next to it the name of the traumatic event, and after these the selected symbol. The size of the letters has to be big enough for anyone to be able to read clearly even in the half dark and without glasses.

For example:

- John's car accident
- Helen breaking her leg while skiing

Now test the subject to find out how many days' repetition will be required for the success of the therapy. We can establish this by counting one by one and watching the indications of the dowsing rod. We have reached the required length of time when it produces a strong horizontal pull. If the rod indicates 12 days, this means the patient will need to repeat looking at the sheet of paper twice a day, morning and evening, for 4 minutes at a time for 12 days. This is done directly after waking up, while still sleepy, and directly before sleep. After the 12 days are up we wait for another few days.

If the patient is able to visit us in person we arrange a personal meeting and retest. This is when we identify how many more days the patient needs to do further consolidating exercises with the Y symbol. So now we change the symbol for a Y. This means that the subject is looking at a new sheet of paper. We now establish how many days of further consolidating exercise are required, putting this into practice by looking at the new figure in the same way as before, morning and night for 4 minutes each time.

If the patient lives too far away and cannot visit us in person, an experienced therapist can identify the duration of the exercises using the Y symbol at the first visit. This operation falls into the category of remote healing. For less experienced therapists a second visit is recommended by the patient – this is what most patients prefers.

These repeated exercises are usually sufficient to neutralize the unfavorable information of the traumatic event.

If the subject has undergone a number of similar traumatic events during his or her lifetime, e.g. had more than one road accident, we choose the most serious one, *adding the exact date to the event.*

For instance:

- John's second car crash, April 9, 1999

If the subject cannot recall the traumatic event and we only know the date judging by the leftward circular movement of the dowsing rod, we always focus on the earliest critical point in time and the related life event. We define the most intense traumatic moment and work on it according to the same method as in the previous case. The only difference is that instead of naming the life event, we find the appropriate symbol for the point in time itself. In the test, the subject repeats the critical date several times over, for instance, 'I am 1 year and 4 months old'. Sometimes individuals undergo intense emotional reactions when recalling such critical points in time, although this is less common. If we manage to find the appropriate symbol with the help of the dowsing rod, the patient will receive a sheet of paper to look at at home for 4 minutes at a time, morning and night for several days, for the purpose of therapy:

- 'I am 1 year and 4 months old' ∿

We determine the number of days and then also define the duration of confirmation with the Y symbol, just as in the previous case.

In each therapy session we only focus on one traumatic event. Once we have checked, a few weeks later, whether the therapy has been a success, we move on to treating the second most traumatic event.

If we fail to find any kind of life event which produces a leftward circulation, and the individual has long been suffering from the disease, we examine the phase of embryonic life. In treating the traumatic points in time, we follow the same routine as in treating current events. This operation also belongs in the category of remote healing.

For instance:

- Helen is an embryo of 33 weeks ∿

The impact of therapy and additional effects

Experience shows that after psychomeridian therapy patients usually undergo a significant change in their psychological and physical condition. They quickly and easily get over their previous complaints. In cases of depression and phobias they might not require any other type of treatment whatever.

We often find that after treatment of the most traumatizing events the information of other critical points in their life also changes in a favorable direction and becomes neutralized by themselves.

Similar changes have been observed after treatment of the earliest trauma, as well. The information of several later life events changes and disappears from the life history of the patient.

In the case of allergies, patients also rapidly get rid of their complaints which had prevailed for many years. In the background of long-standing psychosomatic complaints (e.g. neurodermatitis, milk allergy, asthma) we usually find traumatic events that took place in the years of babyhood or early childhood. Experience shows that the treatment of the symptom soon becomes a success after we neutralize such information. In treating physical symptoms, depending on the complaint, we use a combination of a special diet and soft methods.

Chapter 13

Aura Treatment with Körbler's Method

Perceiving the human energy field used to be the privilege of a select few for millennia. In view of the findings of scientific research in the 20th century, however, a whole line of instrumental measurements have shown and proved the existence of the human energy field and examined its qualities. Körbler studied in detail the qualities of the human energy field and, through this, the possibilities of curing the physical body. In the following section I offer a description of his teachings as he presented them at the third training course he gave for doctors in Budapest (October 1–3, 1993).

Körbler's courses made participants feel as if they were sitting in a magicians' school. He always taught by presenting cases. Even in the case of the simplest complaint (e.g. a common cold), he used to explore all the blocked processes of the organism and their interconnections in order to help us appreciate the complexity and importance of the total web of connections. From time to time he would vibrate his fingers or the palm of his hand 5–10–15 cm from the head, or he would connect two points with the span of his hand or a hair-clip, demonstrating that this gesture equals a line. He would do the simplest things and still find the web of connections in the background of things. He used to emphasize that his method did nothing other than optimize electric aspects in the organism, in this way resolving energy blocks and restoring coherence.

Under circumstances of coherence, energy processes in the body all point in the same direction in an organized fashion; all particles flow in a concerted manner. This latter process is indispensable for the healthy co-operation of all components of the body from particles to organs. If the direction of polarization of a particle, i.e. its direction of flow, in other words its orientation of connection, becomes reversed, the energy flow becomes blocked and the system of co-operation becomes damaged at these points. Consequently, biological processes also suffer a disturbance.

In Körbler's lessons we had the chance to experience how this seemingly trifling disturbance is actually the root cause of biochemical dysfunctions in the electric operation of the body, and how restoring it is the key to continued healthy functioning of the body.

In Körbler's method, aura treatment is an important part of the total 'science of magic'. Its effect is shockingly fast and enduring. We had a chance to gain first-hand experience of this.

With my brother István I was giving a training course in Gut Schlickenried, Germany. At the third seminar of one of the series of workshops, in December 1995, we were presenting aura treatment when the following happened. A lady of 44, who had had hip dislocation since her earliest childhood, volunteered as a test patient. Istvan and I duly carried out the aura treatment and, this being the last point, we concluded the workshop, said our goodbyes and left.

In early January we received a letter in which our student reported her happy experience. At last, her pain had diminished. For the first time in her life she danced on New Year's Eve. As a result of aura treatment her hips recovered. During our work on the present volume in September 2011 we asked her about her condition once more, wondering how long the favorable effect of the aura treatment had lasted. We phoned her and she was more than happy to receive our call. In response to our question she sent us the following letter in late September.

My dear friends,

I am so glad that after many years we are in contact once again. Although I am writing with some delay, I hope this is still all right with you. Thank you for the photographs. Have all those years really gone by? You have both stayed so young. I am also sending a photograph of myself and my friend. If you are ever in Germany again, please do contact me. I would be so glad if we could meet again. We send you all our love.

In 1995 I (Inge Husak) took part in a New Homeopathy Seminar given by Dr Mária Sági and István Sági in Gut Schlickenried. I felt highly privileged that in one of the topics I was able to be a subject of the experiment. This enabled me to get a completely new view of New Homeopathy through a new kind of experience. The instructors giving the course, István and Mária Sági, were very considerate to the participants. In my case, they carried out an aura measurement. I have had a dislocated hip ever since I was born.

As a result of the treatment, my pains have gone; on New Year's night I danced for the first time, and I am still able to dance to this day, which makes me very happy. This has made me appreciate life more.

My pain-free condition lasted until spring 2010 (for approximately 15 years). At present I am having treatment in accordance with what I have learned.

I thank God, my Spiritual Leader, and Mária and István Sagi for their love.

With affection and gratitude,

Inge Husak

According to Körbler, an aura is a system of radiation, a set of waves no different than the set of electric waves which emerges when we draw a certain line on a board.

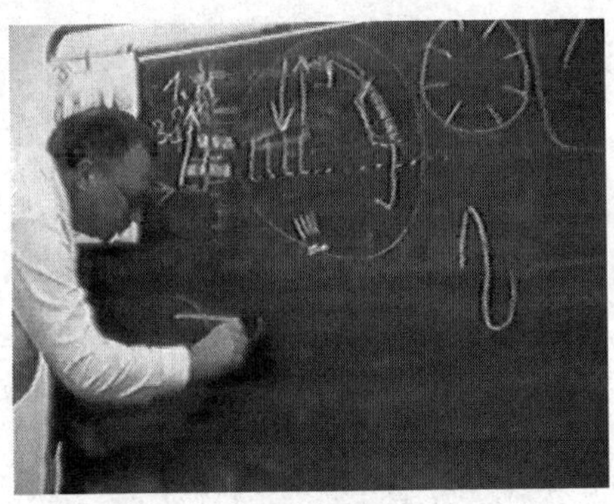

Figure 104

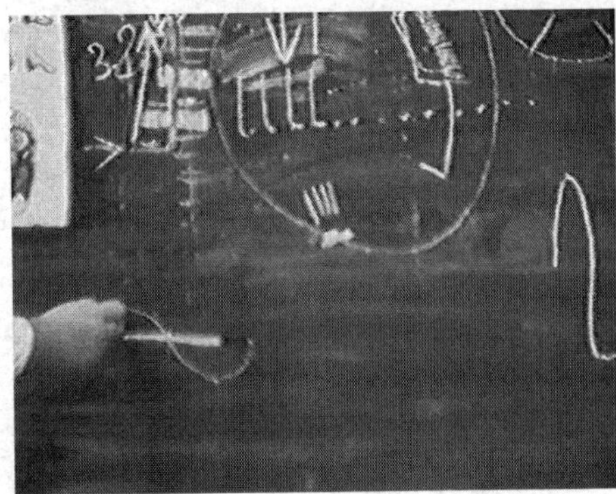

Figure 105

This is presented in the following series of figures *(Figures 104–114)*, based on a video recording produced at the training course for doctors at Budapest.

Körbler drew a line, along with all the relevant electromagnetic qualities which, however, are invisible to us and can only be sensed through the help of the dowsing rod.

As we saw in Chapter 5 (section 'Distribution and polarization of electric and magnetic fields', *Figure 35)*, the dowsing rod swings in opposing ways at the two end-points of the line (A, B). At end-point A it moves horizontally; at end-point B it moves vertically. *(Figures 104–105)*

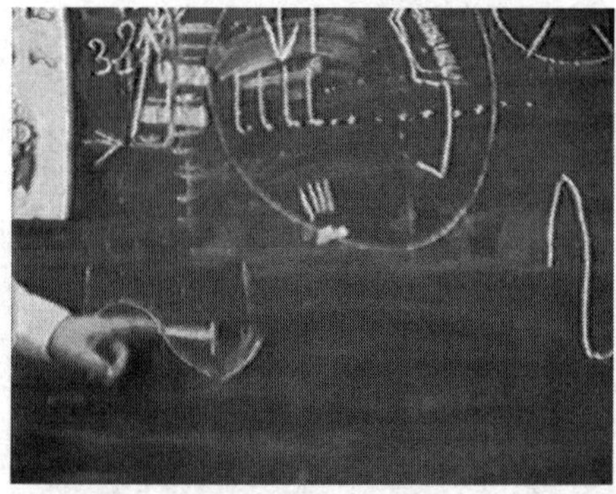

Figure 106

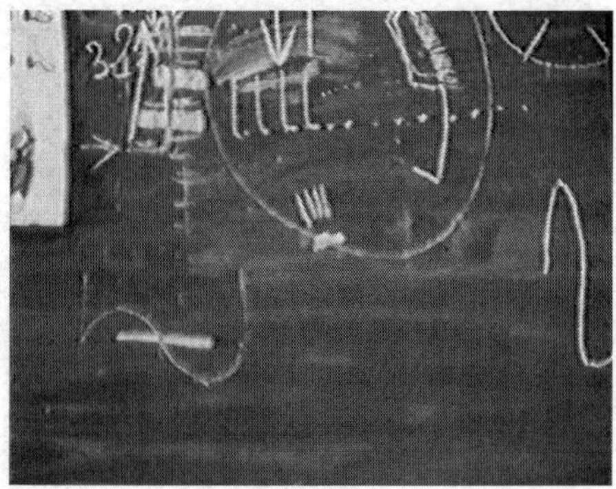

Figure 107

The invisible wave which belongs to this line, however, is only half a wave – the movement of the invisible wave continues on the other side of the line in both directions, thus producing a complete sine wave. *(Figure 106)*

Körbler points out that point 0 in the middle of the line *(see Figure 35)* is the still point of the invisible sine curve. At this spot the swinging of the dowsing rod will stop; it shows no movement. *(Figure 107)*

Körbler also explained that the invisible sine curve meant that the energy starting from the body rises upward from point 0 on and appears almost in its entirety at the height of its inten-

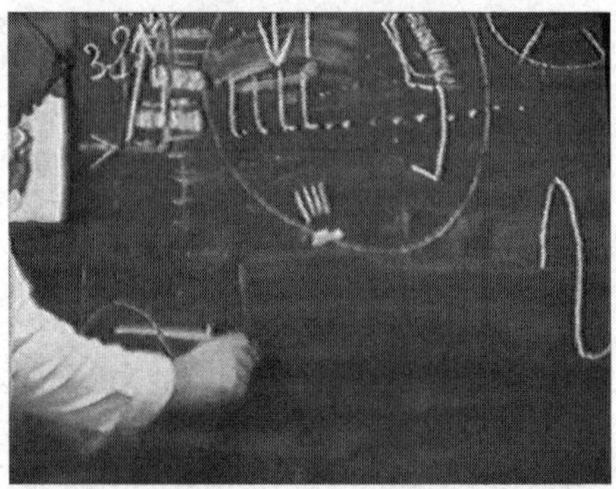

Figure 108

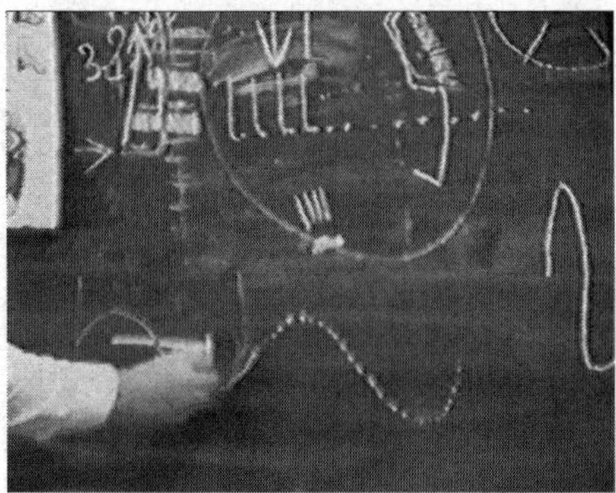

Figure 109

sity, then its energy begins to decline, and it reaches point 0, i.e. disappears. At this point it turns in the opposite direction, its strength begins to grow with an opposing marker and then, again, fully unfolds. The strength of the movement declines once more and reaches point 0 where it disappears again. This is the point where a new sine curve starts, once more flipping in the opposite direction. *(Figure 108)*

In this way, the full wave leads us over into the invisible space where the line continues as an invisible line. Here the same electromagnetic conditions obtain as in the case of visible waves. *(Figure 109)*

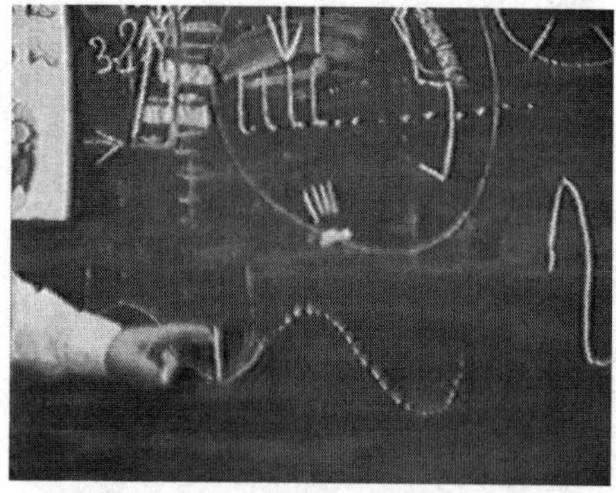

Figure 110

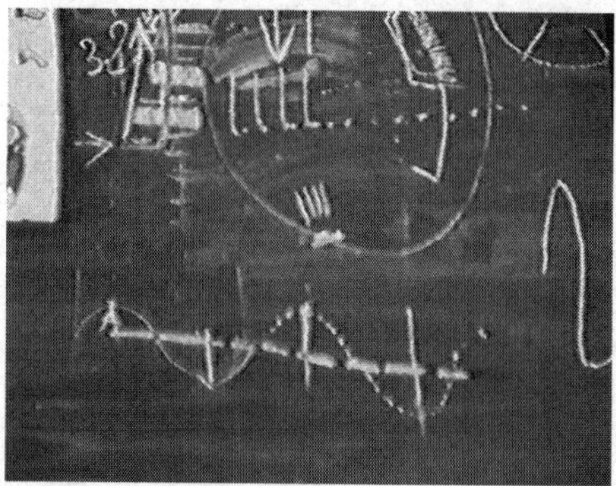

Figure 111

In this invisible space those points of the invisible line where the dowsing rod shows no movement are also repeated. This is the point where the new wave starts. From this point onwards the wave appears as a dotted line in the picture. *(Figure 110)*

The distance of the waves from the current line (whether visible or invisible) will show the quantity of the energy. The point where the energy is at the maximum will become the start of the new imaginary line, which goes on to the point where energy of the opposing polarity reaches its maximum. *(Figure 111)*

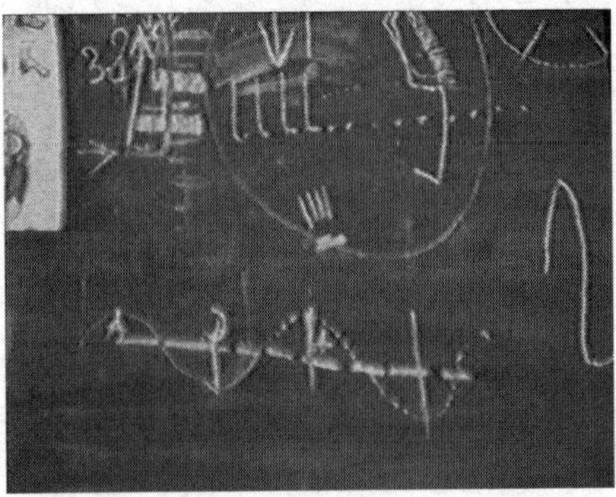

Figure 112

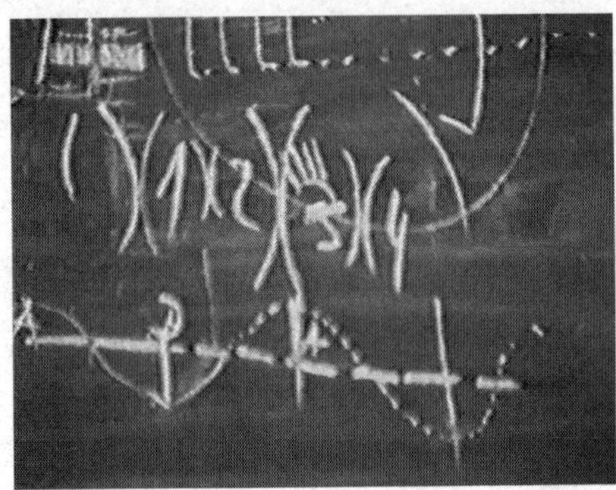

Figure 113a

In this phenomenon we witness the invisible self-repetition of the visible line (indicated by a dotted line in *Figure 112)*, along with all of its electromagnetic qualities. The associated invisible electric wave is just as real as the part which goes with the visible line.

The only difference between the visible and the invisible lines is in terms of polarization. If the first line has an AB polarity, the next, invisible, line, will be BA, the following invisible line AB, and the next one will again be BA in its polarity. The movement of the dowsing rod will follow the changes in polarity precisely and move horizontally at A and vertically at B. *(Figure 113a)*

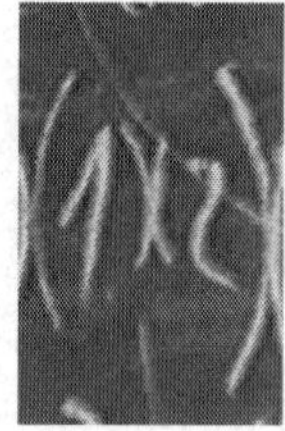

Figure 113b. First aura layer

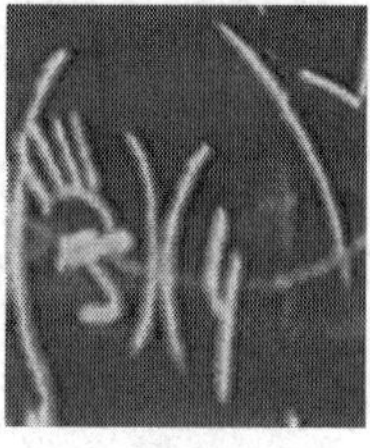

Figure 113c. Second aura layer

The same thing happens with auras. The body has the same kind of radiation as a line drawing. Körbler drew the radiation system of the body over the line drawing. The invisible wave is repeated outside the body. He used to mark the boundary of the aura layers with large brackets and divided this into two parts with smaller brackets:

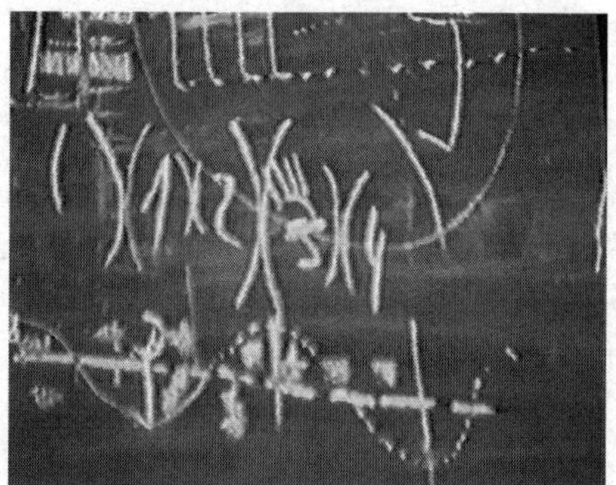

Figure 114

Sections of the aura repeat themselves and remain perceptible until the electric wave issued from the body is extinguished. Körbler marked differences in electromagnetic polarity on the line drawing. He explained that our life is embedded in fields of this kind, connected to similar fields. Since the human eye can only perceive a very narrow spectrum of frequencies, our eyes cannot see the aura. *(Figure 114)*

Testing the Aura

We examine the aura by using the dowsing rod. We define the first four energy layers of the aura, then we examine the areas that correspond to the trouble areas of the body.

Treating the Aura

Treating the aura allows us to *get deeper inside* the body. This technique allows us to resolve blocks, identify and heal trouble areas.

In the aura we find the correlatives to the deep-lying disturbance zones and intervene of this zone of the aura. We generate an 'electric current' by vibrating our hands, and this resolves the deep-lying electrical disturbance. This technique is extremely useful for resolving energy blocks in the head and zones of electrical disturbance. Körbler often used to vibrate his fingers over the top of the head. Within a matter of seconds he could resolve blocks and connect points where energy flow had been interrupted. Naturally, all of this happens in the domain of electrical waves. Körbler repeatedly referred to the fact that vibration produces electricity producing exactly as much as is required at the given spot.

Treatment of the aura also uses the dowsing rod. We identify the direction from which it is best to intervene with the body part which is causing the complaint. The layers of the aura are thinner at the front and back of the body, and they are thicker on the sides of the body. Also, the size of the layers is affected by our physical, emotional and spiritual health.

Lateral aura treatment

If the complaint is related to the hip, we offer lateral treatment. We use a tape measure to identify the distance between the edges of the hips, then, starting from the painful hip, we measure this distance laterally along an imaginary line, in the air. This point will be the first point of the hip bone within the aura. We now test this point with the dowsing rod and if we find any other response than a horizontal movement, we start moving from this point toward the body, looking for the point that has a less favorable vector position than others. This can be any one of vector positions 4, 5, 6 or 7. Now we can start the treatment. We put down the dowsing rod and vibrate both our hands, holding them in front of each other to form a line. We can also vibrate by moving our fingers, or taking turns, using first our fingers then our palms.

After a while we test the imaginary spot with the dowsing rod. We carry on with the vibrations until we find the dowsing rod showing intense horizontal movements.

Once we are done with treating the first layer of the aura we can move on to the next one. We measure the distance with a tape measure, examine the vector position of the place and then vibrate. The examination ends once the fourth layer of the aura has been examined and corrected.

Treating the aura at the back and the front

As mentioned above, the layers of the aura are thinner at the front and back of the body than on the sides. Should the complaint be related, for instance, to the chest, first we define the distance between the point in the chest and the corresponding point in the back; next we measure it along an imaginary line to the front of the body. This imaginary vertical section will be the layer of the aura corresponding to the point in the chest. In this case, too, we find the position with the worst vector position, measure the vector value of the spot and do the vibration. With a child of slender build, layers of the aura may follow on each other at distances of 11–15 cm. In the case of a more corpulent man the layers of the aura at the chest may be as thick as 30–40 cm. With adult women the dimensions of the layers of the aura at the chest depends on the circumference of the bust. This way we can draw the layers of the aura in front, behind and on both sides of an upright body, from head to toe. We use the dowsing rod for testing along the individual layers of the aura just as we would do with the body. The dowsing rod will show clearly the energetic condition of the layers of the aura according to vector values.

If we are examining a human aura, the second, third and fourth auras are significant. We can use the method of aura treatment for purging up to the fourth aura. Thus, for instance, during recovery from a viral infection the information of the virus will quite easily disappear from the second and the third aura. From the fourth, however, it is very difficult to remove it. Thus, the latent condition of a disease will persist.

Viroid Experiments

Everything has an aura – humans, animals, plants, stones and metals alike. Körbler reported on some viroid experiments carried out in the Max Planck Institute in Munich where they tested the aura of plants using a radionic device. The computer of the radionic device gives an accurate representation of the individual layers of the aura of plants, also showing which layer still holds viroid information. In order to remove this information from the aura of plants they tried various gentle remedies similar to tree-blossom remedies but in greater concentration. They found that it was quite easy to remove such information from the first, second and third layer of the plant's aura, but from the fourth it could not be removed or only with great difficulty.

In a series of examinations carried out at about this time, Körbler found that hops grown all over Europe carried viroid infections. The beer brewed using the hops contained the viroid information everywhere. By using the various information remedies, they managed to purge the viroid information from the first, second and third layers of the beer, but they failed to purge the fourth layer. Even though they pasteurized the beer (heating it to 72 °C), the viroid information was still prevalent in the fourth aura. Only after it was heated to 90 °C was the procedure successful, causing the viroid information to disappear.

With the human body, this approach cannot be taken for purging the fourth layer of the aura. Even in high-temperature saunas the heat only penetrates through the skin to a depth of 1 mm. Layers of the aura become purified up to the third layer. Therefore steambaths at a lower temperature are more useful for purifying the human organism. In order to purge the entire aura we need to use other gentle approaches which serve to strengthen the immune system.

Chapter 14

The Diagnosis and Therapy of Mycosis

Today mycosis is seen as an endemic disease. In the past, causes of this condition were, in order of prevalence, bacteria, viruses, parasites and, finally, fungi. In recent years, in developed industrialized countries this order has become reversed and fungi have become the primary cause of disease.

According to certain statistics, some 80% of the population of the Western world suffers from some kind of mycosis. This, however, is still far from becoming common knowledge. As long as the disease causes only minor problems, people pay no attention to it. The mycosis which lingers in the background of chronic complaints is rarely identified. Many people do not seek advice until their complaints or allergies become intolerable or their long-standing, chronic complaints develop into more serious diseases. During medical testing it is often proved that mycosis is the sustaining cause in the background of chronic illnesses or allergies, and thus it is becoming more and more crucial to prevent this condition and find the optimal therapy.

Mycosis is one of the most controversial areas in contemporary medicine. The profession is riddled with differences and alliances, debates and multiple approaches, both with regard to diagnosis and therapy.

In Western medical science we speak of two major groups in the diagnostics and therapy of mycosis. One is academic medicine; the other is holistic, complementary medicine.

Both groups fully subscribe to the view that in the case of a healthy immune system there is no mycosis. They are also agreed about which factors of the modern lifestyle are the physiological causes for people developing mycosis. Both approaches are also agreed that diet powerfully influences whether the organism remains healthy or becomes acidified. They are in accord that acidification helps mycosis develop and become dominant and thus leads on to the emergence of chronic conditions which then remain with us for many years. The profession is also agreed that a radical reduction in the consumption of sugar and simple carbohydrates and keeping the bacterial balance of the intestines healthy actually lay the foundations for microbiological balance and forestall the emergence of mycosis.

The question of acidification as a result of diet has a vast literature in schools of natural healing, addressing techniques and foods promoting alkalization. People suffering from mycosis are assisted by cookbooks, foods, breads and other things to ensure a mycosis diet. A number of best-selling books prove that a candida diet can be successful if one is persistent enough. It remains a question, however, how many mycosis sufferers actually have access to these methods.

Mycosis diagnostics, however, do not have widely accepted and comprehensively practiced methods. Different clinics and groups of doctors apply their own individual methods and procedures; different pharma and other companies offer various diagnostic 'kits'. In the field of research, however, serious efforts are being made to grow different types of mycosis cultures and apply various types of anti-mycotics. There are accurate data showing which type of mycosis is sensitive to which type of anti-mycotics and to what they react, since the various anti-mycotics have different action mechanisms.

1. *Academic medicine* uses bacterium cultures to establish a diagnosis and mostly deploys anti-mycotics to treat mycosis. In order to keep intestinal bacteria in balance they suggest the use of probiotics.

The most commonly used anti-mycotics in academic medicine are (fluconazol, itraconazol, ketoconazol, klotrimazol, miconazol, etc.), N-metil-naftil-amin derivatives (naftilin, terbinafin), poliene-type anti-mycotics (amfotericin, nystatin), while many others are based on single molecules (flucitozin, batrafen).

Different strands of fungi show different sensitivity to anti-mycotics; thus if the wrong drug is selected, the desired effect does not come about. For instance, *Candida kruzei* and *Candida glabrata,* which account for some 25% of infections, are practically resistant to the most commonly used agent, fluconazol.

A seminal study within the current Hungarian literature on mycosis is an article called 'Fungus Diagnostics in the Field of Basic Health Care' [A gombadiagnosztika az alapellátás szintjén] by Gyula Beszedics and Dr Lajos Szolnoki.[1] The authors analyze in detail the social and economic causes which contributed to mycosis becoming such a mass-scale problem, such as the physiological consequences of a modern lifestyle so full of stress and hurry, the widespread use of immune-suppression drugs used in modern medical practice, and the consequences of taking antibiotics unnecessarily. All this is done based on research carried out over 30 years, over 20,000 laboratory measurements, the experiences of co-operating specialists (GPs, dermatologists, gynecologists, gastro-enterologists, nephrologists, microbiologists), regular interviews with patients, co-operation with three Hungarian universities, and a few animal experiments exploring the effect of mycosis infections. They identify the gravity of systemic mycosis infections by doing a serology from a blood serum sample using antigen-antibody agglutination. They produce the phosphopeptid-mannan antigen required for the IgGtyp test by sterile fermentation of candida strands.

2. *The holistic, complementary school of Western medicine* follows a different path in the diagnostics and therapy of mycosis. The point of departure is the microscopy analysis of the living drop of blood which explores the changes and malformations of blood cells, as well as the healthy and pathogenic forms of micro-organisms.

   The method is based on the research carried out by Günter Enderlein (1872–1968), professor of microbiology. His theory of pleomorphism, created in 1925, presented the organic processes taking place in living blood. He pointed out that the different types of microbes, bacteria, fungi and viruses living inside our organism are constantly going through phases of change, and the micro-organisms which become pathogenic in a healthy blood milieu also decompose and may revert back into protein colloids. If, however, the blood becomes acidified, the organic processes which normally take place in a healthy blood milieu become deficient, pathogenic micro-organisms gain dominance and this opens the way to the emergence of various diseases. This method renders latent bacteria, pathogenic mycosis strands and different forms of mycoparasites clearly visible.

   Research done at the Swiss laboratory Ebikon has also revealed that among unfavorable conditions microparasites lose their growth activity and transform into a pseudo-crystal condition. The bloodstream carries them in this crystalline form and as soon as they find an appropriately nourishing milieu they instantly start to grow.

   The method of grey-field blood drop analysis is widely known in Germany, Austria, the UK and the United States, and serves as the basis for the diagnosis and therapy of mycosis at a whole line of clinics. In these countries this is the accepted procedure for medical diagnosis and forms part of clinical diagnostics. The holistic approach boasts some enduring results in healing.

In Hungary and Italy, grey-field blood drop analysis is not recognized as a medical diagnostic method.

Microscopic examination of the living drop of blood after staining was developed by Bruno Haefeli, hematologist researcher at the Swiss laboratory Ebikon.[2] Haefeli was a student and colleague of Enderlein from 1965 till the latter's death in 1968. He made, and fulfilled, the commitment to expand Enderlein's theory of pleomorphism into practical use and introduce it into the daily practice of healing.

These two techniques of examination produce different microscope images of the same pathogenic fungi, since grey-field lighting shows the micro-organisms from a different angle than customary microscope tests.

As regards therapy, both methods which explore the living drop of blood follow the theory of Enderlein's mycosis therapy and aim at restoring the healthy blood milieu. Neither of these methods uses anti-mycotics, since their aim is not to eliminate the fungus but to re-transform it into a useful element of a natural and healthy microflora. They believe that the use of anti-mycotics produces extremely rapid and effective results with regard to treating the immediate symptom, but it does not alleviate the overall load of mycosis on the patient.

Research by Sabina Scheller and Ekkehard Scheller has shown that during the use of nystatin therapy, which does not make its way into the mucous membrane and has therefore been believed to be harmless, what happens is the following. Nystasin destroys the candida fungus, but not its germs. The germs penetrate through the walls of the intestines into the bloodstream and thus make their way into the organs. Six months later they start germinating in the blood in a disguised form which the Schellers call 'molecular mimicry'. This way, candida appears in a far more aggressive form in the blood.[3]

Holistic, complementary mycosis therapy treats dominant pathogenic strands of fungi by isopathic substances. It uses the a-pathogenic stem germs of the fungus strand for making the isopathic substances. The remedy created in this way is suitable for re-transforming the strand of fungi which had become pathogenic into a-pathogenic, symbiotic components of the blood. This kind of therapy is a poison-free and risk-free approach. It intervenes with biological and immunological processes without disturbing their balance, unlike the intense use of medication.

Diagnosis and Therapy of Mycosis with Körbler's Method

Körbler's New Homeopathy, as the method of fungus diagnostics and therapy offered by complementary information medicine, functions by transforming the biofield information of the organism.

Körbler attributed great importance to mycosis exposure in the background of the emergence of tumorous processes. Therefore at the third training course for doctors in Budapest he presented the way in which we examine oncological patients, how we test them to establish their mycosis exposure and how we treat it by the information method of New Homeopathy.

We know that in the case of mycosis exposure the physiological balance of micro-organisms in the internal milieu becomes disturbed and turns pathogenic owing to an over-proliferation of fungi. As a result, the information of the biofield of the pathogenic condition is also altered compared to the healthy information, which is shown by the dowsing rod during testing. The relations of the various geometric symbols inside the living organism may be identified based on the principle of resonance.

Since the size of the geometric symbol is indifferent for the organism from the point of view of resonance (see Chapter 6 on experiments related to the dimension of geometric symbols, *Figures 40–41)*, we can do these experiments by using the geometric symbols of the electron microscope images of the fungi. Körbler tested a series of 24 fungus images produced by Bruno Haefeli in order to establish a diagnosis. If a pathogenic formal structure appears in the organism, during the examination the organism will recognize it based on the principle of resonance and the dowsing rod will indicate the presence of the pathogenic agent.[4]

Based on experiences of the past decades, we recommend that practitioners of Körbler's method use Bruno Haefeli's fungus images for testing and also for therapy, since the organism recognizes these visual structures both as regards diagnosis and treatment.

Since it is important for the diagnostician to know the pathogenic fungus strands, we asked Bruno Haefeli to present his method and his research findings. This section can be found at the end of this volume, in Appendix II.

In the following section we present the procedure for testing for a diagnosis of mycosis and establishing therapy by presenting photographs taken at the training course for doctors that Körbler offered in Budapest.

Diagnosis of mycosis

The diagnostic points for mycosis are the following:

1. on the left hand side of the chest, the interspace of ribs No. 2 and 3, medially from the axis of the nipples *(Figure 115)*;

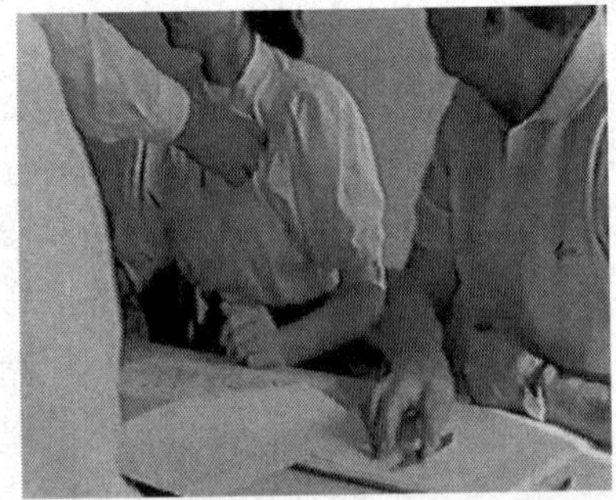

Figure 115

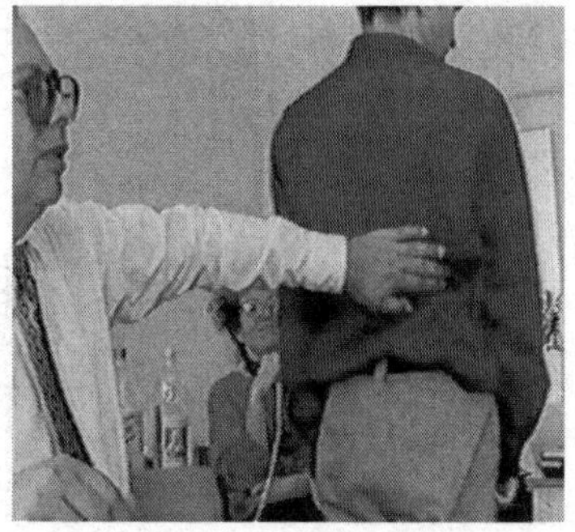

Figure 116

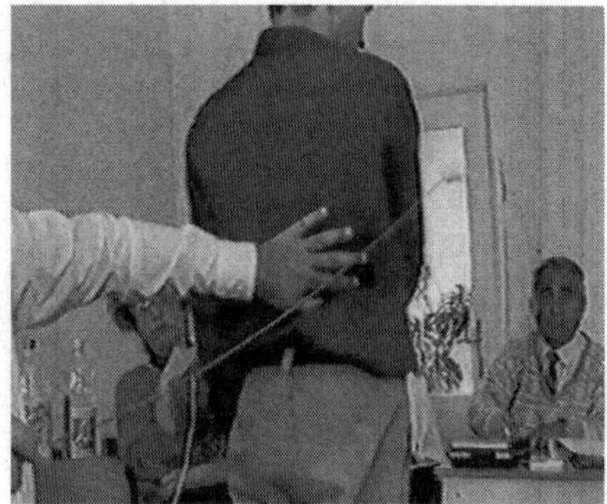

Figure 117

2. the bottom section of the back of the right lung *(Figures 116 and 117).*

If we press the mycosis point on the left-hand side of the chest gently with our finger we get two kinds of reactions: the patient will reveal intense sensitivity, possibly even pain; and the dowsing rod will move vertically. If we examine the base of the lung on the right-hand side, the rod will again show intense movement vertically or circle to the left, as shown by *Figure 117.*

Whether these two points are connected may be tested in the following manner: if the dowsing rod shows mycosis exposure at the base of the right lung, we place a coin on the mycosis point on the left-hand side of the patient's chest and retest the base of the right lung. If the dowsing rod is swinging horizontally, we are indeed testing the right point and are dealing with a case of mycosis exposure, since the coin has reversed the information of the mycosis point. In this way, testing the base of the right lung will also show the right type of information, i.e. the dowsing rod will swing horizontally.

If previous testing has already told us which organs or sets of organs showed unhealthy signals, we identify mycosis exposure with a copper coin. If, for instance, the dowsing rod makes a movement of vector positions 4–5–6–7 at the large intestine point, it is a good idea to examine whether this signal also con-

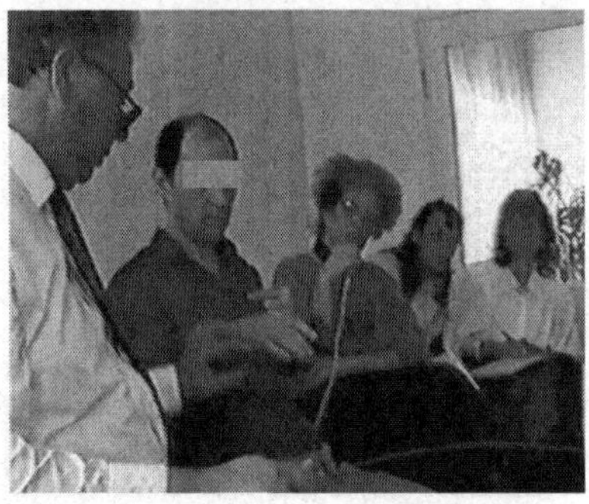

Figure 118

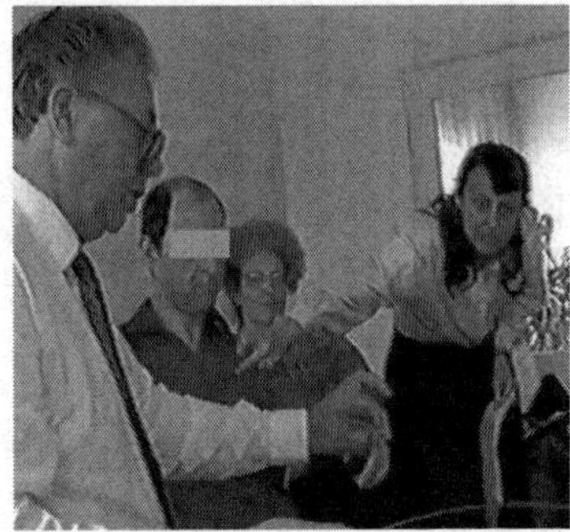

Figure 119

tains mycosis exposure. We can identify this by placing the coin on the mycosis point on the left-hand side of the chest in the interspace of ribs Nos. 2–3 and then retesting the large intestine point. If the movement of the dowsing rod changes in a favorable direction, we have a case of mycosis exposure. If the dowsing rod continues to move in vector positions 4–5–6–7, the problem is caused by a different type of microbiological background cause.

In *Figure 118* Körbler is testing small intestine point 3 of the patient while the latter is holding the coin over the mycosis point with the left hand.

In *Figure 119* Körbler is testing large intestine point 1 of the left hand, while his helper is holding the coin over the mycosis point. Naturally, in practical terms the test may be arranged in different ways; for instance, we can use adhesive tape to affix the coin to the clothing of the patient for the duration of the testing, which leaves them freedom of movement during the procedure.

The next step is to identify the type of mycosis present.

Identifying the type of mycosis

The type of mycosis is identified with the help of the dowsing rod. We hold the various fungus images opposite the patient, at chest height, facing the mycosis point; at the same time we hold the dowsing rod between the patient and the fungus image *(Fig-*

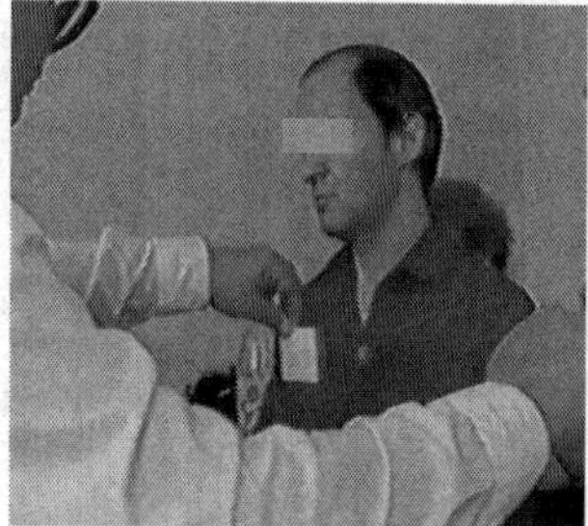

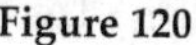

Figure 120

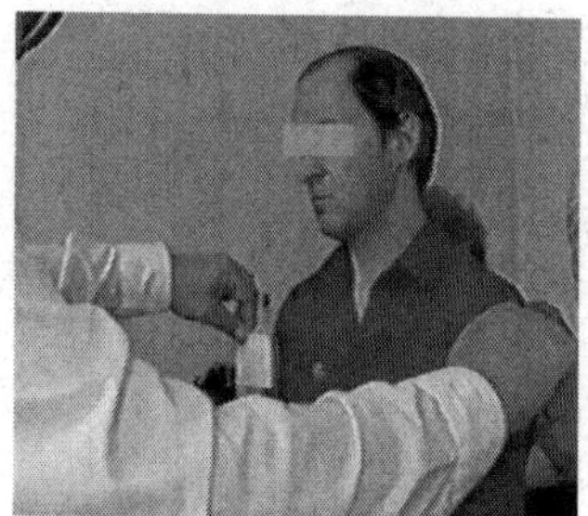

Figure 121

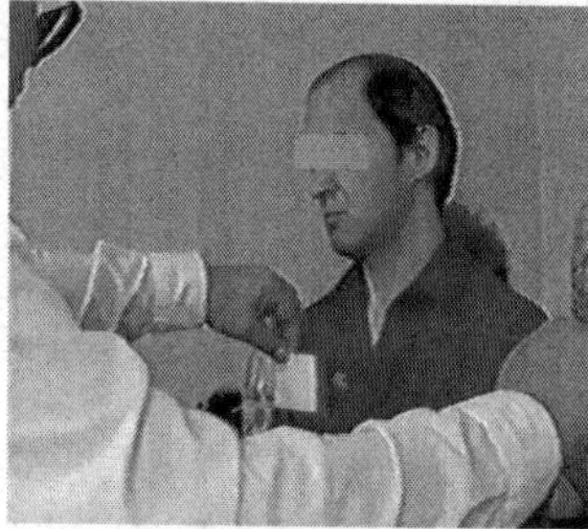

Figure 122

ure 120). Wherever the dowsing rod swings horizontally, the image of the mycosis is provoking a reaction from the living organism; in other words the same geometric form may also be found in the body. This is why the dowsing rod swings horizontally *(Figure 121).* Where the dowsing rod does not move at all, the geometric form of the mycosis image does not provoke any reaction from the living organism; in other words that particular geometric form is not to be found in the body *(Figure 122).* In the case of mycosis exposure we may come across several different types of mycosis during testing.

It is important also to point out which organ or set of organs contains the mycosis. This is identified in the following manner. We test the various mycosis images by holding them against the various organs. While testing his patient, Körbler established that the pathogenic fungus types shown in Figures 123–125 may be found in the organism of the patient. Then he went on to examine

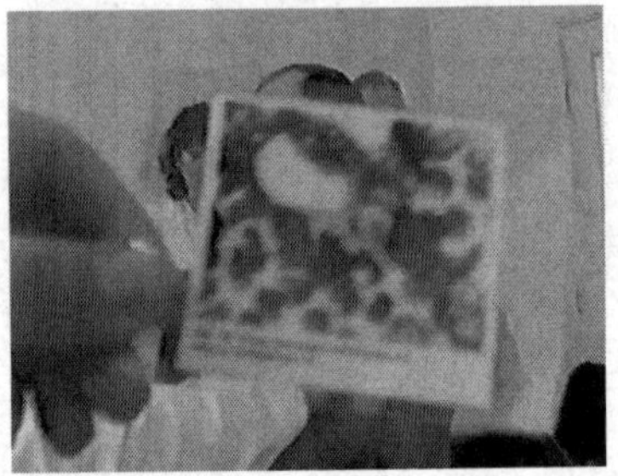

Figure 123

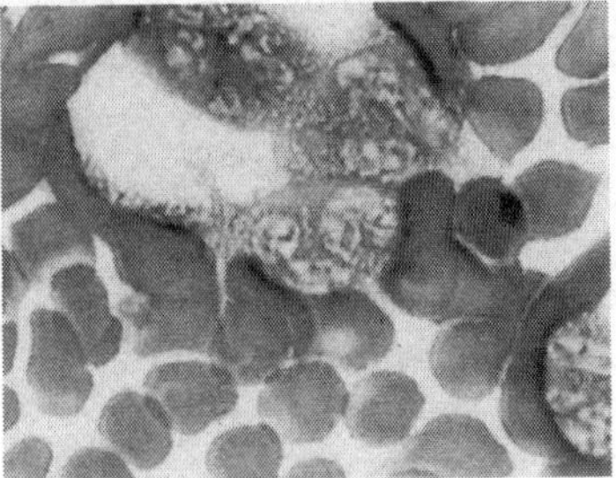

Figure 124

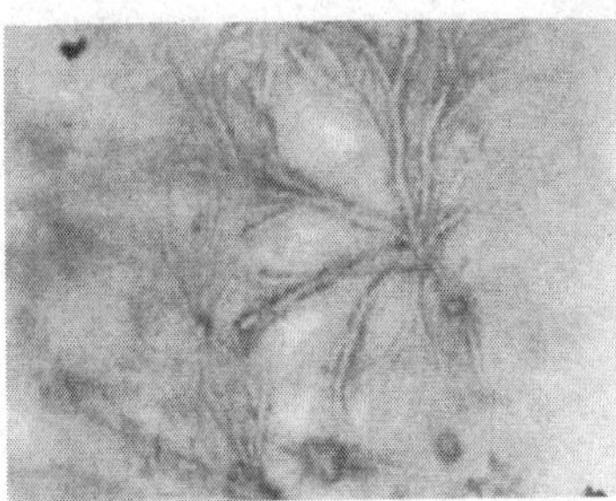

Figure 125

the degree of mycosis exposure in the case of the various organs.

The pathogenic fungus types shown in Figures 123 and 124 reveal the over-exposure of the thyroid gland. The pathogenic fungus type seen in Figure 125 shows the over-exposure of the intestinal tract.

Preparing healing information for mycosis exposure

We use the dowsing rod to select the geometric symbol which is able to alter and eliminate the information of the mycosis exposure. In the process of selecting the optimal complementary geometric symbol, when the patient is looking at the image of the fungus and the geometric symbol at the same time *(Figure 122)*, the dowsing rod will swing horizontally. Figures 126 and 127 show two electron microscope photographs of the same fungus, with the sine curve underneath, which Körbler had placed on his knee for the patient.

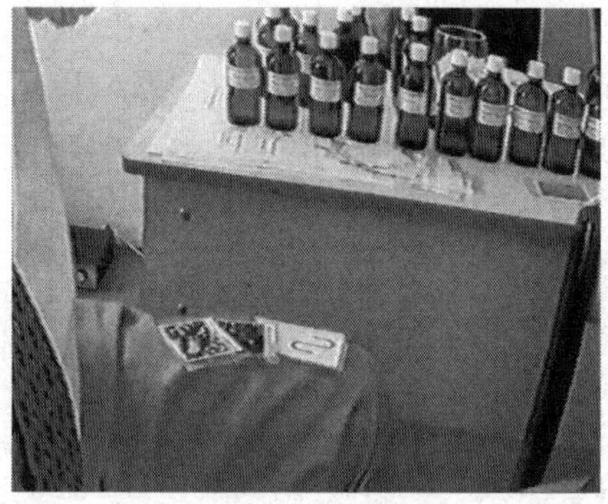

Figure 126

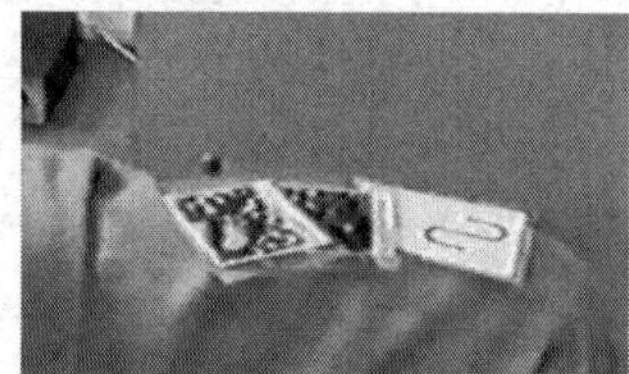

Figure 127

Next, we anchor the healing information for the patient in a suitable carrier. For this information carrier we may use a quartz crystal or a copper coin. The patient is requested to hold a quartz crystal or a copper coin in his/her right hand while looking at the image of the pathogenic fungus for 4 minutes together with (for instance) the sine curve drawn underneath. After 4 minutes the informed quartz crystal or coin will contain the healing information which will enable the patient to make their own informed water.

Now the patient is asked to hold the quartz crystal or coin in their left hand, while in their right they hold a glass of water for 4 minutes and then go on to drink that water. Patients will make informed water for themselves three to four times a day. The advantage of this method is that the organism creates its own healing information, the basis of which is always the biofield information of the given condition. This is why it is crucial to make the informed water anew each time.

By testing we can identify how long the patient needs to use the healing information.

If there are two types of mycosis present, we prepare healing information for both fungi separately. We follow the same procedure in the second case, too. The healing information of the second informed coin will be transferred by the patient to the already informed water in the following manner. In their left hand they hold the second informed coin for 4 minutes, while in their right they hold the water that has once been informed already. This way, the informed water will now contain the healing information of both types of fungus.

In the case of three or more types of mycosis, first we treat the one or two types that show the most intense reaction. If the condition of one or both has become normalized, we move on to treating the remaining mycosis types. We never treat more than two types at any one time.

At the same time when we prepare the healing information we draw four parallel vertical lines on the skin over the mycosis point, which the patient will redraw repeatedly. This acts as an additional support in restoring microbiological balance.

A male patient aged 36 had undergone two operations. On March 24, 1993 (Dg: Semicastratio propt. neopl. l.d.), and on April 29 for extensive retroperitoneal metastases of the lymphal glands (Dg: Lymphadenectomia retroperitonealis radicalis). He contacted me 3 weeks after his second operation, looking for alternative therapeutic suggestions for his recovery. Based on his own decision he did not take part in chemotherapy and radiotherapy. He knew our profile in which, as complementary treatment, we applied a macrobiotic diet, piantobiotic nutritional supplements and the method and techniques of New Homeopathy. The patient only wished to take advantage of the complementary methods.

After 4 months of macrobiotic, piantobiotic and New Homeopathic treatment, the third training course for doctors offered an occasion for Körbler to examine and advise the patient personally. As a result of his examination Körbler found that one of the main causes for the development of the oncological condition had been mycosis exposure in the intestinal tract, primarily in the small intestines. His proposed therapy was to prepare in-

formed water for the two types of mycosis exposure. By way of supplement he also chose two tree-blossom remedies which granted a higher level of energy for the cells. The patient made 1.5 l of water solution using 30–30 drops of this remedy each day. This he consumed over the course of the day, distributed between waking up and going to sleep. He used the tree-blossom remedy to make informed water three times a day, morning, noon and night, to eliminate his mycosis-related condition. For this he used the coin which he had supplied with information under Körbler's instruction (Figure 127). He held the coin in his right hand, while he kept looking at the selected images of fungi, together with the sine curve underneath them, for 4 minutes each. After 4 minutes the informed coin came to contain the healing information which the patient had used to prepare the informed water.

On top of all this, the patient was given a vertical line followed by a sine curve: |∿ drawn to fill the whole of his right palm for a duration of 40 days. Living in the countryside, he came for a check-up once a month. It was 3 months after Körbler's treatment (October 2–3, 1993) in the following January that we shifted to using the customary therapy by geometric symbols at the end-points of the meridians. After 1 year of treatment starting from the second surgical operation, the medical check-up established his full recovery. Today, 22 years later, the patient is still in good health.

In the service of the progress of science and the recovery of other patients, this ex-patient, now a healthy person, has kindly given us permission to divulge his photograph, diagnosis and the course of his treatment and recovery. We take this occasion to thank him very much in the name of all of us concerned.

Since that time, we have successfully used this type of therapy on a number of occasions. Its success is explained by the fact that the living organism is able to re-transform currently pathogenic fungi to an a-pathogenic form by altering the information of the biofield.

Körbler's therapy does the work of re-transformation by altering the information of the biofield. Joint application of the wave information of the pathogenic fungus and the sine curve jointly enable the organism to produce healthy wave information and thus sustain health.

Modulation of the information of the pathogenic biofield may be combined with any kind of gentle therapy. We can apply supplementary health-sustaining diets, microbiological roborative therapies (for restoring the balance of vitamins, minerals and probiotics, etc.), blood milieu correction, homeopathy, isopathy, Bach flower therapy, Körbler tree-blossom remedies, essential oils, herbal tinctures, etc. It is important, however, to use the dowsing rod to decide which set of tools to apply as therapy.

As we have seen in Körbler's example, he also used a complex of tree-blossom remedies, the symbol of a vertical line followed by a sine curve: |∿ in the palm of the hand, the sine-informed water for modifying pathogenic fungi, a macrobiotic diet, and piantobiotic roborative food supplements.

Part III

Articles Published by the Authors after Körbler's Death

Chapter 15

Diagnosis and Therapy of Allergies[1]

Food allergies have become one of the endemic diseases of our age with an increasing percentage of the population suffering from one or other of its types. Symptoms range on a wide scale, involving the digestive and respiratory system and the skin, to mention just the most salient few. Food allergies are also becoming more and more common among small children, but some forms have existed for 20–40 years. In 50% of cases food allergy causes skin complaints, in 20% it affects the intestinal system, in 20% the respiratory system while the remaining 10% of cases cause complications in the circulation. This is no wonder, since the food industry, growing at a breathtaking pace and showing little sense of responsibility, does all in its power to make sure that the quality of food on people's tables on a mass scale declines in quality continually.

The chain begins with the low level of nutrients and trace elements in the soil, with artificial fertilizing and chemical spraying; it continues with the practice of harvesting unripe fruit, storage and industrial processing; and finally ends with cooking in aluminum and Teflon dishes and reheating in microwave ovens.

Declining industrial quality affects meat, dairy products, vegetables and cereals alike. It is no accident that people who work at dairy plants would not drink a single gulp of milk, as they know all too well the production process it goes through. Anyone who has ever visited a poultry-processing plant or a slaughterhouse develops the same detestation for consuming eggs, poultry or red meats.

As long as our industrial-scale food supply is organized by an increasingly profit-oriented value system, there is no reason for hope.

There are many (mostly economic) counter-arguments to these proposals – the current method of production is certainly more lucrative and, indeed, not all people become sick, and when disease does finally arrive there are drugs to treat it. Looking at it from the angle of the sick individual, however, we get to know the flipside of things, too. Food allergies that have prevailed for many years and have resisted modern therapies are part of our day-to-day experience. The solution requires a change in attitudes, both on the patients' side and within the medical profession.

Modern Mainstream and Alternative Explanations of Food Allergy

Modern Western medicine views the human organism as an isolated, omnivorous biochemical machinery which contains the necessary biochemical processes for digesting and breaking down all types of food. If there is a flaw in this process, all they need to do is find the faulty link in the biochemical chain and supplement the missing element or destroy with allopathic drugs the pathogens which prevent healthy biochemical processes.

The alternative approach of natural healing, by contrast, considers the human organism an interactive system within an energy field. In Körbler's view, all living things are a part of their environment and can only be examined in unity with that environment, since their existence (as open dissipative systems) is based on the constant exchange of energy with their environment. The process of energy exchange varies from individual to individual, since the bio-energetic field of every individual preserves the information of its inherited characteristics and all life events of its current life. Naturally, this also makes itself felt in their diet. There is little exaggeration in the saying that 'One man's meat is another man's poison'.

The alternative healing approach is explained by the latest scientific findings. Since the 1980s, based on biological experiments and the latest theories, scientists have started to claim once more that the subtle fine-tuning of the organism is the work of the bio-energy field. This concept once enjoyed popularity in the 1920s in the wake of the theories of A. Gurwitch and P. Weiss, but at that time they were not able to define the exact physical nature of these fields. Therefore, from the 1950s onwards, biologists tried to explain all living mechanisms on a molecular, i.e. genetic, basis. Describing the coherence of the organism presented a similar challenge. Today's biophysicists are aware that sustaining coherence in the living organism cannot be explained unless we resort to the emergence of quantum action. This is also clear from the fact that the molecules which constitute the basis of coherence connect with each other so rapidly and so extensively that describing them inevitably requires assuming the connection of wave function phases. David Bohm described the possibility of fields carrying extremely fine and constant connections within the physical world as a holo-field. According to the latest theories of Ervin Laszlo, this phenomenon may be observed not only in physics but also in biology and cosmology; therefore he named this holo-field a 'psi-field', in connection with the energy at vacuum zero point.[2]

Körbler gives us a tool which enables us to perceive these otherwise imperceptible subtle interactions and individual characteristics. The human nervous system and human brain, being a far more sensitive instrument than any that man has been able to construct to this day, perceives and is actually able to read subtle-energetic radiations.

On the Origins of Food Allergies

Besides genetic determinations, there are two important factors that play a part in the emergence of food allergies. One is the psychological factor; the other is the 'toxin content' of the food.

The significance of the psychological factor may not be sufficiently well known, even though it plays a decisive role in the development of food allergies. For instance, difficult mother–child relations or harmful external circumstances (e.g. babies born during wars) play a far greater pathogenic role than one would think.

As regards the 'toxin content' of food, what justifies the inverted commas is that it is clear that food and poison are mutually exclusive terms; nevertheless, either owing to its character or its industrial production much of the food we eat may contain substances (artificial fertilizers, pesticides, etc.) which will be perceived as poison by the given organism at the given time.

How is this possible? Every living organism is a unified system structured in a complex manner; it is a bio-energetic field in which the immune system integrates all of the cell and organ functions in such a way as to enable the total system to sustain itself, to harmonize in a flexible manner the internal connections with external impulses and to eliminate those which are harmful. Naturally, its capacity changes from culture to culture and also between individuals, as well as over time.

Thus, biochemical processes are determined by this integrated bio-energetic field. Tolerable or favorable impulses from the outside world affect the totality of the system in a direction of better co-ordinating all of its functions. Intolerable and unfavorable impulses, on the other hand, such as chemically treated food, disturb the integrated function of the field, and this manifests in various symptoms.

In Körbler's approach, in patients suffering from food allergy the bio-energetic system is constantly under such heavy pressure that the integrity of the biofield becomes damaged, the capacity of the immune system declines and thus the organism begins to manifest symptoms. This load is usually complex; it is a summation of all impulses reaching our organism, such as those coming from the quality of our foods, the harmful effect of the electromagnetic fields coming from the products of modern industrial civilization, and the super-subtle energy fields of psychological and mental factors.

Diagnosing Food Allergies

a) First we map out the patient's bio-energetic field with the dowsing rod on the top of the head, along the psychomeridian and the following meridian points: large intestine 1; small intestine 3; kidneys 3; spleen 6; stomach 36; gall 40; lungs 1; Körbler's mycosis point on the left-hand side of the chest and the area of the thyroid gland.

b) The healer examines the sensitivity of the organism to any substance (medicines, chemicals, cosmetics, etc.).

c) The healer uses the dowsing rod to test the food list (this contains some 250 types of foods in subgroups); and examines the interactions of various foods and the organism to establish which foods are favorable, which are unfavorable and which are clearly harmful and allergenic. The same kind of testing is carried out with regard to combinations of foods. If the dowsing rod produces an elliptical movement to the left or circles to the left, we can be sure that the food is harmful and allergenic.

d) The healer uses the dowsing rod to identify which foods and combinations of foods put a pressure on which organs.

e) The healer also identifies when the allergy in question began and what sort of psychological trauma or what person or persons it can be associated with.

The final point is one that requires special attention. Allergenic foods can be tested by a number of modern mainstream medical and alternative healing methods (e.g. the bicom machine). Where Körbler's method is unique, however, is in testing food combinations and food components, the date when the allergy began and the related psychological component. It allows us to identify accurately the extent to which the flesh of an apple and its skin are allergenic; or, if we are talking about milk, which is the component (lactose, casein or the mixture of the various protein molecules) which is causing the allergy. Before Körbler's work, the origin of the allergy and its connection with psychological factors could only be identified in very complicated and time-consuming ways (exploration of the past, hypnotherapies, radionic devices, etc.).

Körbler discovered that the totality of the information stored by the organism, including that on interpersonal relationships, may be tested along the psychomeridian and over the right hemisphere. As we saw, the psychomeridian is a line that runs along the back of the head, in the middle, and connects the Atlas (birth point) and the crown of the hair (present age). Along the psychomeridian we can test quite clearly at what age the trauma took place and who it was related to. Experience shows that the psychological component is at least as important in the development of allergies, if we are talking about food and not poisonous substances, as the compatibility of the person and the food. The treatment of allergy cannot be successful unless we identify and remedy the psychological trauma, too. In such cases we identify to the day when and at what age the food became allergenic for the person and with whom is this associated with emotionally.

The Therapy of Food Allergies

The healer selects the method or combination of methods to be used in healing with the help of the dowsing rod. Körbler's diagnostic approach can be used extremely well even if we eventually use a different energetic approach for the therapy. It is important, however, that regardless of which energetic method we use, the dowsing rod needs to move horizontally, as this is what indicates that our choice was correct.

In the case of more serious illnesses a combination of several energetic methods will deliver us the expected results, and these need to be tested both separately and together. Such methods may include Körbler's geometric symbols, Körbler's tree-blossom remedies, substances used in classical homeopathy, special diet (macrobiotics, etc.), nutritional supplements (minerals, pianto, etc.), the use of Körbler-symbols in psychotherapy, etc. The quality and order of combination will be shown by the dowsing rod.

1. As the first step of therapy we change the information of the poisonous substance in question with the help of a symbol, depending on the vector position shown by the reaction of the dowsing rod. We do this with the help of the left–right meridian and measure the result through the right hemisphere. In severe cases we transfer the new information onto a precious stone or gold object and recommend wearing it for 4–6 weeks. If we are talking about poisonous substances, e.g. the kind of cytostatic drugs used in the past for oncological patients, after changing the information the dowsing rod will first show an unfavorable reaction and accordingly swing vertically. Now the patient's immune system is not as heavily challenged with this information as it was in the past. Nevertheless, the therapy needs to be continued until the dowsing rod starts responding positively even to the previously mentioned cytostatic drug. This is when the load on the immune system is over; yet we must emphasize that this only happens on the information level.

   If we are talking about food, the test must show a clear

positive with horizontal swinging. This, however, does not mean that the patient is free to eat the type of food in question or use the cosmetic or chemical substance. It is important to wait until the allergenic information changes into positive information in all the units of the storage system of the organism which consists of thousands of subunits.

2. We eliminate the use of unfavourable drugs and cut out from the diet all unfavourable or harmful foodstuffs for a period of at least 6 months.

3. As a next step, it is important to identify the reasons and consequences of food allergy to find out what sensitivity to flour, milk, meat, eggs, or, for that matter, fructose allergy, mean for that particular organism.

   The food list will help explore the causes. The test result of one young woman, for instance, showed allergy to carrots, vitamin A and cow's milk products. As soon as we eliminated milk allergy, the dowsing rod produced a vertical movement in response to vitamin A, proving it to be unfavorable; while it clearly showed carrots to be favorable. This means that the carrot allergy was caused by allergy to cow's milk and the two were connected by vitamin A and carotene.

   As regards conclusions, the response would again be coming from results of different vector positions found by testing on various organs. Experience shows that in the case of food allergies we often find disturbances of varying degrees in the energy supply of the large and small intestines and the liver. The reduced energy supply of the disturbed organs or sets of organs may be changed with the appropriate symbols, while in more serious cases we propose the consumption of informed water once or even several times a day, as a remedy made by the patient.

4. We assemble a diet of foods favourable to the organism.

5. We treat the information of the psychological factor which is causing the allergy with the Körbler method. Thus, for instance, in the case of a young man, Z. B., aged 21, rashes due to milk allergy first appeared on his neck, shoulders, arms and legs when he was 3 months old and have persisted ever since (for 20 years). As a result of complex treatment with the Körbler method they disappeared in 6 months while all we eliminated from his diet was milk and sugar. During the first session it turned out that the patient had only been breastfed for 2 weeks, after which he was given another woman's milk and formula. Although the rashes did not appear until he was 3 months old, the testing showed that the allergy actually started when he was 23 days old. In this way, during the first two sessions we treated the psychological cause alone, and only then did we transfer to the homeopathic treatment.

6. We strengthen the immune system by homeopathic remedies and other alternative treatments. Full recovery, however, takes longer than we would like.

   If we eliminate allergenic foods and drugs from the diet, acute symptoms will disappear very rapidly, possibly within 5–6 days, but the full regeneration of the organism and the strengthening of the immune system will take between 6 and 12 months. If it is not possible to eliminate allergenic foods and drugs, symptoms will not vanish for 5–6 months.

   Strengthening the immune system requires a complex approach. Besides adapting the right diet and treatment, the patient must have sufficient light, fresh air, exercise and sleep. It is fortunate if we can eliminate unfavorable electromagnetic effects from the environment (water veins, hubs of earth radiation, etc.) and install adequate compensation for harmful electromagnetic field effects from the electric equipment of modern technology (e.g. old-fashioned computer screens producing an exposure of 10–15 mG). It is important to make sure that at least our home should provide a truly favourable environment for our organism.

The Körbler method enables us to compile a customized diet which is in harmony with the client's current condition, and to adapt by constant testing to subtle-energetic changes taking place in the body.

Experience shows that a food which was selected carefully for the patient always proves tasty and pleasant in the event. This apparently trivial detail is actually highly significant because if someone begins the therapy with a very tasty and enjoyable food, their recovery will also be quicker. To quote Hippocrates, 'Every single component of one's diet has an impact on the body and changes it in some ways – and life depends on these changes.'

Chapter 16

Diagnosis and Therapy of Milk Allergy[1]

One of Körbler's excellent inventions is that the dowsing rod he developed enables us to detect the presence of allergies and even differentiate regarding the quality of these allergies and the time when they started. In Issue No. 1/1994 of *Természetgyógyász* we describe the full course of allergy testing. In the present chapter all we wish to focus on is milk allergy, as this affects a great many people these days.

As I mentioned before, for identifying an allergy in the case of adults it is sufficient if the patient keeps repeating the name of the food out loud while the healer holds his/her left palm over the patient's right brain hemisphere. This way the movement of the dowsing rod will reveal the attitude of the person toward the food in question. The case is the same if we test the patient's relationship to milk.

Our information storage system stores all information from the whole of our personal past, and all that is required is a trigger for a summary of all the information related to that particular stimulus (in this case milk) to become active again. If the patient repeats several times out loud the phrase, 'Cow's milk, cow's milk, cow's milk', we will be able to read off the summation of their entire attitude to cow's milk from the movement of the dowsing rod.

It is enough to consider how many times we come in contact with cow's milk over the total course of our lives, since it is a staple from earliest childhood. Most of us, when we were children, consumed it fresh, boiled, preserved, fermented (yoghurt, cheeses, cream cheeses); blended with other ingredients and cooked; with and without sugar, with coffee, cocoa, in puddings, cakes, creams, mousses and ice creams, and even in creamy liqueurs, to mention just a few of the truly innumerable examples. There are also countless cases where we consume various dairy products. These occasions vary in terms of time, season, the age we are, the other foods that provide the context, and even our own mental and physical condition is different each time. We have consumed milk in health and in sickness; during work, half unaware, or sitting in a café and perceiving it as a luxury.

On each of these occasions our body encountered milk as a slightly different stimulus and information, depending on its condition, and reacted accordingly. Sometimes milk was good for us; at other times it was bad; this was a result of the interaction between the quality of the milk and the momentary condition of our organism. One thing is certain: our information storage system registered and evaluated each encounter with milk as information. Each new piece of milk-related information was added to the sum of all previous information and modified it. If, for instance, milk was unfavourable for a child for a long time, after a while the body becomes unable to compensate this unfavorable effect and further doses of unfavourable milk become a harmful factor. In terms of Körbler's vectors this corresponds to movements 6–7–8 of the dowsing rod. In other words, when we test milk samples, the rod will usually circle to the left. It is possible that when the first allergy reaction emerged, the quality of the milk was no worse than that of any milk consumed earlier; only the condition of the immune system was different, i.e. weaker, until finally it could no longer cope with the milk.

The condition of the immune system depends on many factors:

- First and foremost is the *psychological factor.* If our spirit is happy and content, positive, cheerful and forgiving, the immune system is able to perform at a much higher level and the coherence of the organism is of a far higher quality. In a state like this 'you could eat iron nails', nothing will make you sick. If, however, you happen to be tired, despairing or unsatisfied, the performance of the immune system is far lower and the coherence level of the body declines. At times like this even good-quality food is more likely to cause damage.

- The *physical condition* of our body also matters a great deal. A sporty, strong and healthy physique will tolerate even poorer-quality food, while a tired and sick body is more sensitive to uneven standards of food.
- It is natural, however, that the *quality of the food itself* is also a decisive factor. In our current industrial society, sadly, poor-quality food of little value is very common, since most of what you get in the shops has been treated with chemicals, filled with preservatives; it is mostly mass-produced and packaged, 'dead' food.
- The condition of the immune system is also influenced by the *environmental pollution* which is present as a consequence of industrial civilization. We must stress specially the role that aluminum, so widely used, plays in modern large-scale industry, whether it crops up as packaging, as window blinds or as central heating radiators – all of which explains the spreading of aluminum sensitivity.

The eating habits and lifestyle of modern man (fast food, high sugar consumption, too little exercise, etc.) lead to an increased prevalence of diseases of the digestive and intestinal system. Even in the healthy population we find very few people whose intestinal tract proves to be in an optimal energetic condition when tested with Körbler's method. This condition is bound to lead to dysfunctions and organic malformations in due course.

If a weakened digestive system and poor-quality, harmful food occur simultaneously and for an extended period of time, it is natural that the body should start signaling this unblissful state by producing symptoms.

Milk allergy may occur in a number of forms, and can have several factors in the background. The cause may be lactose sensitivity, casein sensitivity or sensitivity to the chemical structure of cow's milk.

The medical profession is finding that the vaccination system is becoming a crucial factor these days. Genetic factors may also play a part since people of yellow and black skin color cannot digest cow's milk and thus avoid its consumption. Therefore dieticians also usually advise people from the Far East to avoid cow's milk (e.g. macrobiotics). Hungarian genetics expert Endre Czeizel reported that 33% of the Hungarian population is sensitive to cow's milk for genetic reasons and thus milk consumption is responsible for a great deal of digestive disorders (bloating, wind, diarrhea, etc.).

My own professional experience shows that the chemical structure of cow's milk may be one of the factors causing this sensitivity, as cow's milk contains L-lactic acid, while the consumption of ewe's or goat's milk, which contains D-lactic acid, causes no problem whatever. The simple fact that industrially produced milk and dairy products are of poor quality and a risk for our body may, however, also be playing a part.

What Can We Do in Daily Practice to Avoid the Symptoms?

Lactose sensitivity may be eliminated if we only consume milk in fermented forms. In the case of casein sensitivity, however, the entire digestive system requires treatment. If problems with the digestive system go back to sensitivity to amalgam or heavy metals, it is almost impossible to restore the digestive system and eliminate milk allergy without homeopathic treatment. Cases of amalgam sensitivity need homeopathic treatment even if the patient no longer has amalgam fillings. Toxic factors caused by vaccinations also need to be eliminated by homeopathic means. Moreover, medical experience shows that if we eliminate sugar consumption (white and brown sugar alike), milk allergy usually stops.

It is worth exploring whether milk from one single cow is also harmful for the body or whether it is merely the commercially available industrial milk. It is a known fact that each individual cow produces a different protein structure. It is possible that milk from a single cow proves favorable for a person, while mixing the milk of a number of animals is unfavorable.

People with that kind of sensitivity find no relief in drinking organic milk if it comes from a number of cows. In the best case it influences the degree of harm; in other words the dowsing rod will only produce vertical movements (vector position 5) and not circle to the left (vector positions 6–7–8).

It is a commonly known fact that the quality of industrial milk is also greatly influenced by the drugs and hormones that the animal receives, as well as the production processes of the industrial milk. We tend to ignore this fact, since taking it on board would mean giving up advantages in quantity in exchange for quality and for our own health. In fact, even in the case of good-quality organic milk, if it is produced in industrial conditions we need to consider the following factors, not to mention non-organic milk.

According to Hungarian regulations, for instance, all dairy products are made from pasteurized milk. The milk is skimmed by skimming machines and the 30–40% cream which results is then homogenized; in other words the little balls of fat inside it are dispersed by mechanical collisions. The homogenized cream is then re-added to the milk in the required quantity. This is how milk with 1.5% or 3.6% fat is produced. This is followed by pasteurization, which means that the milk is heated to a temperature of 86 °C for a duration of 1–40 seconds and instantly cooled off. This amount of time is short enough for the milk sugar not to caramelize and for the proteins not to coagulate. Ultra pasteurization (ultra heat treatment), however, means that the milk is heated to 126 °C for 1 second, resulting in a bacterium-free milk which does not contain a single living germ. This is why UHT milk can be kept for a long time without refrigeration. It is hard to tell, however, how our digestive system can cope with a milk of this kind.

As regards fermented milk products, these are also first pasteurized, then cooled to 30–40 °C and injected with various cultures. Cheeses are matured for varying lengths of time. Mature cheeses are favorable for the body and easy to digest, while unripe cheeses are unfavorable. Consuming them over a long time turns cheese into an allergenic factor.

Identifying Milk Allergy with the Method of New Homeopathy

Knowing all this, the question remains whether Körbler's method enables us to examine such a multitude of factors. The answer is a clear yes. On April 29–30, 1995, we gave an advanced course in *New Homeopathy* in Gut Schlickenried, Munich, Germany. We demonstrated testing for milk allergy on the 37 students present. We acquired the necessary samples of organic milk from a homestead farm in Lochen. Complying with our request they provided us with some newly acquired, hand-milked fresh milk from one single cow, as well as machine-milked organic milk from several cows. We also curdled some of both kinds of milk, without any heat treatment. Thus we used the following milk samples for our experiments, in glass containers:

1. homogenized milk in tetra packaging (3.5% fat);
2. Meggle factory-made coffee cream (10% fat);
3. fresh organic milk hand-milked from a single cow;

4. fresh organic milk hand-milked from a single cow, curdled;
5. fresh organic milk machine-milked from multiple cows, curdled.

Naturally, students did not know which bottle contained which milk sample. The course of the testing went as follows:

1. Testing in pairs over the right hemisphere

Students tested each other in pairs (hand held over the right hemisphere, using the dowsing rod), and identified the persons who showed an allergic reaction when pronouncing the phrase 'cow's milk' out loud. Guidelines for evaluating test results are as follows:

- If the dowsing rod swings horizontally, the cow's milk is favourable to the organism.
- If the dowsing rod swings vertically, there is a case of milk sensitivity and the cow's milk is unfavourable to the body.
- If the dowsing rod circles to the left in any form, consuming cow's milk will produce an allergic reaction in the organism. Allergy manifests itself in many different ways varying from person to person.

Out of 37 students, 11 showed an allergic reaction to milk upon testing. We then went on to examine all of the 11 students in the following manner.

2. Testing individuals

a) We test the top of the head and the psychomeridian to find out whether the individual is testable or not. If not, we correct this condition using the methodology of New Homeopathy.
b) We test the allergy point used in kinesiology, which is in front of the right ear.

- If the dowsing rod moves horizontally, there is no allergy.
- If the dowsing rod moves vertically, we are witnessing a case of milk sensitivity which has not manifested in symptoms.
- If the dowsing rod makes any kind of circling movement to the left, the performance of the immune system is feeble and this is expressed by various symptoms such as digestion problems, frequent infections of the upper respiratory tracts, asthma, neurodermatitis, etc.). Experience shows that in cases like this the body shows an allergic reaction to certain foods and chemicals just as when testing the allergy point.

c) We test the amalgam point used in kinesiology, which is between the right wing of the nose and the upper lip. Movements of the dowsing rod are to be interpreted in the same way as when testing the allergy point:
   - If the dowsing rod swings horizontally, there is no amalgam sensitivity.
   - If the dowsing rod swings vertically, there is a case of amalgam sensitivity.
   - If the dowsing rod circles to the left, we are witnessing a case of allergy, which usually manifests in dysfunctions of the digestive system. This reaction is possible even if the person has had no amalgam fillings for years, but it can also occur if fillings, false teeth and inlays are made of various metals.

d) We test the milk samples by having the subject touch the samples with his/her left index finger, while the tester tests the reaction over the right hemisphere and records the movement of the dowsing rod.
   - If the dowsing rod swings horizontally, the milk sample is favourable.

- If the dowsing rod swings vertically, the milk sample is unfavourable.
- If the dowsing rod makes any kind of circling movement to the left, the milk sample is evoking an experience of the organism whereby cow's milk consumed in the past proved to carry harmful information; therefore we call this an allergic reaction.

The results of our tests are shown in *Figure 128.*

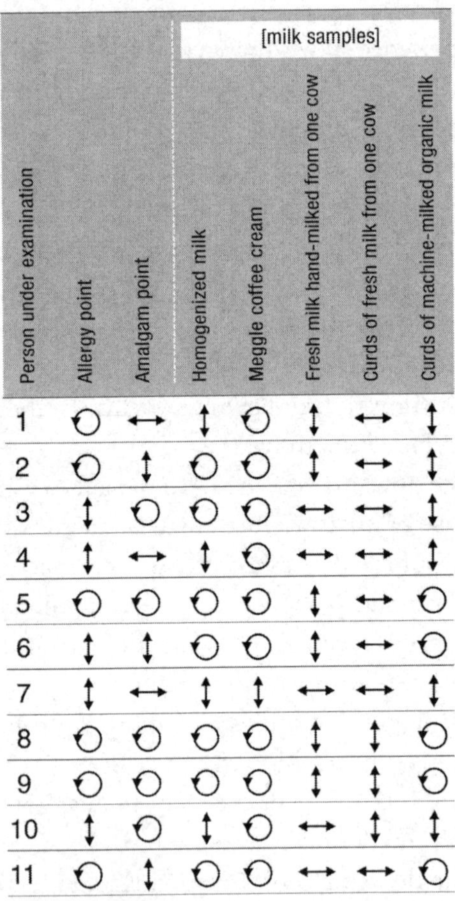

			[milk samples]				
Person under examination	Allergy point	Amalgam point	Homogenized milk	Meggle coffee cream	Fresh milk hand-milked from one cow	Curds of fresh milk from one cow	Curds of machine-milked organic milk
1	↺	↔	↕	↺	↕	↔	↕
2	↺	↕	↺	↺	↕	↔	↕
3	↕	↺	↺	↺	↔	↔	↕
4	↕	↔	↕	↺	↔	↔	↕
5	↺	↺	↺	↺	↕	↔	↺
6	↕	↕	↺	↺	↕	↔	↺
7	↕	↔	↕	↕	↔	↔	↕
8	↺	↺	↺	↺	↕	↕	↺
9	↺	↺	↺	↺	↕	↕	↺
10	↕	↺	↕	↺	↔	↕	↕
11	↺	↕	↺	↺	↔	↔	↺

Figure 128. Milk allergy

If we analyze the table we arrive at the following results:

- Out of the 11 persons testing themselves and each other there was only one who showed no allergic reaction to any of the milk samples, only an 'unfavourable' response.
- All other persons (10) showed an allergic reaction to Meggle coffee cream.
- No one proved allergic to hand-milked fresh milk from a single cow; nor to the curds made from this milk.
- The organic curdled milk from several cows was not favourable to any of the persons; it was either unfavourable or provoked an allergic reaction.

In each of the tested persons we found sensitivity at the allergy and amalgam points or at both. If we compare these results with those of the milk samples, we get closer to the root cause of milk allergy.

1. As regards the first person tested, the allergy point produces an allergic reaction, and the amalgam point shows a good reaction. Of the milk samples, only Meggle coffee cream produced an allergic reaction. Curds from a single cow are favourable to the organism; the other milk samples are unfavourable. The person proves sensitive to both lactose and the mixture of several protein structures.
2. In the case of the second person tested, the allergy point shows an allergy, the amalgam point only a sensitivity. As regards milk samples, both types of industrial milk provoke an allergic sensitivity, while in the range of fresh samples the curds from a single cow proved favourable to the organism, and the other two samples prove unfavourable. The tested person proves sensitive to lactose and to heat treatment.
3. As regards the third person tested, the allergy point shows only sensitivity, while the amalgam point shows

allergy. Of the milk samples, industrial types of milk provoke allergy; organic types of milk do not. Fresh and fermented organic milk from a single cow proved favourable; the mixed fermented milk proved unfavourable. The tested person is sensitive to mixing various protein structures and to industrial types of milk. Thus it is probable that in the absence of milk cultures which become lost during the heat treatment of industrially produced milk, the intestinal system debilitated by amalgam allergy is no longer able to process these types of milk product.

4. The fourth person showed sensitivity at the allergy point but not at the amalgam point. Nevertheless there was an allergy to Meggle coffee cream, while organic fermented milk from several cows proved unfavourable. The two milk samples from single cows both proved highly favourable. It is likely that the disturbing effect comes from a mixture of various protein structures.
5. As regards the fifth subject, despite the fact that the allergy and amalgam points showed allergy, in terms of milk samples the fermented fresh milk from one cow proved favourable, fresh milk from a single cow merely unfavourable. In this case the causes in the background of the milk allergy are the mixture of different protein structures, lactose sensitivity and the production of industrial milk. All of this becomes clear if we are talking about an organism burdened by amalgam sensitivity and the resulting condition of the digestive system.
6. The sixth person we tested showed sensitivity at the amalgam and allergy points, yet produced the same reaction to milk samples as the previous (fifth) person. This means that this person's organism has a more unfavourable relationship to milk than the previous person.
7. With the seventh person we found no allergic reaction to any of the milk samples; the industrial milk and the or-

ganic fermented milk proved unfavourable. Both milk samples from a single cow proved highly favourable.

8–9. Persons 8 and 9 both showed allergies both at the allergy and the amalgam points, and the same happened upon testing industrial milk samples and mixed organic fermented milk. Milk from a single cow proved merely unfavourable. It is probable that in both cases we are talking about casein sensitivity, the cause for which can be explored through further testing.

10. The tenth person we tested showed an allergic reaction at the amalgam point and only sensitivity at the allergy point. Nevertheless, Meggle coffee cream provoked an allergic reaction. Fresh organic milk from a single cow proved favourable to the organism. In cases like this it is probable that if we manage to eliminate the body's exposure to amalgam, further testing on a similar milk sample will produce a more favorable result.

11. In the case of the eleventh person we tested, the allergy point, as well as the testing of industrial milk samples and mixed organic fermented milk, provoked allergic reactions from the body; while testing the amalgam point showed a mere sensitivity. In spite of all of this both milk samples from a single cow proved favourable. The problem in this case probably came from the treatment of industrial milk and the mixture of different protein structures.

This means that not a single one of these cases was genuine milk allergy, since the samples of fresh organic milk from a single cow did not provoke allergic reactions in any of them and only proved unfavourable to two persons (Nos. 8 and 9). The other nine persons examined found at least one of the fresh milk samples favourable to their organism, while four of them found both fresh samples favourable.

Testing for the Root Cause of Milk Allergy

If we wish to get an exact understanding of the cause of milk allergy the procedure starts by

1. asking the person to repeat out loud the name of the possible causes, for instance,
   - 'lactose, lactose, lactose';
   - 'mixture of different protein structures';
   - 'heat treatment of the milk'.

These provide us with answers in the same way as during testing when the person repeats the phrase 'cow's milk' out loud.

2. Next we need to identify what other food allergies are combined with the cow's milk allergy. Experience shows that it practically never stands alone. It is a good idea to test the entire food list in the way we described in Issue No. 1/1994 of *Természetgyógyász.* If there is not enough time to test through the entire food list, we at least need to test cheese, fats, meats and even vegetables such as carrots and different types of beans.

3. As a next step, we need to test the organism of the person under examination, to find out what sort of functional or possibly organic disturbances (e.g. of the large intestines, small intestines, pancreas, liver, gall, etc.) may be in the background of the difficulty in processing milk.

4. The following step is to explore the psychological factors that led to the food sensitivity we are dealing with, which means exploring the subject's interpersonal relationships by testing the psychomeridian.

5. Finally, we need to establish the date when the milk allergy started, also by testing the psychomeridian.

   In the experiment described, we established that in the case of the eleventh person the milk allergy started when the person was 27 weeks old. For the age of 24 weeks the testing only showed an unfavourable reaction to cow's milk.

Eliminating Milk Allergy

Putting an end to milk allergy always requires a complex approach. We need to attend to both psychological and physical factors, since the current symptom is the result of a long process. It may have prevailed for years or even decades and, as such, it may be extremely deeply ingrained in our information storage system.

Stages of the process of recovery are the following:

1. Consuming the foods which produce an allergic reaction (milk, butter, yoghurt, kefir, cheeses, etc.) must be avoided during the period while we modify the harmful information about cow's milk in the psychological and physical domains of the body and rectify the functional and organic disturbances which developed as a result.

2. We can find the healing symbol that is best suited for modifying the harmful information associated with the time when the milk allergy started. We must always reckon with the earliest time in question. If the milk allergy started
   - at the age of 3 years, that is what we reckon with;
   - at the age of 6 months, we reckon with that;
   - at the age of 3 weeks, that is the age we work with.

We also use testing in order to find out how many days of practice are required to modify the harmful information. For instance, the subject needs to look at the symbol of a vertical line followed by a sine curve |∿ for 4 minutes a day for 9 days and repeat out loud 'I am 3 months old' if that was the age when the milk allergy developed.

The eleventh person who took part in our experiment, for instance, needed the symbol of two vertical lines followed by a sine curve ||∿. He was 27 weeks old when the trauma happened. He had to look at the symbol ||∿ and the words '27 weeks' for 21 days.

3. We must use the method of New Homeopathy, i.e. geometric symbols, to correct the energetic state of the organism.

4. We must apply natural substances to help purify the body (Bio-St. Joseph products, minerals, etc.).

5. We must apply substances which carry higher-level information (homeopathy, Körbler tree-blossom remedies) in order to support optimizing psychological and physical functions.

6. Once we have successfully completed processes 1–5 we may retest the previously tested foods. If the reaction to the foods is clearly positive, we can start returning to consuming the food in question, but always paying attention to the quality of the food and to moderation.

7. Obviously we should only eat the foods which prove favourable to the body upon testing. It is possible that, for instance, Meggle coffee cream will never be favorable for the organism even after its recovery, so its consumption must be avoided. (It is worth finding out the mechanism by which it is produced, which would explain why.)

On this occasion we test not through the right hemisphere, since after correction all milk samples should be favourable by this time, but through the right hand of the subject. If in this case the food provokes an unfavourable or harmful reaction, the result is clearly due to the quality of the food. We must not expect our organism to welcome food which is harmful by its very quality. In fact, Körbler's wonderful invention teaches us to take into account and follow the reactions of our body, since our organism is always 'smarter' than we are. Our body is never mistaken.

Chapter 17

The Impact and Measurement of Harmful Influences in the Everyday Environment[1]

Although different types of earth radiation have been empirically identified through the history of radiesthesia, contemporary science still does not look on them as real, due to the fact that they cannot be measured by instruments. In fact, empirical observations about their effect have been present throughout time.

Spiritus Loci – the Spirit of the Site

Examining people's living environment is not a modern invention. People have always been interested in 'the spirit of the site'. The profession of the contemporary experts in radiesthesia has also been known for a long time; these experts were simply called by different names. In fact, in ancient cultures this knowledge was part of the common stock of knowledge – people would not build a church or a temple unless the spot was proven to be a 'power place'. The building process itself often followed rules which have been lost by now and which make their impact felt in the cultural treasures of humanity to this day. (See e.g. the internal force-fields of cathedrals, pyramids, etc.) The ancient Romans used to rely on ant nests to determine where a house was to be built (wherever an ant nest stays together, the place is unsuitable for building), even though the environment was simpler at that time as regards harmful environmental effects. It was common knowledge for ordinary people that a place where a dog will lie down is a good spot to sit around, while a spot where a cat will lie down is best avoided. Animals sense accurately the radiations of their environment and a good master will build his sties or stables with the same care as his own house. Only contemporary man believes that all of this is superstition. In fact most of us know very well how certain spots make one feel sleepy, tired or unhappy. Different places can be favourable, unfavourable or expressly harmful for us and this is a common truth, similarly to what we know about food, clothes, cosmetics or chemicals.

As regards surveys of this phenomenon, the most remarkable is, to mention just one example, Gustav Freiherr von Pohl's research done in 1929 in the Bavarian village of Vilsbiburg, Germany. Pohl examined every single house of this village, no fewer than 565 buildings. With his magic rod, and in the presence of official witnesses, he was looking for signs of earth radiation. He marked the spots in the ground plan of each house which he believed could be bad for people's health. After the survey, the village doctor compared the data with the contents of his own files on his patients and found, to his astonishment, that Pohl marked exactly the spots where people over the previous 25 years had suffered from or died of cancer.

How Do Plants and Animals React to Geopathic Radiation?

The literature of radiesthesia gives detailed attention to the sensitivity of both plants and animals to geopathic radiations. In the following section, we present a few examples based on Czeslaw Spychalski's work.[2] Although in previous times this property of plants and animals was common knowledge for people living close to nature, modern people have lost this knowledge, due to their urban lifestyle.

It is a good idea to observe which plants find it harmful and which ones find it favorable if they grow over a water vein. In the same way, it is interesting which animals avoid and which ones like water veins.

Reaction of Various Plants to Geopathic Radiation

Trees sensitive to geopathic radiation

Most trees develop better in areas free of geopathic radiation; in fact they only show optimal development in such territory. These trees include birch, silver fir, lime trees, elms, chestnuts, scots pine, silver birch, hazelnuts. Fruit trees of this kind are apple, pear, plum, cherry, sour cherry, apricot and peach, while berries include gooseberries, currants and grapes.

There are many fruit trees which become seriously sick if they grow above water veins or at the intersection of such veins. Their yield goes down, their branches dry out and at the same time they develop thick sections, cracks and growths on their trunks. These extra-thick tree trunks are characterized by a disorganized tissue of tree fibers which is extremely valuable for furniture-makers, particularly in the case of silver birch trees. Cracks on the branch of young trees, often attributed to frost, are particularly common on trees which grow over water veins. The extent of the sickness depends on the intensity of the radiation of the water vein. Peach trees are the most sensitive – in fact they will not put down a root over a water vein at all. If the trunk stands next to an area which lies over a water vein, i.e. a part of the crown of the tree bends over the water vein, it will not yield fruit despite a profusion of blossom. Another part of the crown of the same tree, which stands over an area free of geopathic radiation, gives a rich harvest and yields fine-quality fruit.

An experiment with sour cherry trees has revealed that the position of the growths on the tree trunk betrays the depth of the water veins underneath them. If the growth is, say, 3 m above ground, the water vein is around 10 m underground. The closer the growth is to the ground, the deeper we find the water vein.

Plants particularly sensitive to geopathic radiation

As regards common vegetables, the following are particularly sensitive: beetroot, peas, cucumbers, leeks, lettuce, sorrel, potatoes, cauliflowers, kohlrabi and rosemary. Peas are very sensitive, but cucumbers are even more so – planted over a water vein they will soon die. Cauliflowers develop small flowers on long stems despite the most attentive care, and kohlrabi will crack, no matter how well we tend to it.

Gooseberries and currants are also very sensitive to water veins. These bushes rarely grow over water veins at all, but if they do, their leaves go brown around the end of May or June and then drop off. This means that by the time their little berries ripen, there are practically no leaves left on the bushes.

It is quite common in orchards and glasshouses, or even in cultivated fields, to see strips of land covered in plants which are not as well developed as the rest, even if the entire field received the same kind of treatment. The common belief is that the quality of the land is inferior along these strips, whereas in fact the reason for poorer development is that underneath the strip there is a water vein of the same width.

Further plants sensitive to geopathic radiation are evergreens, roses, marigolds and tobacco.

Plants favoring geopathic radiation

Trees which show a healthy development over water veins and even at their intersections include oaks, weeping willow, red pine, maple and walnut trees.

Vegetables of this quality are radishes, onions, garlic, chives, celeriac, beans, carrots, tomatoes and rhubarb.

Plants which flourish under circumstances of this kind include oats, clovers, lilac, elderberries, hawthorn, ferns, viscum, foxglove, *Atropa belladonna,* autumn crocus, hemlock, pink morning glory *(Ipomoea),* cow parsley, buttercups, thistles, mugwort, narrowleaf plantain, various mosses and lichens. Stinging nettles and shepherd's purse also grow best at the intersection of water veins. Mushrooms also like water veins.

Reactions of Various Animals to Geopathic Radiation

Animals avoiding geopathic radiation

Animals in this category find water veins harmful. The first signs are usually loss of appetite and lethargy, as well as swollen legs. Animals move about restlessly, but refuse to lie down even though they are apparently tired.

Cows get cramps, spasms; they become infertile or frequently miscarry. Occasionally their uterus becomes malformed or their udders develop inflammations. In summertime their hair becomes long and shabby, their milk yield is low, and in the fields they chew at the remains of burnt-out grass as if they did not notice the nearby lush vegetation which grows over the water vein. Calves are born underweight and often rheumatic. Mortality rate among calves is high under such circumstances.

Pigs develop a cough and do not gain weight even if fed on the best fodder. Medical treatment by the vet remains ineffectual; pigs perish one after the other.

If you herd sheep into a pen which is over a water vein, they will stop at the gateway. If forced to move on, they will quickly leap over the radiation streak and conglomerate in one corner even if the whole pen is free.

Hens in a roost will choose to sit on the ground, free of radiation, rather than on a beam which radiates.

In cases like this it is crucial to build a new pen, sty or stable in an area which we examine beforehand; or we need to implement devices which neutralize geopathic radiation and eliminate disturbance zones that could cause disease.

Dogs tend to avoid areas over water veins and radiation hubs. Birds (except for magpies) build their nests on trees which are in areas free from radiation. Houses and trees with a stork's nest on them are never struck by lightning. It is widely known that lightning usually strikes at the intersection of water veins. Rural wisdom has it that you should build your house where the stork makes her nest and look for water where the magpie makes hers.

Animals favoring geopathic radiation

Cats tend to look for intersections of water veins and spend long periods of time there. Bees are also quite happy close to water veins. Beekeepers take advantage of this and build their hives over water veins. This way they get at least twice as much honey as at other places, and also create better life conditions for the bees. Similarly, wasps, mosquitos and different types of flies, ants and termites also favor a habitat near the intersection of water veins.

Earth Radiations and Electrosmog from a Scientific Point of View

As regards earth radiations, scientific forums studying their impact on living organisms began to appear in the 1980s. In Munich, for instance, 12 noted scientists of Ludwig Maximilian University, headed by Professor Dr Betz, carried out investigations in this area. They proved that the living organism does indeed 'notice' water veins, i.e. there are measurable reactions in 'biological macrosystems'.

With regard to electrosmog the question is not whether it exists or not, since all scientists are agreed about that. What is debated is whether our body perceives it and whether it has any harmful effect on us. Research began as far back as the 1930s. During World War II, science was enriched with a multitude of experience and ideas in this respect, too. Then, from the 1980s onwards, to this very day there has been an increasing number of research projects in developed countries which clearly prove the unfavorable effect of electrosmog on the living organism. However, daily practice habitually ignores this kind of information, due to the advantages which modern technical civilization affords. It is enough to think of the enhanced exposure to electrosmog in urban settings. Throughout the 1990s, a number of biological research findings came out which used experimental evidence to prove that living organisms are in close interaction with the surrounding electromagnetic and quantum fields. A collection of papers edited by Ho, Popp and Warnke[3] presents results which demonstrate such sensitivity of living organisms in all fields of life. Ulrich Warnke, a scientist at Saarbrücken University, describes the results of many years' research in chapter 15 of this collection, headed 'Electromagnetic Sensitivity of Animals and Humans'.[4] He highlights the following. It is a self-evident fact that in the course of phylogenetic adaptation the natural magnetic fields of the Earth have acted as important information carriers for the creatures living on Earth, with different species sensing it in different ways. Species on the lower rungs of development have special receptors and sensory organs for absorbing the signs of magnetic and electromagnetic fields.

Fish, for instance, are guided by magnetic fields in the sea. Termites build their hills along the North–South axis of the Earth. Carrier pigeons can sense fluctuations in the magnetic field amounting to no more than a few nanoTesla (nT), and bees also orient themselves and communicate with the help of the Earth's magnetic field. Migrating birds tend to fly parallel or at a right angle to the force fields of the magnetic field. Whales also sense the Earth's magnetic field.

The human organism is so sensitive that even without dedicated receptors our nervous system absorbs electromagnetic impulses of the 10–50 kHz range. These affect our body directly. The photon–photon system which transmits and stores information directly perceives the frequencies absorbed in the electromechanical process. For instance, the magnetic effect of the Earth influences our sleep, enzyme metabolism, daily biorhythm, the hormone secretion of the central nervous system, the levels of vitamin B1 and iron in the blood serum, the average temperature of the skin and our twilight vision.

The problem begins when artificial magnetic and electromagnetic fields begin to interfere with the natural magnetic fields of the Earth. The human organism can sense these and reacts to them. We live our modern life amid artificial magnetic fields with an intensity ranging from a few nT to about 1 million T. As a result, some of the neurons in our brain become synchronized and this effect continues even when the outside influence has ended.

In this synchronized condition the excitatory post-synaptic potential (EPSP) of the cells becomes multiplied. If, for instance, only 1% of our cells become synchronized, the voltage of their EPSP will be ten times higher than the total EPSP of all the rest of the cells. In other words, from this time on, the oscillatory cells of the organism work with the new resonance information. This has a great many harmful consequences for the body. For instance, the cell receptors in the walls of the blood vessels undergo a reduction in receptivity due to the fact that secretion of adrenaline, noradrenaline and cortisone goes down. Free nerve endings become more sensitive to stimuli by virtue of the fact that the frequency of the oscillator cells in the brain is altered, as are insulin secretion, insulin reception and the breaking down of fatty acids.

Artificial magnetic fields also influence the quality of our sleep. The pineal gland is sensitive to their effect. When our nervous system resonates with the natural magnetic fields of the Earth, i.e. in the normal waking state, it does not produce melatonin. At night, when our brain is in a theta state, it switches off these resonances, in order to guarantee the healthy hormone chain reaction required for good sleep (tryptophan–serotonin–melatonin–vasotocyn–somatropine). If in the course of sleep our head is exposed to high- or low-frequency magnetic transmitters such us magnetic irons, iron shelves or spiral staircases, radiators, small household appliances that run on direct current, mobile phones, televisions, power transformers for halogen lamps, high-voltage electric cables, or 50 Hz frequency power supplies and their harmonics), and to this the oscillatory activity in the brain may respond by increases in frequency, and thus a resonance develops or is preserved between the brain and the magnetic space. This will disturb the functioning of the normal hormone chain reaction and will not produce enough melatonin for deep sleep. The most recent cancer research has shown that the presence of melatonin in the organism is required for preventing and blocking carcinogenic processes. Very low-intensity magnetic fields which appear around 50 Hz actually stimulate the multiplication of cancerous cells.

Identifying and measuring harmful radiation

Körbler developed his own theory and practical method for both defining and neutralizing geopathic radiations and artificial electromagnetic radiations. Where his method differs from previous methods of radiesthesia is that he could identify in detail the effect of harmful environmental radiation on the body of individuals. A site that is tolerable for one person may well be expressly harmful for another person. Besides being able to measure individual geopathic impulses separately, he treated them in the same category as harmful artificial radiation and explored their total effect.

In *Chapter 4* we described in detail Körbler's method of exploring water veins, geological fault-lines, lateral radiations, hubs, and the testing of satellite broadcasting stations and electric cables in the wall.

Körbler used a trifield meter[5] for measuring electrosmog. The aim of the trifield meter is to define the electric, magnetic, radio and microwave qualities of a place. In an optimal case the value is 0 mG. A healthy average adult person can tolerate up to 1–3 mG, although for small children even this level can be dangerous. According to Swedish research, children sleeping under such conditions run a 4 times higher risk of cancer. For all that, electromagnetic exposure can be 10–20 mG when sitting in front of a computer; 25–100 mG on an international train; and 100–1000 mG near electric meters, high-voltage cables or poorly mounted electric networks.

Besides his own experimental data Körbler was also well acquainted with the latest scientific findings. It was in line with all of this that he developed his diagnostic method and his techniques for screening. He discovered that unhealthy radiations in the nanometer range can be modified by geometric symbols that act as antennas. In frequency zones higher or lower than the said range this method will not work. Therefore he always began the environmental exploration of the living organism, i.e. the living space and the workplace, with instrumental measurements.

If the needle of the trifield meter sways, first you need to get technical help or switch off the machinery. If the needle of the trifield meter stays on zero, next comes the use of the dowsing rod. This instrument will indicate results in the same way as in all other examinations. If it swings horizontally, the quality of radiation is acceptable.

The Body's Reaction to Harmful Radiation – Testing with the Körbler Method

The present authors have carried out a number of experiments to demonstrate how the dowsing rod indicates the effect of geopathic radiation and of satellite stations on individuals.

If you choose a point on your body which has a good energy, and then test it as you stand over a water vein, you will find that the same point now provokes the dowsing rod to swing vertically. If you once again stand over a good spot and choose a point on your body which has an unfavorable energy where the dowsing rod moves vertically, and again examine this spot standing over a water vein, the energetic condition of that point will also shift to its opposite and move horizontally. The experiment shows quite clearly why it is tiring for the organism to sit for a long time over a water vein (say, in the workplace), or to sleep in a spot which is over a water vein. Owing to the coherence of the organism, in the case of a more or less healthy organism we always find that the greater part of the energy supply of the organism is favorable, i.e. the dowsing rod swings horizontally upon examination, and only at certain spots do we find areas which are less favorable than required. We can define the quality of these with the help of Körbler's vectors. We find signals circling to the left or right or swinging vertically, depending on the quality of health.

If someone spends a longer period of time over a water vein, the organism's level of coherence descends. This means that the healthy parts of the body are shifted into a negative energy condition and previously negatively charged parts of the body become favorable. They are now in a positive energy condition. However, the positive energy condition of smaller parts of the body is not sufficient to sustain the health and coherence of the organism. In a situation like this, parts that were previously negatively charged fail to recover, since the otherwise healthy organism has now become negatively charged and the previously healthy parts fail to provide energy for the recovery of the parts that are poorly energized. In places like this therefore it is not surprising if at first we feel tired and experience a bad mood or exhaustion. After a while diseases begin to appear.

In the case of lateral radiations, as well as near electric cables, if we test the healthy parts of the body, the dowsing rod will show an ellipsoid movement or swing horizontally.

At intersections of radiation, if we test the healthy parts of the body, the dowsing rod will show an ellipsoid movement to the right, while places with a previously disturbed energy will circle to the left.

What is most unfavorable for the organism is to spend time in the vicinity of a satellite station. If we examine an organism with a previously healthy energy supply in a spot like this, we find that the dowsing rod will circle anti-clockwise, i.e. to the left. This means a heavy burden on the organism at first, and after a long time it may lead to the emergence of disease.

Testing the effect of geopathic radiations: some examples

The processes described above refer to healthy organisms. If we perform the above experiments with sick organisms, we get different results. Reactions of the body differ widely, depending on the extent of health or sickness, as well as on age.

The test procedure was the following. The subject was tested first in a favorable site, then over a water vein and finally at an intersection point, in the following order: top of the head; psychomeridian; meridian points kidney 3; large intestine 1; small intestine 3; spleen 6; and then lungs 1 and stomach 36 as required.

According to our experience, it is the testing of the top of the head that shows the overall condition of the organism, while testing the psychomeridian shows the quality of the functional problems in the organism.

We present a few examples below:

> **A 40-year-old man.** *A strong and healthy man of 40, who is practically never ill, came to us with a rash which appeared on his chest as a consequence of sunbathing. His test results were as follows.*
>
> *In his intestines the energy supply diverged from the healthy state. The dowsing rod showed an ellipsoid movement to the right at points large intestine 1, small intestine 3 and spleen 6. It moved vertically upon examining the psychomeridian but was*

favorable for the overall energy condition of the rest of the body. The overall condition was shown by a horizontal movement over the top of the head.

When the subject stood over a water vein, kidney point 3 provoked the dowsing rod to make an ellipsoid circling to the right, while at spleen 6 it swung horizontally, and circled to the left when testing the intestines. When we examined the psychomeridian it showed an ellipsoid movement to the right. Testing the psychomeridian caused it to move along an ellipsoid to the right, while the overall condition was shown by horizontal movement found at the top of the head.

If the same person stood at a radiation hub the previously favorable kidney point 3 now made the dowsing rod circle in an ellipsoid shape to the right; at spleen point 6 it moved horizontally and circled to the left when testing the psychomeridian and the intestinal system. Over the top of the head, however, the dowsing rod still swung horizontally. In this man's case, therefore, the result of testing over a water vein and a radiation hub only manifested itself when testing the psychomeridian. Certain details of the measurements at the three different spots differed, but the total energy condition of the body was favorable at all three spots. It must be noted that cases like this are quite rare, but they do exist, which is why we decided that it was worth presenting. (Figure 129)

	good spot	over a water-vein	in a radiation hub
top of the head	↔	↔	↔
psychomeridian	↕	↻	↺
kidney 3	↔	↻	↻
large intestine 1	↻	↺	↺
small intestine 3	↻	↺	↺
spleen 6	↻	↔	↔

Figure 129. 40-year-old man

56-year-old man. *This man came to me with a long-standing digestion problem. When I examined him, points of the intestinal system, lungs and stomach meridians showed dysfunctions.*

With the patient standing over a water vein the same points caused the dowsing rod to circle to the left, while upon examining the top of the head the rod swung vertically. When testing kidney point 3 the circling of the dowsing rod became reversed and it swung vertically. The energy condition of spleen point 6, on the other hand, became normal.

When the patient stood in a radiation hub, the dowsing rod moved along an upright ellipsoid to the right when testing the psychomeridian and kidney point 3, and only spleen point 6 remained favorable in its energy. The totality of the organism reflected this situation by a circling movement of the dowsing rod to the left over the top of the head as well as points of the intestinal system, lungs and stomach meridians. (Figure 130)

	good spot	over a water-vein	in a radiation hub
top of the head	↻	↕	↺
psychomeridian	↻	↕	↻
kidney 3	↔	↕	↻
large intestine 1	↻	↺	↺
small intestine 3	↻	↺	↺
lungs 1	↻	↺	↺
stomach 36	↻	↺	↺
spleen 6	↻	↔	↔

Figure 130. 56-year-old man

8-year-old boy. *The experiment was also carried out on some completely healthy children. In the case here presented we measured energy radiation of a height of 1 m which is characteristic of healthy children, while at other spots we tested, the dowsing rod also swung horizontally. When the child stood over a water vein, with the exception of the top of the head, the dowsing rod* *swung vertically at all tested points, including the psychomeridian. The healthy energy level was still measurable at the top of the head but its size had become reduced to one fifth, i.e. to a mere 20 cm. At the radiation hub the dowsing rod moved in an upright ellipsoid to the right. The total energy condition of the organism was reflected in the vertical movement shown over the top of the head. (Figure 131)*

	good spot	over a water-vein	in a radiation hub
top of the head	↔ 1 m	↔ 20 cm	↕
psychomeridian	↔	↕	↻
kidney 3	↔	↕	↻
large intestine 1	↔	↕	↻
small intestine 3	↔	↕	↻
lungs 1	↔	↕	↻
stomach 36	↔	↕	↻
spleen 6	↔	↕	↻

Figure 131. 8-year-old boy

The superaddition of disturbing radiation in our environment

The results described above only inform us about the effect of geopathic radiations selected for this purpose. In daily practice one rarely comes across such 'pure' cases. This is because the effect of all other harmful environmental radiations becomes superadded, such as the already mentioned artificial electric and magnetic radiations (mobile phone, computer, household machinery, electric motors, power transformers, energy-saving light bulbs), the radiation of the building material (panel, cinder concrete), etc. In this way, the unfavorable overall effect and presence in the affected spot for a longer period mean a considerable burden for the regulation mechanism of the organism.

Modern architecture and interior design present a number of stumbling blocks as regards harmful radiations on the subtle-energy level. The quality and position of the building where people live, as well as the objects they use, all modify the nature of the original effect of water veins, Hartmann webs, etc. which finally reach the organism. Since Körbler's last stay in Budapest (1993), the subtle-energetic pollution level of our homes has changed fundamentally. The main harmful factor now is electrosmog. Thus the complex effect of unfavorable subtle radiations immeasurable by instruments has become multiplied.

Over the past 20 years, electronic technology has developed by leaps and bounds. As electrosmog increases, various instruments for measuring frequencies and analyzing electrosmog have also started to appear. Today you can buy, in normal commercial practice, anything from simple household electrosmog meters to the most complex devices for measuring any kind of electrosmog. If we only look at the range offered by a single company, for example Gigahertz Solution, Germany, there are 19 different frequency meters and electrosmog-analyzing devices advertised on their homepage, but you can also choose to buy from other manufacturers.

The situation is similar as regards research into measuring the health impact of electrosmog. Reports and warnings from developed countries appear one after the other. From the research findings of the recent years, we selected a few important facts based on reports published in the periodical *Naturartzt*.[6]

Of all the common practical objects we use, mobile phones and smartphones are the most intense source of radiation. A survey financed by the European Union has shown that the ultra high frequency radiation emitted by mobile phones is as harmful as X-rays.

The transmitters of mobile telephone networks pollute not only our own space but also the shared space of all of us, since they produce a far more intense force field than the mobile phones themselves. If there is a transmitting station of this kind on top of our building and the data and electric cables have not been screened, they also operate as radiating antennas. The various stories of the building are thus exposed to radiation, less and less powerful as we move down through the building. If you have any doubts about the antennas, certainty can only come about through adequate instrumental measurement.

Digitally enhanced cordless telecommunication (DECT) devices[7] also emit constant radiation and operate through microwaves of approximately 1900 MHz frequency. Devices like this continue to radiate even when we are not using them for conversation, and even if we did not buy a cordless supplement for the basic equipment. Every electric part related to the base station, including the receiver of that base station, acts as a radiating antenna. Cordless telephones work excellently, because their ultra high frequency radiation penetrates through roofs and walls unobstructed. Thus the cordless device of our next-door neighbor represents a more serious hazard than our own. If the neighbor is helpful, the best idea is if they can be persuaded to replace their outdated device. Should your neighbor be less cooperative, the best thing you can do is have your home tested by a professional specializing in electrosmog.

It is not for nothing that flight attendants ask us to switch off any devices that emit electrosmog. Such devices include mobile phones and smartphones, walkie-talkies, CB radios, pagers, AM/FM radios, cathode ray tube televisions, computers, printers, scanners, cordless computer accessories such as a cordless mouse, CD/DVD/M2 players with USB storage, portable electronic games, professional digital cameras and video cameras.

Lighting bodies also emit harmful radiation. During one of his stays in Budapest Körbler visited Hungarian manufacturer Tungsram's showroom in order to choose lighting bodies for the Natural Healing Hospital then under construction. He took this occasion to show us the energetic impact of various lighting bodies. He tested the series of light tubes exhibited, as well as all the bulbs that are in commercial circulation. The results were sobering and served as a warning. Even the most carefully assembled lighting tube has a highly unfavorable energetic effect – even a healthy person when standing under a light tube will provoke the dowsing rod to circle to the left. This is sad, since even the most modern hospitals have light tubes in metal casings over the heads of their patients. These people spend hours each day lying underneath these lit-up light tubes, particularly through the winter months. The same effect is responsible for the sensation of tiredness and lack of concentration which pupils experience in schools where the light tubes are positioned low in the classroom. The situation is similar with energy-saving compact bulbs.

In 1993 Körbler stated that the only lighting body with favorable radiation was the traditional pear-shaped bulb, which only produced a small electric field and practically no magnetic field at all. This is what he recommended, particularly if used close-up for extended reading, such as in a desk lamp or a bedside lamp.

However since September 1, 2009, the EU has started to gradually withdraw traditional light bulbs in order to save energy. Since that date, it is illegal to sell lighting bodies of 80 W or more. Even bulbs of a lower wattage have gradually disappeared from the shelves in stores within the EU. By 2012 all bulbs with a performance exceeding 7 W are supposed to be withdrawn from commercial circulation.

Instead of traditional lighting bodies, the customer will need to make a choice from a range of modern halogen lamps and energy-saving lighting bodies. This transition again inspired a series of studies analyzing the qualities and health effect of traditional bulbs and energy-saving lighting bodies. In the following section we present some of the most important considerations.

Energy-saving bulbs produce electrosmog, their light vibrates, and their light spectrum and colors are less favorable than those of traditional bulbs. Their only advantage is low consumption.

The electronic parts incorporated into the stem of some energy-saving bulbs produce such intense high frequency electromagnetic fields, even using the normal low frequency fields of the electric network, that even at a distance of 30 cm they strongly exceed the limits defined for low radiation screens.

The light of energy-saving lighting bodies vibrates at high and low frequencies because of the inbuilt electronic parts, and thus produces a 'dirty' light. Although our naked eye does not notice this vibration, its frequency is harmful for the eyes, the brain, our brain processes, our hormones, our nervous system, our neural processes, co-ordination, metabolism, glucose use, capillary blood supply and even the quality of our sleep. It can cause migraine, headaches or epileptic seizures. The degree of health hazard posed by a light body depends on how far its spectrum is removed from that of natural sunshine. The light spectrum of energy-saving bulbs is way below that of natural light because of its higher blue and UV content. They produce an unpleasant, strange, 'cold', bluish light. Those with a compact structure do not even attain the standard of the traditional light tubes.

Energy-saving compact light tubes contain poisonous substances, heavy metals, plastic and glue. They also contain an average of 2–5 mg of mercury each. Under the effect of heat they issue harmful substances and unpleasant smells.

Of all lighting solutions currently available, modern halogen lamps have relatively the most favourable effect on our organism, due to their strong heat and low blue light content. However, exposure to the power transformer of old-fashioned halogen lamps which operate with a transformer is equal, as Körbler pointed out, to having a rest underneath a 400 kV high-voltage cable. The electromagnetic field of a 400 kV high-voltage cable is still less harmful than being next to a power transformer.

LED-lights available today produce a cold, blinding and unnatural light. The voltage-regulating unit which is indispensable for their operation may also result in powerful vibration and electrosmog. Therefore they are mostly recommended, for the time being, for outdoor lighting.

Design lighting and light rails placed close to each other are similarly harmful, as they create a powerful magnetic field.

Besides the degree of lighting, the distribution of light also plays an important part in lighting our living environment. It is crucial that the light should have a balanced composition, containing sufficient long-wave red and infrared rays which have a regenerating effect. This requirement is met by traditional light bulbs and by halogen lamps without transformers which use network voltage. These provide a balanced light spectrum close to the natural range, as well as an almost continuous, harmonious distribution of light. In our living and working spaces, particularly over desks, it is recommended to use traditional bulbs of a light color or halogen lights without transformers.

As we have seen, results of contemporary scientific research confirm Körbler's findings and proposals from 20 years earlier.

Once we eliminate electrosmog measurable by instruments, we also need to pay attention to the unfavorable, harmful radiation disturbance zones which might result from the position and furnishings of our living space. Most people are familiar with the experience of a work space or living space which makes one feel tired, sleepy or stressy. There are cases when a place seems fine according to our measuring instruments, although this is becoming increasingly rare due to the high electrosmog level of our cities; nevertheless the experience of being present at the place is unfavorable and unpleasant. In cases like this we need to reckon with the unfavourable subtle-energetic radiations which are only sensed by living organisms. Since the extent of electrosmog coming from the outside decreases in proportion to the distance, it often happens that the instrument shows nothing in particular near a radio or television station but our organism can sense the disturbance zone.

German physician Dr. Aschoff developed a blood test which allows us to measure the damage which our body suffers due to environmental factors. He discovered that there are crystals which can divert the microwave radiation of disturbance zones. These diverted rays can penetrate through walls but are reflected by mirrors or window panes. This is what we call 'Aschoff's mirror phenomenon'.[8]

Who would believe that the sloping windows of an attic space, a badly placed mirror or a piece of metal furnishing, a lamp or a bookshelf, can cause a disturbance zone?

As an example, Körbler demonstrated that a circular plastic or metal waste-basket or a plastic bucket used for the same purpose can actually make people working in that office feel uncomfortable and restless, and the same can happen to a crowd of schoolchildren. The cause is that these objects reflect a combination of water veins and electromagnetic radiation and can thus create a most unfavorable radiating environment.

Exploring the combined effect of unfavorable and harmful radiations

The way in which the combined effect of geopathic and other harmful radiations can show up in our testing is by the dowsing rod producing an ellipsoid movement to the right whenever we test the usual acupuncture points. In cases like this we need to examine the places where the patient or subject usually spends his/her time, particularly the place where they sleep. If they sleep next to a radio or television station or inside its emission zone, the dowsing rod will clearly circle anti-clockwise. When we test a person in a place like this, just as in the case of being inside geopathic zones, the dowsing rod will indicate the condition of the person.

If the person is living in an environment with a high artificial electromagnetic force field, testing with the dowsing rod will reveal this, as described in the following passage.

> *It was with a German female patient that we first noticed that the dowsing rod was circling to the right when testing the usual acupuncture points. When we found the same reaction at all acupuncture points we tested, it became clear that the cause of this strange phenomenon had to be found. During the anamnesis we only recorded the usual data and questioned the patient about her complaints. Therefore we knew that she was a pharmacist by profession, but we were not acquainted with her life conditions. So now we asked her to tell us where she lived, how she spent her time and what her work was about. We soon found out that both her home and the pharmacy where she worked were alongside the suburban railway line, one on either side of the tracks. This meant that she was living in the same highly intense artificial electromagnetic field almost all of the time. Her organism had become so saturated with the harmful effects of this force field that she was impossible to examine, despite the fact that in our surgery she was in a favorable environment. Therefore we first had to eliminate this effect, to create the possibility for the dowsing rod to show the energetic qualities of the organism.*

Since that time we have experienced the same phenomenon repeatedly. An intense artificial electromagnetic force field produces a negative reaction which is indicated by the clockwise circling movement of the dowsing rod.

Our examinations show clearly that the organism perceives the totality of radiations in the environment and evaluates them in a unique manner in line with the state of the organism.

Neutralizing Harmful Environmental Effects

We have seen how Körbler's vector system can change the information of harmful electromagnetic waves. The essence of this is that the use of such geometric symbols allows the electromagnetic radiation to keep its energy but its quality becomes compatible, i.e. useful for the living organism. An electromagnetic wave which has been filtered through an interposed geometric symbol will not have a harmful effect on the human organism, even though it remains a wave, as long as the geometric symbol is actually present between the electromagnetic wave and the organism. This remains valid even if we are exploring the effect of harmful electromagnetic waves arising from the external environment (soil, neighboring building) and wish to neutralize their harmful effect.

There are several ways in which geometric symbols can be introduced between the human body and the places, devices or equipment which emit electromagnetic waves. It can be as simple as drawing the geometric symbol on a piece of linen and placing it over the body. It can be used as protective clothing, a bedsheet, wall hanging or underneath a carpet, etc. There are also numerous other ways of using geometric symbols – carved into wood, painted on a wall, etc. The result will always be the same, as geometric symbols placed in the way of radiation operate as antennas and neutralize the quality of radiation which would be harmful for the living organism or modify it to become positive.

There were three geometric symbols that Körbler used to neutralize harmful environmental effects:

- the equal-armed cross;
- a variant of five parallel lines *(Figure 132);*
- the Y symbol.

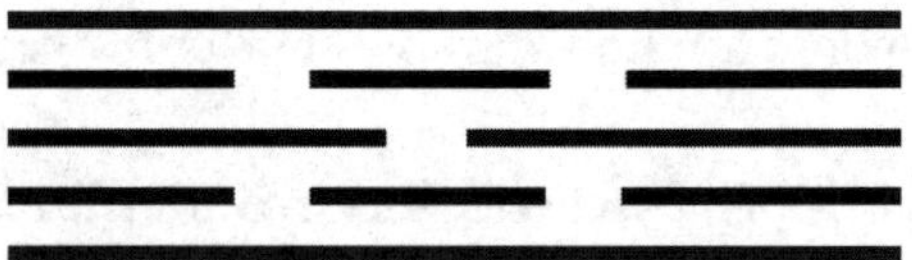

Figure 132

These were the symbols that proved most effective as shown by his experiments.

The first time I met Körbler he was sitting behind his desk in his office. During our conversation I noticed that on the wall behind him, at about the height of his head, there was an A4 sheet of paper fixed to the wall, showing five horizontal lines underneath each other, and the three in the middle were discontinuous. I asked him about the purpose of the sheet of paper. In response he showed me the effect of the five lines, which were neutralizing some lateral radiation. At the same time, he pointed out to me that a sheet of paper with a figure drawn on it should only be used for a few days at a time, because the paper would become filled with electrostatic charge and once that happens it would do more harm than good. If, however, we draw the geometric symbol on a piece of linen, that can be used for any amount of time.

Körbler often gave simple, easily executed practical advice also on how to improve the energetic qualities of the place where we spend our time, as well as those of our own body.

Below we list a few examples:

- You can draw a Y on the window pane with chalk or the edge of a bar of soap.
- You can cover your mirror with a sheet of cloth or raw silk for the night; while for the daytime you can draw a large equal-armed cross or Y on it.
- Wastepaper baskets of plastic or metal can be replaced by others made of natural material, and their position needs to be carefully chosen.
- Television sets and HIFI centers need to be turned off entirely for the night and not left on standby; and it is a good idea to cover them with silk or a piece of linen.

When you cannot improve your environment any further, you can examine whether you might be able to modify your dress habits.

- People who wear glasses should pay attention to the material and shape of the frame.
- Jewelry should be chosen so that the material and the forms are favourable to the organism, and it should only be worn for short periods at a time. In necklaces you should always insert one ring of plastic. Body piercing, however trendy with young people today, should most definitely be avoided because it is extremely harmful for the energetic condition of the head and the body.
- Your watchstrap should be made of leather rather than metal and instead of battery-run quartz watches you are better off with a traditional wind-up wristwatch.
- You should avoid using different metals and amalgam for fillings and also false teeth or bridges which are a combination of several metals. Women should avoid IUDs.

Outdoor Screening

If there is a larger outdoor area which needs to be freed of disturbances, the best solution is to construct an equal-armed copper cross, with arms 40 cm in length. We use two copper bars 3×5 mm in diameter. The size of the protected area grows in proportion to the size of the equal-armed cross. A 40 cm cross protects against earth radiation in a circle with a radius of 5 m. Equal-armed copper crosses are also extremely well suited to screen gardens.

If you wish to use geometric symbols inside your home, the best idea is to use an equal-armed cross made of the same material as the dowsing rod. This should be placed under the bed, but recent experience has shown that it is most effective if it is fixed to the wall at a right angle to the water vein, standing directly on the floor at the point where the water vein leaves the room. The size of the equal-armed cross can be 15–25 cm in each arm, depending on the place where it is used. When building a new house, the best idea is to incorporate it in the plaster or the foundation.

Indoor Screening

Indoor screening is more significant than outdoor screening. Inside the rectangular architecture used in our modern world, i.e. inside a closed system, lateral radiations are more intense, due to constant reflection, than they are out of doors; indeed, this leads to the emergence of artificial radiation networks. This can cause biological systems (humans, animals and plants) to overheat, and this will result in a decline in the function of the immune system.

There are two geometric symbols used for screening both geopathic radiation and lateral artificial and satellite radiations. One is the equal-armed cross; the other is a combination of the equal-armed cross and the Y.

As we have already mentioned in the Preface, this is the principle Körbler applied when he created his two types of transformer sheets which made him internationally acclaimed. The transformer sheet was made using a combination of equal-armed crosses, while the energy-building sheet used combinations of equal-armed crosses and Y-s, both printed in red ink. Both the pattern, and the production process, are under copyright protection.

The present authors have developed a screening device based on a combination of equal-armed crosses and Y symbols. It can be used both when an apartment is in construction and after it is finished.

The right instrument to use is selected by careful testing on each occasion.

Instruments for Screening

The equal-armed cross is 25 cm long on each arm and is made of the same material as the dowsing rod, which is thin PVC fiber 3 mm in thickness.

The material of the geometric symbol combining the equal-armed cross with the Y is the same. In the fields of the equal-armed cross we have placed two V symbols facing each other; in other words we omitted the leg of the Y. This geometric symbol is highly energizing and is suited for screening intensely unfavorable radiation. In the case of intense geopathic radiations it can be used just as well as for lateral radiations. Depending on the quality and intensity of the radiation, it may be used for screening a living space of 10–50 m^2. The combined geometric symbol is produced in two variants: one is a 'picture' in which the combination of geometric symbols has been placed between two sheets of cork. In the case of lateral radiation this is hung on the wall like a painting. It is suitable for screening satellite radiation and other combined harmful radiations if the angle at which it is suspended is accurately defined.

The second variant of combined geometric symbols may be incorporated in its elements in the plaster of a house or the foundation underneath the floor covering. This technique is presented below, under the heading 'Screening walls'.

Constructing our Home Following Körbler's Energy Considerations

As we have already mentioned, the most important consideration is the choice of site, both as regards earth radiations and artificial electromagnetic force fields. In other words, we should always avoid building next to high-voltage lines, television transmitters, etc. If there is a tram or trolleybus in the street, or even if it has a stop nearby, make sure that the house you build is as far from the street as possible.

If your home is satisfactory in this respect, the next things to reckon with in the planning process are the principles related to screening electrosmog, in other words artificial electromagnetic fields. Remember that Körbler's screening methods are only applicable in places which have no measurable electrosmog. Living spaces should be positioned in a way which enables you to avoid harmful influences related to modern heating and electric equipment. Since walls and ceilings are no obstacle to artificial radiation, a living, working or sleeping space is best positioned if it is as far removed as possible from the electronic equipment used in the service of the modern lifestyle. For instance, desks or couches should not be placed on the far side of a wall with the kitchen worktop next to it. Particular attention must be paid to the setting of children's rooms and beds. If a child's bed is on the far side of a wall behind a television set, computer or printer, the child will be sleeping or playing in electrosmog the whole time whenever these devices are used. If the electricity meter has not been screened you must make sure that you do not arrange any space where you spend considerable amounts of time (bedroom, desk, dining room, etc.) within a circle with a radius of 1.5 m around it. If this is not possible, the best idea is to screen the entire wall *(Figure 133)*.

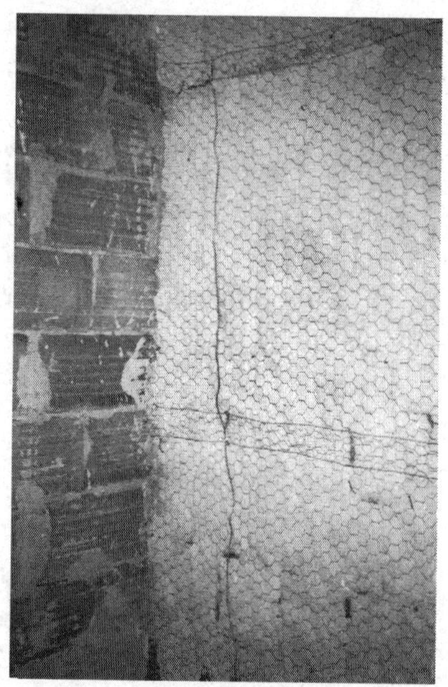

Figure 133

When creating the architectural plan it is important to pay attention to the architectural forms and the way they are executed. Even a space of optimal energy may be disturbed, for example by a reinforced concrete banister around a semicircular terrace.

The ceiling of boiler houses must be screened for electrosmog. Persons who are particularly sensitive to subtle energies should avoid using underfloor heating. When designing the pipework of your central heating, you must bear in mind how you are to design the interior later on, and leave resting and sleeping spaces free. Aluminum radiators should be avoided. When you design the interior you should also consider that sleep and work spaces should not be within 1 meter of your radiators. The same applies to spaces next to chimneys and gas convectors.

The electric network of your house should be designed with special care. The best idea is to follow the more elaborate guidelines for organic architecture which are in place in Western European countries.

Here we recommend an English and a German book on the subject[9] as manuals for screening electrosmog. They offer relatively simple and low-cost tips and shortcuts which, together with a well-designed electric plan, can help you forestall later problems.

The way you position electric cables and sockets is also very important. While the force field of electric cables and equipment declines in proportion to distance, the same is not true of sockets. If sockets are placed at the height of your bed, this will render it difficult to choose a good spot for sleeping, since no matter where you put the bed, it will be within the radiation zone of sockets from one side or more. The radiation of the socket crosses the entire room and the distance makes no difference in this case.

In the same way, it is not a good idea to place your mattress directly on the floor since if you are in a multistory building, or even on the ground floor with a cellar underneath that has lighting, there will be electric cables running inside the flooring which have a force field extending to around 50 cm. Since average modern reinforced concrete roofing is around 17 cm thick, and even with the flooring materials laid on top of it it rarely exceeds 25–28 cm, a body sleeping on a thin mattress will still be inside the force field of the cables.

If you wish to make your living space free of electricity at night, you can use a special switch which limits the voltage to 3 V.

You should use as little metal for building and furnishing as possible. Metal doors and windows should certainly be avoided.

Once you have taken all these considerations into account, the next step is to use good-quality natural building material and competent, knowledgeable builders. This is not easy, because in the wake of the spreading of industrial techniques a great deal of important knowledge and acumen has sunk into oblivion.

Builders in times past used to know that every piece of stone and every brick has a positive and a negative pole and they would fit building blocks together using their own instinct. Contemporary builders have never even heard of such a thing. If we use the dowsing rod to test the walls of churches built hundreds of years ago, the pendulum will swing intensely in a horizontal direction. If you examine a brick wall built today, you will get a very different result even if the materials are favorable when tested one by one. The case is the same as regards church mosaics created a thousand years ago. Even though a great many people have been walking on them for a thousand years, they are still intact and motionless, despite the fact that glues and cement were not known at the time when they were constructed.

A case in point is the Cathedral of Münster. Damaged during World War II, the walls were restored using the same natural stone from which they were originally built. However, the newly inserted parts soon perished. For a long time this seemed inexplicable, until the answer finally came from the old 'expert' building masters. They said that in bygone times stones used to be inserted in the wall the same way as they had been quarried, i.e. they retained their original North–South polarity. If stones are inserted haphazardly, free electrons will gradually rearrange themselves in line with the Earth's magnetic field, resulting in a depolarization which entails a loss of energy and so rocks will corrode more easily.

By using and further improving on Körbler's method we can grant good energetic conditions to our walls and flooring even under conditions of modern architecture. Interventions need to start at the plastering stage.

Screening walls

1. If you mix zeolite into the plaster, this eliminates the unfavorable effect of the unevenness of the building material and the plastering. It is useful to test the quality and grain size of the zeolite first, so that you can choose what is best. (As we have already mentioned, grain size plays a great part in healing, with everyone finding zeolite of a different grain size remedial.) Our experience shows that the energetic quality of a cellar, used as an underground storage space, can be improved adequately by mixing small to medium grain size zeolite into the plaster. The energy quality of living spaces can be improved by mixing zeolite into the last, fine layer of plaster. In cases like this it is best to use a small grain size, applying about 1.5–2 kg of zeolite for a room 4×5 m in size. *(Figure 134)*

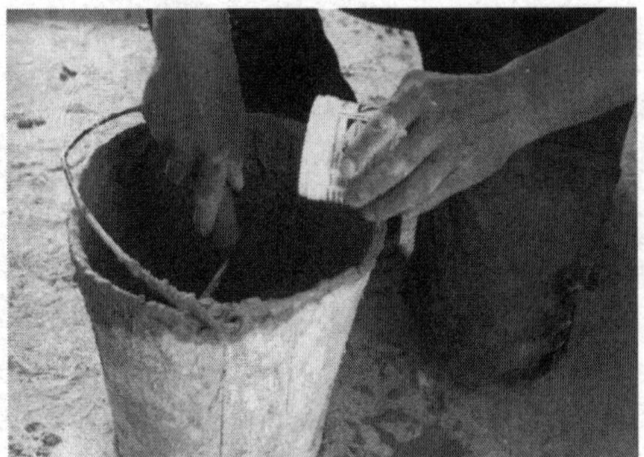

Figure 134

2. When the last layer of plaster has had 24–36 hours to dry, depending on the weather, test the energy quality of the wall surface *(Figure 135)*.
3. You only need to do more work on wall surfaces which cause the dowsing rod to produce something other than a horizontal swinging motion, such as vertical swinging or any circular

motion. At spots like this you need to test in order to find the geometric symbol that *re-informs* the energy of the spot.

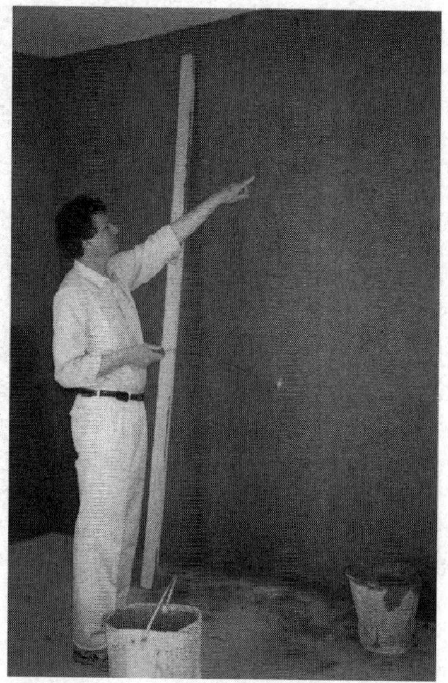

Figure 135

4. There are two types of geometric symbols you can use: one is the equal-armed cross; the other is the combination described earlier – that of equal-armed crosses and V symbols.
5. We start testing with the equal-armed cross and identify how many crosses and of what size we need to place on the given wall surface. At spots where using an equal-armed cross does not bring the desired results, you test the combination of symbols and the orientation of the V symbols. You also need to identify how many and what size you need and then measure out exactly the required arrangement of these symbols.
6. Special attention must be paid to the distance between geometric symbols. You can place up to three crosses on a wall 4–5 m long, where each arm of the cross is 25 cm long. You need to leave a space of at least 25 cm next to doors, windows or arches. You also need to test to identify the distance from corners. Experience shows that it is good to leave 25 cm at corners, too. Open stretches of wall have different dynamics than corners or wall surfaces. The same applies to the meeting of walls and floors. If you need to place several geometric

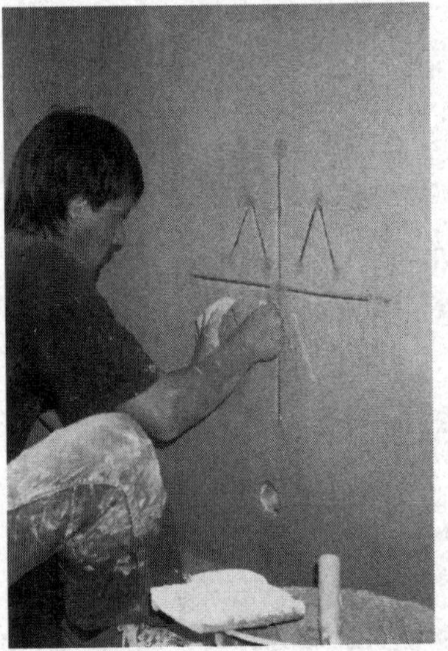

Figure 136

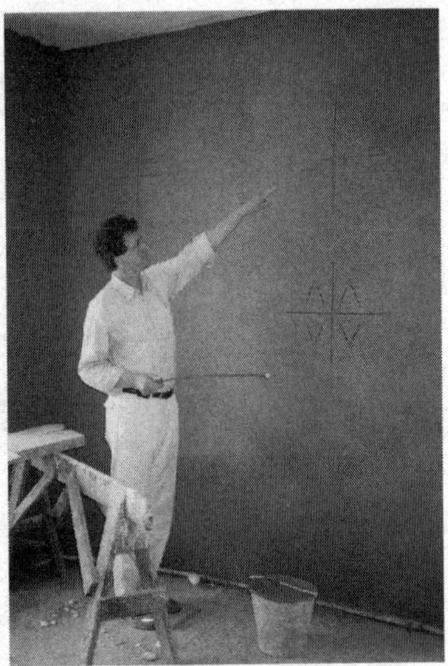

Figure 137

symbols on a wall surface, it is best to create rows or columns of them.

7. By way of control you scan the wall with your left palm held about 50 cm from the wall itself. If the dowsing rod clearly swings horizontally all over the wall surface, this shows you have done good work.

Practical implementation

1. Use cardboard to create the negative of the geometric symbols. *(Figure 139)* First draw the symbol on the cardboard in the chosen size. The width of the lines should be between 3–4 mm. Cut the symbols out with a razor blade or a sharp knife.
2. Mark the place on the wall where you want to draw the symbols, you may want to use a water level to do that. Draw a horizontal line to guide you, then at the midpoint, another line perpendicular to that.
3. Place the cardboard on the wall with the help of the „guide

lines". Using a nail, draw the symbols on the wall, remove the cardboard and widen and deepen the cuts to 3 mm. *(Figure 136)*

4. Once you have traced all the geometric symbols, you can test the surface. The dowsing rod will clearly show you the results and at this stage you still have a chance to make alterations. *(Figure 137)*
5. If the test result is clearly positive, place the prepared geometric symbols inside the traced lines.

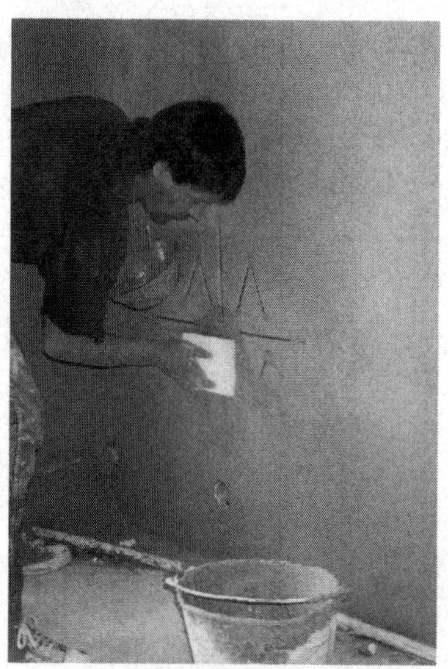

Figure 138

6. Renewed testing will cause the dowsing rod to swing more intensely in a horizontal direction.
7. As a last step, the builder smooths the geometric symbols over with the plaster containing the zeolite *(Figure 138)*.

When it comes to painting the walls, you also need to test the material of the paint. Several plastic paints have highly unfavourable radiation even after drying. The same applies to wallpaper glue. If you choose to paint the walls it is a good idea to mix zeolite into the wall paint.

Screening the flooring

Whether it is parquet flooring or stone flooring, several factors need to be taken into account. You need to test the radiation of the covering material, the substrate and the glue. In all cases it is the quality of the room which determines, for instance, what size of tile to use and what pattern to create. In some rooms it is better to use relatively small flooring panels, say 10×10, 15×15 or 20×20 cm; in others a larger kind of tiles, starting from 30×30 cm, might be more favorable.

It is also important whether you lay the tiles diagonally across or in a straight web. Whether you are using tiles or other flooring blocks you need to pay attention to the pattern even if this is seemingly insignificant, since every tile or mosaic piece also has a positive and a negative pole, just like natural stone.

If your flooring material is adequate and you have also chosen the pattern, next comes the job of screening the floor. The equal-armed crosses or, whenever necessary, the combination of symbols previously described (equal-armed crosses and V symbols; see *Figure 136)* are pressed into the base, and the mosaic or tiles are laid on top. The procedure is the same with parquet flooring.

The most effective solution is to use traditional parquet or floorboards laid over solid timber. In cases like this you insert your equal-armed cross or combination into the sand between the solid timbers. If you are fitting glued floorboards it is very important to choose the right glue. In this case the geometric symbols are inserted into whatever material you are using for leveling your base. In choosing the material for your floorboards or parquet you must reckon with personal preferences. Some people find beech wood most favourable; others prefer oak or ash. It is also crucial to test the substance you use for treating your surfaces. Even though there are a number of different lacquers and varnishes you can use today, the most favorable substance to use is beeswax. Avoid using plastic floors and fitted carpets, because they collect electrostatic charge.

When you are painting doors or windows it is important to test the paint before use, since paints with an unfavorable information content retain this content even after drying.

If you manage to make the right choices producing favorable information, the completed home will have such a good 'spirit' that it will be worth the effort of all your testing.

Appendix I

An Interview with Erich Körbler by János Déri[1]

Of all the episodes of our TV show *Close Encounters of Type Zero,* the one we created in Austria turned out to be perhaps the most controversial. Whether the subject under discussion here is pure science or a heap of well-constructed charlatanism is, unfortunately, something that everyone will have to decide according to their own convictions and desires. Passing judgment of that kind is not one of the missions of this show, nor do we have the means required for proper scientific verification. What we do know is that Erich Körbler won Eureka and Albert Schweitzer awards for his research, and the Thomas Steinmann laboratory receives a fair amount of external business commissions. Please, make your own judgments.

Who are you really, Dr. Körbler?
I am the CEO of COB Innovation. This is a company dedicated to the methodology used for developing new industrial products. Ten years ago something completely unexpected and strange happened to me. We were working on measuring the conductivity of supra-conductors when one day I noticed a diversion in measurement. What happened was that I picked up an apple and this apple noticeably altered the relationship between me and my environment. Naturally, this intrigued me. I am quite a curious soul, so I started looking for professionals near Vienna who worked with dowsing rods and perhaps could enlighten me regarding the explanation. But I could not find anyone. This meant that no one gave me an explanation of the fact

that the radiation of an apple altered our test results through one's person. What we needed to identify was: What were these radiations coming from different substances which affected the human body?

Could you explain to us what these radiations are?

Certainly. You see, all living beings absorb and emit energy. This has been shown by physical research. Communication inside our body is an electromagnetic system. All regulation in our body happens through electromagnetic waves. This is a new discovery validated internationally and this is what my work is based on.

I was looking for a type of plastic with a special conductivity and through my experiments I added copper ions, i.e. negative ions, to this plastic. This resulted in a very special conductivity. This plastic vibrates in a unique and characteristic way in the hand of every individual, reflecting the radiations affecting the person. This is a very simple tool, a modern rediscovery of the ancient dowsing rod. It has a given length and a weight at the end of the rod. It also has a set degree of flexibility and conductivity. If I pick up this tool it measures my relationship to my environment.

Give me your hand and you will also notice the horizontal swinging.

Let us perform a simple experiment. Pick this thing up in your hand – see, the movement is vertical, which shows that the thing you are holding in your hand is intolerable for both of us. This brings us to a very important point, namely that of tolerability and intolerability. It appears that people are affected by electromagnetic waves from all directions. If this is true, these influence the function of our organs, i.e. the entire human organism. In the same way, humans also emit electromagnetic waves, because it is a basic law of physics that energy is never lost. Since the human organism cannot absorb infinite amounts of energy, it also needs to emit energy. The organism works like an antenna which absorbs and emits energy.

Can I ask you a question? What are electromagnetic waves?
This is a very important question. Lots of people who work with dowsing rods and are involved in these phenomena confuse electromagnetic waves with magnetic and electric fields. These are completely different things. Magnetic fields, such as the magnetic field of the Earth, are a natural given. During our evolution we have become adapted to it. This is not harmful. The only exception is if other factors cause these fields to change. The same is true of electric fields. Measuring these fields requires no special instruments – you can measure them with completely ordinary, cheap instruments. What does affect our body are electromagnetic waves. Electromagnetic waves move; they have a certain frequency and radiation.

What is this frequency?
The frequency which affects us is higher than that of microwaves, including light frequency, infrared and UV frequency. These are the communicational frequencies of our organism. We sense the impulses which surround us within this wave band, and as a result the human organism cannot be examined individually, in an isolated manner, as it has been by medical science for centuries. To the contrary, people need to be examined within their natural setting. In other words, my organism is not just me, but me plus my environment. I demonstrate this phenomenon through a simple antenna. The antenna is a simple line on a piece of paper. The reason this works is because the conductivity of the material of the line and the conductivity of the paper are different. Therefore, within a certain frequency domain the line behaves like an antenna which receives and emits. The kind of charge pattern it emits depends on the form of the line. Let us look at this step by step. I noticed that the sides became polarized near the line. I now place my fingertip to the left of the line, my

left, and this way my instrument produces a horizontal swinging motion. When touching the right end, the instrument shows vertical motions. If I place it in the middle, the rod will stop.

The cause for this phenomenon is a static electric wave that emerges in the center line of the antenna and spreads further in the room.

However, it is not only electric fields that are produced along the antenna, but also magnetic fields which are at a right angle to it.

By using this rod, I can point out quite accurately which things are favorable or tolerable to my body and which things are not. To be sure, this is not quite the same as other people will find for themselves. But you can identify preferences for everyone, case by case.

For testing, I place the experimental material in my left hand which has a negative effect. Put it in your left hand and now give me your right hand. Now put it down. Now pick it up again. The rod will show the change instantly and this works for everyone, not only me. With a little bit of practice you can try it, too, on a person of any training or occupation. So, I look at humans not on their own, but in their natural setting, and because the environment changes all the time, you also need to examine people differently each time. This applies most of all to people who influence the health of others. This means doctors, healers, people who advise and counsel others.

We must make sure, and, of course, these persons must make sure for themselves, that they live in the most tolerable environment possible. This is the principle of preserving health – the main principle of New Homeopathy. Fundamentally, Hippocrates had already discovered New Homeopathy 2500 years ago. He wrote that disease can be best conquered by the factors which caused the disease. Today we know that, thanks to this guiding principle, the diseases do not even need to develop, provided that we just take into account the first half of the Hippocratic tenet and keep looking at the factors which provoke disease. If we explore them from the electromagnetic point of view, we need to intervene in good time and the organism will never develop the disease. In other words, the immune system which has already been weakened by harmful environmental factors will not be dealt that final blow but, to the contrary, we can strengthen our immune system once more.

This is something that all people can do for themselves, as you yourself can test whether a particular substance is favourable to you or not. You can start with the food you eat, the clothes you wear, the bed you sleep in, the building material that you use to build your house. If intolerability has become ingrained in a product, you can never remove it. It consistently makes its way into the organism through the foods, the cleaning chemicals or in any other form, and this way the radiation affecting the body becomes all-encompassing. Radiation of this kind affects us from practically everywhere and, of all of us, children are the most sensitive to it.

Why children, exactly?

Because children get an overdose of ever increasing environmental impulses and they don't get time to adapt gradually.

In everyday life we can establish which substance or textile is tolerable for us. Horizontal swinging indicates tolerability.

Now I take another substance – see, here it is in my hand, and it seems that for me it is intolerable. The active substance in one fabric strengthens my organism, while the substance of another weakens it. I have done the same test on jewelry, on everything that surrounds us, and if you wear it all the time, you need to get rid of half the things that most people like, and just live on with the rest that are healthy.

By the way, besides objects, we are also affected by what is called 'earth radiation'.

Could you tell me what earth radiation is?

These are electromagnetic rays of unknown origin. But we can influence these radiations. In order to demonstrate this, we produce artificial earth radiation in that we place in front of us an object with a negative radiation. See, the rod swings vertically, showing something negative. But what can we do against this? Again we draw a line, and another one across, and place this over the object under examination. The dowsing rod stays steady; the radiation has disappeared. If we remove this little piece of paper, see, the dowsing rod begins to move again, up and down.

Fantastic! But what does that mean?
This means that this geometric symbol can screen the radiation of this negative object. Why does this happen? Because if a line functions like an antenna – we spoke about this a little while earlier – then this cross behaves in the same way with earth radiation as the so-called Faraday cage does with radio waves: it blocks them or at least weakens them beyond all recognition.

So it neutralizes the radiation?
Yes, this is the symbol we use for eliminating or disempowering radiations of this kind. But of course you cannot just switch off any impulse just like that. This requires deeper attention. On top of all this, different symbols produce different effects. For instance, with a Y you can reverse the effect, i.e. turn something negative into something positive. As the test has shown, the material is negative. Now I place a Y over it and – see? – the intolerable radiation has become tolerable. You can attain this kind of reversal with another symbol as well, and this is a sine curve.

Knowing all this, how can you strengthen the immune system?
By making sure that your body gets only positive impulses; in other words you need to avoid all intolerable impulses. This can be a kind of food, building material or a flower that you put in a vase in your room. But the same applies to certain people, too. Before you get married, for instance, you need to check this – at

least, people should. There are intolerabilities and these intolerable impulses damage the immune system. In fact the condition of the immune system is actually the very foundation of health preservation. This means that this new form of medicine, New Homeopathy, focuses on the preservation of health.

As far as I know, intolerability has not only physiological, but also psychological effects.

That is right and this is a very important point. People seem to have found radiations at the scene of accidents at certain spots on motorways, and experts on earth radiation do all they can to eliminate these. Experiments of this kind have been going on for many years, for decades in fact.

If you are interested, I can tell you about a new experiment that I myself also took part in. In a school near where I work there was a point in the stairway where children kept having accidents. No one could tell why. We examined the spot and found a very, very high vertical radiation. Within 2 minutes we eliminated this radiation with a similar symbol. Since that time there has been no accident there. But colors also have a huge impact on our organism. If I place a color card in front of me and examine it, I can tell you exactly which colors are intolerable and which ones are not. You will see that there are two or even three colors which are negative for all organisms. But in fact everyone needs to choose the colors they find tolerable. If you keep wearing the wrong color or sit next to a wall which is the wrong color for you, this will have a negative influence on your health.

I heard that one can also use colors to protect against earth radiation.

We developed combinations of symbols and colors for this purpose. We mounted them on simple sheets and received really quite excellent feedback from the doctors and institutions involved in this kind of energetic examination procedure.

As you can see, we did this with a combination of crosses, colors and symbols and quite simply put the new sheet underneath the ordinary sheet that people sleep on. This sheet will protect a sleeping person without him or her sensing anything at all. The sheet helps physicians by enabling the drugs they prescribe to produce their optimal effect for the patient.

If earth radiation is too strong, even the best of medicine remains ineffectual, because the co-ordinates in the body, which always arrange themselves in line with external influences, will fit the external impulses instead of the drugs and so the treatment remains powerless. This is something that many doctors have admitted and they realized, along with me, that 'symbols' can often actually replace medication. Of course, this is only true in certain cases.

For instance, if someone feels pain, you can intervene with symbols. You don't need to take medicines or drugs, which are often very strong. It is worth a try. For this experiment I suggest the sine curve. This is what everyone should try when they have a mosquito or bee bite.

I don't have either kind of bite at this moment.

Not now, but when you do, if only you draw this symbol on your skin, the pain will go away instantly. Some people have pains in their knees or their elbows or have other dull aches – it is always worth experimenting with this symbol. New Homeopathy is not a treatment to counter an existing effect. It actually belongs to the sphere of communication in that it is related to the outside world but the effect is based on feedback produced by the body itself.

This means that I can produce certain impacts in the body through the symbols I draw on people's body, on their skin. However, it is important that anyone who works with these symbols should be a medical doctor or have medical training, because one can achieve not only positive, but also negative results.

Appendix II

Theses and Hypotheses Regarding Connections between Fungi and Cancer

by Bruno Haefeli
Dedicated to the Present Volume

Introduction by Mária Sági

Bruno Haefeli (1928–2012) was a Swiss medical researcher in the field of hematology. By a special gift of fortune, 6 months before he died I was lucky enough to meet him personally in his Swiss laboratory where he presented his methodology for hematological diagnostics and therapy. True to the spirit of our co-operation, he committed himself to write a paper for our book describing his method, since we practice Körbler's mycosis diagnostics and therapy based on his fungus images.

Haefeli had been working in hematological research and therapy as a student and colleague of Professor Dr. Günther Enderlein (1872–1968) since 1965. He is one of the few hematologist researchers who consistently carried through Enderlein's legacy after the latter's death. He continued to elaborate on the early insights before and the consequent insights after Enderlein's time and used both the new and the traditional methods of blood mycosis analysis to identify parasites in the blood. On this basis he developed new methods of treatment.

In the wake of his activities a new area of analyzing and imaging of the blood appeared in medical research and therapy which presented entirely novel considerations. This is due to the fact that instead of exploring the parameters customary in clinical and medical practice he actually examined the biological process in the very way in which it takes place in our body. Lacking clear and definitive results, he went beyond the grey-field technique and used what is called a differential interference contrast microscope and a light-field procedure.

His hematological research was based on cyclogeny, understood in Enderlein's sense, and the recognition of mycosis in the blood, including the visual imaging of mycoid forms. He developed a technique for staining blood which he termed HAE blood staining. This enabled him to identify parasite germs in the blood, more precisely pleomorph active pre-mycostases (the earliest visible developmental forms of fungi) and their final forms, i.e. fungi themselves (Mycota). *He set up a new system for classifying pathogenic processes and their indications which has proved useful in medical practice. Terms describing his reactive agents are the ERY method (1968), HAE II (1976–1983) and HAE III (2003). His publications and books, including the volume on pleomorphism* [Pleomorphismus] *co-authored with Jost Dumrese, serve as a seminal work and a point of reference for experts in the field.*

Blood Mycosis – Fungoid Infection in the Blood
BHS Laboratory, Microanalytic Blood Mycosis Research

How Fungi Operate as Parasites, How They Conquer and Hollow the Tissue Cells of the Organism, How They Reprogram Them into Cancer Cells and Disintegrate Them

Parasites in the Blood

It is becoming more and more clear that the cause of clinically proven cancerous processes could be clarified by *blood mycosis analysis.* I treated my patients with *isotherapeutic anti-mycotic therapy* custom-selected specifically for each individual. During these therapies I observed that atypical cells go through a morphological change, in other words that the cause of cancer is related to the effect of one or more fungi related to obligatory fungi such as *Mucoracae* and *Ascomycota* (the latter group includes, for instance, *Aspergillus* and *Penicillium).* Several decades of experience have shown that targeted analytic processes can render fungi present in the blood identifiable.[1] This fact confirms the hypothesis that in a pleomorphic sense cancer is one of the end products of the activity of fungi.

I studied this area for over 50 years. Based on my therapeutic findings I have come to the conclusion that in order to prevent the emergence and proliferation of cancer we need to carry on exploring the role of blood mycosis. My experience in therapy has led me to the firm conviction that if we find fungi in the blood our most important job is to reduce them to the most primal form of their existence and grant the conditions for the self-regulation they carry out in the service of their own survival. If we eliminate the disharmonious conditions in the blood which emerged due to an unhealthy diet and led to the appearance of a number of diseases by introducing a new, healthier diet, our immune system, i.e. the self-defense mechanism of our body, becomes more effective. Once that happens, fungi discontinue their parasitic way of life and return to their normal, healthy and balanced life-functions, entering a functional symbiosis with the host organism. Only now can they start fulfilling their role in defense against diseases in the service of the host organism. The previously hostile attitude of the fungus to the host organism is replaced by a symbiotic, co-operative relationship.

During the years when I was actively involved in treating patients, I examined every single patient entrusted to my care in the most thorough manner possible concerning the presence of fungi in the blood. If I detected one or more species of fungus in the blood I injected the dominant type of fungus, using a diluted solution of the type in question, and soon found that as a result of this treatment the fungi and mycelia found in the blood earlier were now declining, perishing and the organism was voiding them. Patients only became free of symptoms in the presence of low concentrations of self-regulating, 'tolerable' fungi in a self-promoting form, and only this condition could provide protection against disease, including colds, flu, inflammations and other assaults weakening the immune system. Therapy was particularly successful in patients who suffered from chronic diseases with regular flare-ups. Based on analyses of therapy, I can report that the fungus treatment I propose is not only useful in the treatment of degenerative diseases, but also, as a kind of 'side product', it allows us to arrest and modify the proliferation of cancer. In many cases the tumor vanished entirely.

During the course of therapy, just as with a healthy normal lifestyle, we need to pay special attention to diet. It is particularly crucial to avoid foods and drinks which provide fungi with sustenance. Certain drugs are also a source of food for fungi and support their growth and proliferation.

During the course of treatment, because of cell acidosis, we must provide for adequate detoxication, voiding through the required organs, and for restoring conditions for normal cell functioning, such as pH conditions or basic functioning by Pischinger's cell model. All foods which promote over-acidification must be eliminated. By following this method we deprive fungi of their source of nourishment.

It has long been known that mold fungi such as *Mucor, Aspergillus* and *Penicillium* live on the materials produced in the body and partly demand a heightened input of protein and partly, in the case of *Candida,* induce patients to consume all manners of sugar, including the immoderate consumption of sugared delicacies.

Rapid proliferation of fungi in the blood is prevented by the customary defense mechanisms of the immune system. The proliferation of fungi in the circulation is a very slow process. Therefore the patient senses no pain for years; they feel generally good and energetic, until at one point the morpho-pathogenic modification of cells sets in. In order to stop the process of the emergence of cancer it is important to have regular blood check-ups regarding blood mycosis.

Analyzing old case histories has shown that nosodes created

from mold fungi cultured in vitro can effectively counter pathogenic processes. These nosodes are the following: Erycin, Erymykin, Erymykin-forte, Erycetan and Candida-forte.

The unstoppable blood mycosis

Over the past years we have seen a sharp rise in the number of diseases that go back to harmful environmental influences and defects of the immune system. These include cancer, problems of blood-clotting and the resulting diseases such as thrombosis, heart attacks, strokes and arteriosclerosis. The same is true of chronic rheumatism, fibromyalgia syndrome (muscle pains), Type II Diabetes (diabetes mellitus), multiple sclerosis, skin eczema, stomach and intestinal complaints, immune deficiencies, low resistance to infections, sleep problems, allergies, osteoporosis, etc.

The microflora of the blood

Before causing symptoms, most diseases develop unnoticed for long periods of time. The environment and microflora of the blood influenced by that environment both play a decisive role in this process.

This is due to causes which we have not really taken into account before. The present study will help connect results and understanding from this entire range of areas and rule out a whole set of misunderstandings.

Areas in question are the following:

- extracellular and intracellular acidosis;
- vacuolization of red corpuscles;
- rigidity of erythrocytes;
- pre-mycotic systases (the earliest developmental stage of fungi).

A sense of sickness without any apparent cause

Many people today feel that they are inexplicably tired, listless, and their capacity to perform has declined. More and more people complain of headaches, dizziness, nausea and a general feeling of ill health. Unpleasant symptoms include digestion problems such as too much acid, bloating, constipation and cramps. Even young people complain of pains in the joints and rigid muscles, while sciatica is almost a common condition. No matter what the complaints are, however, doctors stand baffled, because lab findings of these patients, coming with such diffuse complaints, show no sign of disease, gastroscopy shows nothing out of the ordinary, and the intestinal system also proves normal and offers no cause for alarm. From the point of view of modern mainstream medicine the patient is completely healthy. Now the doctor goes on to question the patient about the degree of stress they are experiencing and will conclude by referring to the psychological and social causes of the disease.

All of this, however, is unlikely to help the patient, so the question is justified whether any other reasons ought to be considered.

Factors affecting the blood's microflora

In this day and age we are all exposed to heavy environmental load. Our food is poisoned by a multitude of chemicals; our cosmetic products, clothes, furniture and building material all contain substances which represent a load on our body. Our food chain contains a growing amount of residual drugs, pesticides and anti-mycotics and we are also increasingly exposed to load from electrosmog and artificial electromagnetic fields. The consequences that all of these factors will have on our organism cannot be predicted at this moment. At the same time, every single individual also contributes to weakening their own body by their own behavior, eating habits and lifestyle. Eating too much poor-quality food, consuming stimulants and consumer products without moderation, shortage of exercises, and stress at work and in the family all might provide sufficient ground in itself for the development of some chronic disease or other.

Effects of a derailed, pathogenic microflora

Microbiological research of the past hundred years, which has not found reception within modern mainstream medicine to this very day, has led to recognitions about the 'microflora' of the blood. Changes in this microflora are presumed to be in direct causal relation to the emergence of various chronic and degenerative diseases. These include cancer, blood-clotting problems and resulting diseases such as thrombosis, heart attacks, strokes, arteriosclerosis, rheumatoid dysfunctions, Type II Diabetes (diabetes mellitus), multiple sclerosis, and many others (see above).

Changes taking place in the microflora of the blood can be detected and made visible by BHS mycosis analysis. This provides us with information about the degree of load the blood is exposed to. From this we can, in turn, draw reliable conclusions about the patient's state of health. We can also establish early diagnoses from signs of disease. Early recognition is a crucial question from the point of view of preventing these pathogenic processes and sustaining health. Early recognition allows us to identify various tendencies, weak points and defects in good time, in order to restore the normal balance of the organism by regulation through natural products such as ERY or HAE III diagnostics or homeopathic or isopathic therapies.

Disturbances of regulatory processes

Cells and organs develop diseases when regulatory processes in the body suffer chronic or abrupt, acute and intense disturbances. Disease emerges at points of disturbance in the supply of nourishment and in the voiding of harmful substances, and where information transmission is no longer possible. All of this together leads to the enfeeblement of the immune system. The organism becomes sensitive to infections, and chronic and degenerative diseases.

Lasting acidic exposure causes the human organism to develop a milieu which modifies the microflora of the blood. It loses its natural self-regulatory qualities and allows the development of various modified, pathogenic formations.

Over-acidification – the beginning of a health problem?

We should never belittle the significance of the over-acidification processes taking place in our body. To the contrary – they should be taken into account in all our diagnoses and therapies. Over-acidification should never be considered a harmless circumstance; it requires the full attention of both therapist and patient.

Noted researchers and doctors have proposed the theme of over-acidification over the last few years and come to contradictory conclusions. It is surprising in the context of the theme of 'acid' that, probably for want of alternatives or sufficient knowledge, over-acidification is described as a dysfunction of the connective tissue. In fact, over-acidification should not be curtailed to such a narrow understanding. We must pay special attention to the over-acidification taking place inside and outside the cell which was revealed by Haefeli, particularly as regards the vacuolization processes inside the cells. My latest findings show that although the connective tissue absorbs acids, the blood shows pathogenic diversions from normal if the pH is constantly acidy. The structural image of erythrocytes (red corpuscles) shows increasingly distinct, if previously unknown, morphological alterations.

Latent acidosis of the connective tissues

The concept of the 'latent acidosis of the connective tissue' was proposed by Friedrich F. Sander. It encountered controversy in professional circles right from the start. His statement referred to the condition where the alkaline reserves of the blood have been partially used up, but its pH has not changed. This is the point at which the body begins to rob its own alkaline reserves, entailing the dissolution of mineral salts from bones, cartilage and teeth.

Scientific antecedents

The essence of Franz Xaver Mayr's method is to clear the acidified organism of its waste, which is done by a starving diet and alkaline powder. Considering the time in which he lived and worked, in 1953 Friedrich F. Sander gave a very accurate and instructive explanation of the problematic of acidification. Professor Alfred Pischinger from Vienna, an expert in histology, studied the (patho) physiological role of the connective tissue in even more profound detail. He created the concept of the 'connective tissue matrix' and described its impact on cell metabolism. Pischinger's work was transferred to clinical application by Perger and Wendt. Many years later these insights were carried forth by Hartmut Heine at Witten University, and later Stossier, Witasek and Wortlitschek published articles on the principle of the acid-alkaline metabolism.

General acidosis

It is most thought-provoking that the number of patients suffering from acidosis has gone up and is still on the increase. In the case of general acidosis, modern mainstream therapies remain ineffective unless accompanied by changes in lifestyle and eating habits. The consequences of acidosis are an entire complex of chronic diseases where we observe the development and over-proliferation of primitive organisms. They not only flood the tissues and cells, but are also present in all the bodily fluids of the organism. These observations have led to the creation of the term 'humoral pathology', i.e. the study of the pathologies of bodily fluids.

The cell as a source of over-acidification

The regulation of pH is a very complex process which takes place under strictly determined conditions, particularly in the blood. It is the result of the co-operation of various buffer systems. At present we talk about intracellular and extracellular acid exposure.

Extracellular and intracellular acidosis

It is extremely important not to focus exclusively on extracellular acidosis (of the intercellular stock or matrix) but also to consider the over-acidification of the blood's pH. As soon as the buffer capacity of the body and the blood, serving to keep the latter's pH within the right band, is exhausted, it starts withdrawing alkaline substances from the tissues and even the bones. Compensatory mechanisms only become active when the blood's pH fluctuates, first through breathing and then through the vacuolization of the red corpuscles. The aim of all prevention and therapy is to strengthen and harmonize the supplying and purifying system of the body, since the secretion of fluids is fundamental to health.

The acid–alkaline balance

In the blood itself, fluctuations of pH are balanced out by the bicarbonate and protein buffers, as well as by hemoglobin.

Some 75% of the acid exposure is compensated by the bicarbonate buffer. This reaction produces carbonic acid which decomposes into neutral water and carbon dioxide and exits through the lungs by exhaling.

The more acid the organism is exposed to, the heavier the burden on the buffer systems. For want of more accurate knowledge, the hypothesis at the moment is that in the case of over-acidification the surplus acids are drained by a regulatory process through the connective tissue which also serves as a storage space for all acids, poisons and waste material.

Where do acids go?

Up till now the generally accepted view had been that a bad diet over a long period of time causes the latent acidification of all tissues and organs. Acids conglomerate in the connective tissue that is found everywhere in the body. It has been commonly agreed that the functionality of the connective tissues is the basis of all regulatory processes of the body, ranging from breathing through maintaining the acid–alkaline balance all the way to regulating recovery processes.

A healthy regulation system consists of constant transitions between the parenchyme, the interstitium (the substance among the cells) and the blood vessels. An acid level which is higher due to a bad diet becomes reduced due to this set of filters and passes in an intravasal fashion (i.e. within the blood vessels) through the kidneys, the bladder, the intestines and the skin, as well as through the lungs in gaseous forms.

Animal proteins, carbohydrates (sugars) and the acidic environment

Acids are produced in the breakdown of certain animal protein and refined carbohydrates (sugars). By contrast, the breakdown of vegetable foods has an alkalizing effect on the body. Fats and oils behave in neutral ways in our metabolism.

Enzyme over-load

The metabolism of the cells participates to the greatest possible extent in the production of acidy metabolites (poisons). As the concentration of acids from the metabolism increases, an overly high need emerges for enzyme production, which the secreting organ cannot fulfill after a while. If the performance of enzyme production declines, this function becomes relatively overloaded, consequences of which include hyperuricemia (a pathogenic increase in the uric acid content of the blood, also related to the emergence of gout) and lactacidosis. This means that the source of the 'acidosis' is the cell itself, even though the pH value is measured outside the cell, in the blood.

Diet – Vital nutrients and ballast materials

Today it is clearly known that crucial nutrients as co-factors of cell enzymes have a decisive influence on channeling away cell acids into the body tissues and the spaces between the organs, as well as into the blood, also meaning that they strengthen the operation of the buffer system.

Consuming vegetables, potatoes and wholemeal cereals every day can replenish the body's storehouse of vital nutrients which in turn can optimally support the production and secretion of enzymes. Buffer capacity is further enhanced by introducing alkaline electrolytes. This is served by using alkaline powders as a dietary supplement.

Measuring alkaline buffer capacity – attempting the impossible

Laboratory diagnostic measurements of pH values show only the momentary state of reduction potential, i.e. of the buffer capacity. We can only assume what goes on in the background. Pure vitamins, anti-oxidants, vitamin combinations or natural vitamin complexes only yield uncertain data regarding 'redox values' and alkaline buffer capacity. Naturally, pH values can also be accurately measured by the available modern methods at individual points, e.g. in the blood, in the interstitial space, the inside of the cell and the components of the cytoplasm; at the same time it does not provide adequate information about the capacity of the organism to absorb acids as determined by the buffer capacity. (Sanders also made attempts to analyze buffer capacity through urine. Jörgensen defined 'alkaline buffer capacity' by titration – using volume analysis – from the total blood. These and similar methods are still used in medical laboratories, even though they have never been validated.)

Acidosis and the connective tissue

The connective tissue has long been known to be a deposit of various metabolites produced during the metabolic process. If intake of proteins and carbohydrates from food is excessive, the buffer capacity of the connective tissue becomes insufficient after a while. This does not directly influence the pH value of the interstitium (the substance filling the intercellular space) but it does affect the level of the buffer capacity of the connective tissue to serve as an intermediary depot for acids produced from the metabolic process. This 'waste depot' becomes filled up and unusable after a while.

Acidosis and the structural changes of red corpuscles

Neutral pH is usually defined at 7.0. In a normal case, the blood's pH is between 7.35 and 7.45. Experience shows that if the pH is outside of this zone, the first digressions from normality become recognizable – being clearly visible morphological changes in the structural image of red corpuscles.

If the pH is solidly between 7.35 and 7.45, this shows that there is an efficient, self-regulating mechanism in place. If this mechanism starts to fail in playing its part in the metabolic processes due to abnormalities, and acids or alkalines are flooding into the blood to an overly high degree and the blood's buffer function is compromised, the pH value may shift in one or the other direction.

This may seem paradoxical, but the antagonism between acid and alkaline will only stay within the frames of the functioning system until the buffering in the blood collapses. The reaction between acid and alkaline, in other words the balance of the two, is extremely significant for the totality of the organism.

When enzymes, hormones and vital nutrients can not act

Enzymes can only remain optimally active within a certain level of pH. They react most sensitively to changes in pH and so even the most vital nutrients can only be fully active if the selection of foods is satisfactory, i.e. the combination of foods eaten is harmonious from the point of view of acid-alkaline balance. Both extreme opinions are wrong – either if you think that you don't need to worry at all about the acid-alkaline balance, or if you think that all acidy foods are the work of the devil. As usual, the truth is somewhere halfway: the body needs both acid and alkaline substances – in the right balance!

Often it is not quite clear what we mean by acid-alkaline balance. The main reason for this is that we do not distinguish between blood pH and tissue pH and do not differentiate between extracellular and intracellular pH, either.

The vacuolization of erythrocytes (red corpuscles)

Due to constant flooding by acids, the connective tissue becomes overburdened and the superfluous acids leave the tissues through the lymphal passages and pass into the blood serum. In these cases the first thing that happens is that the body mobilizes all of its alkaline reserves. When this is no longer sufficient for restoring the extremely sensitive pH value, the superfluous acids in the red corpuscles use the last and only possible storage resort: the vacuole of the red corpuscles. This, however, considerably reduces the performance of the red corpuscles and the membrane structure changes visibly. This phenomenon is also called *the rigidity of erythrocytes.* This fact was highlighted by Dr. Berthold Kern, and Haefeli managed to demonstrate it through his blood analyses (Haefeli's ERY method). If there is a prolonged import of hydrogen ions from the serum, in the final stage these overused vacuoles can also void their content into the intercellular space and introduce acid inside the cell which, eventually, will lead to damaging the cell (hemolysis).

If there is a heightened influx of acid into the blood, in an effort to secure the pH balance of the circulation the alkaline reserves are exhausted. Although the antagonism of these two values is visible, most routine measurements do not reveal this difference and the acidosis is not betrayed by any sign. Measuring pH only allows for identifying a combined measurement, since in most cases all that is measured is the extracellular environment. Besides the early recognition system developed by the present author, there seems to be no other simple and low-cost method for identifying existing acidosis.

Haefeli's BHS analytic

In a blood picture made by the Haefeli method, formations damaged by acids can be well distinguished from cells unaffected by acids. This proves that acidosis of the blood can indeed be identified and imaged through a simple staining technique. Although the blood's pH value is subject to the constant fluctuation between acidosis and alkalosis, the pH balance is constantly restored in an autonomous fashion by the vacuolum mechanism which I discovered. I have demonstrated through laboratory experiments that tendencies for over-acidification may manifest in the blood through highly specific mechanisms. At the same time, over-acidification can be clearly and spectacularly rendered visible by the vacuolization of the red corpuscles and the proliferation of pre-mycotic systases.

New hope

The 'acid-alkaline balance is influenced by the introduction of both healthy and unhealthy foods and micronutrients. If we examine this process merely through the laboratory methods known today, we do not get a full understanding of this complex question. Therefore we need to introduce new and different diagnostic methods, such as the Haefeli HAE III analytics.

This is a blood test which, besides allowing the user to identify imbalance in pH, also gives an optical representation of the vacuole appearing in the red corpuscles, the deformation of these corpuscles and the consequent rigidity of the erythrocytes. We can also see the development of pre-mycotic systases and the mycotic infections (mycetosis) in the blood. This method can then lead to a reinterpretation of acidosis and clarify the connections between problem areas that mutually influence each other.

HAE II staining technique, a new technology offered by BHS-

Labor Schenkon, is excellently suited to identify blood mycosis, so much so that the result becomes visible on the mount within a matter of minutes. This is a decisive step in diagnostics and therapy alike.

'I am happy and grateful that by means of the BHS analytic diagnostics I have been able to contribute to the early recognition and therapy of chronic diseases.'

Bruno Haefeli

The total colored photographic documentation comes from earlier publications of BHS-Labor. Data of the corresponding pathologies was derived from longitudinal check-ups of the blood, while the various developmental stages were traced from the medical anamneses.

Blood smear stained with HAEIII testing solution

R: The entire image under the microscope is intertwined with fungoid filaments.

Diagnosis
This blood smear documents a strained immune system to the degree which Enderlein called 'gigatovalent', entailing damage of vitally important organs. In the case of fungal infections this usually means latent diseases which remain undetected in the course of normal examination.

This is an 82-year-old male patient with the following complaints:

- angina pectoris
- diabetes
- prostate problems
- muscle and joint complaints (rheumatism)
- feebleness of muscles when walking
- deterioration of vision and hearing.

Blood smear HAE III testing solution 231010

Fungal filament
(stained yellow)
Genuine long-branch mycelium, micro-recording 1000 times enlargement.
(Figure 139)

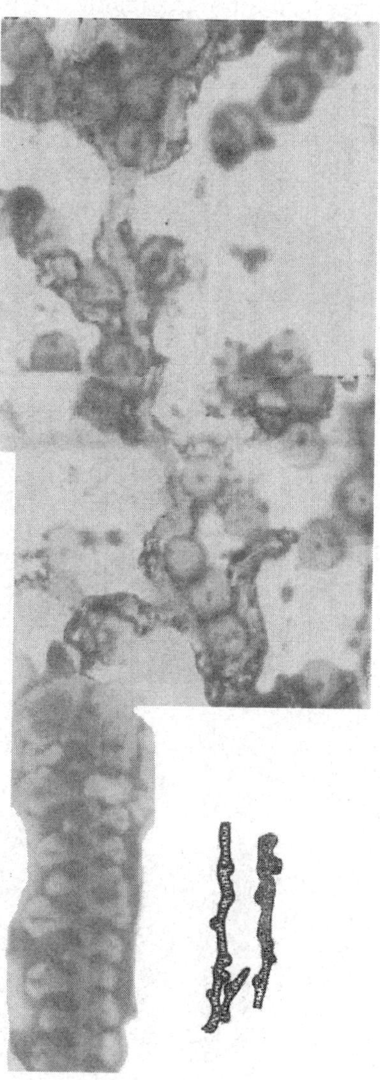

Figure 139.
Archive images of giant mycelia

Giant-scale development of fungal asci in blood and tissue under gigatovalent acid exposure. Processes of this kind, if untreated, may lead through organic dysfunctions and damage to death. The blood contains several types of parasitic fungi. *(Figure 140)*

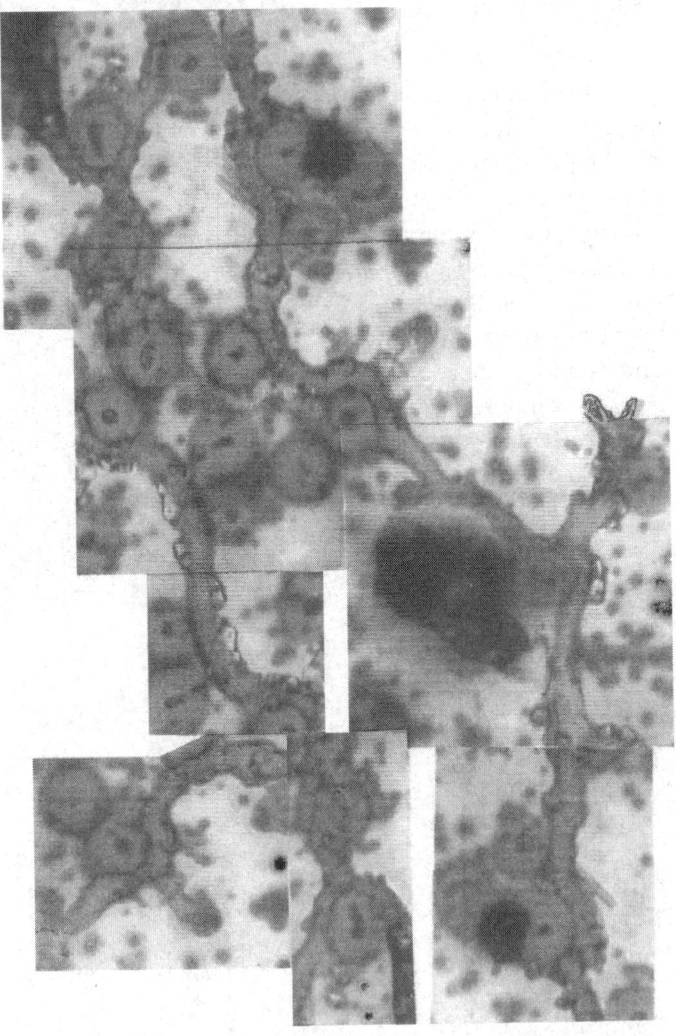

Figure 140. Parasitic fungal sacs

To ensure a better understanding of the cyclogenetic development of fungi over time we present pre-mycotic systases, the earliest developmental formations of genuine fungi which may colonize the blood and any tissue of the organism. *(Figure 141)*

Primitive fungal germs on the erythrocyte membrane, arranged between the layers.
Healthy finding.

The first developmental phase of the mycelium, germinating from the vacuolum.
Acceptable finding.

The mycelium growth shows heightened activity and spreads over the edge of the cell.
Slightly pathogenic finding.

The mycelia colonize the two red corpuscles, partly rounded; they are squeezed out of the cell into the blood serum and start a cycle of aggressive growth.
Greater pathogenic finding.

Owing to aggressive mycelium growth, the fungus colonizes further blood corpuscles. The infection usually covers large areas of the field under the microscope and offers a wide range of medium to highly pathogenic conditions.
A highly pathogenic condition.

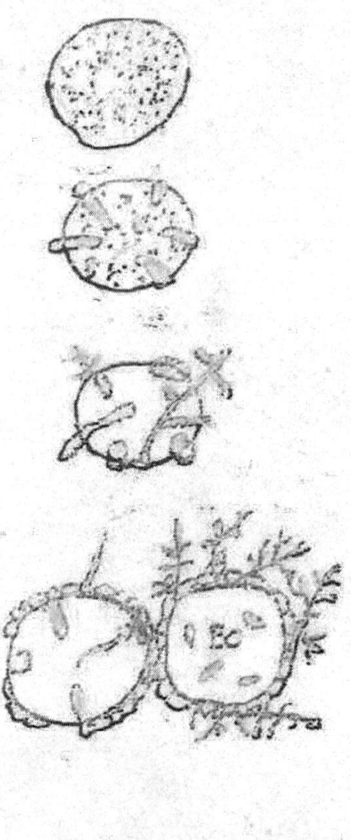

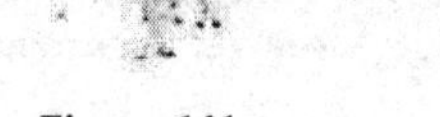

Figure 141

Haefeli mycosis

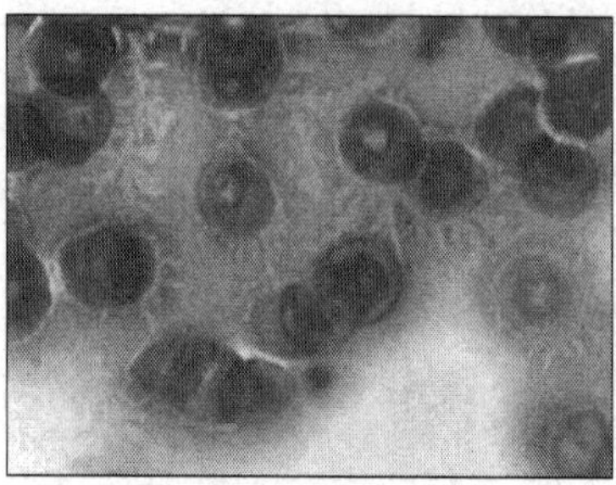

Figure 1. Mucor – mold fungus in grave arterio-venous diseases

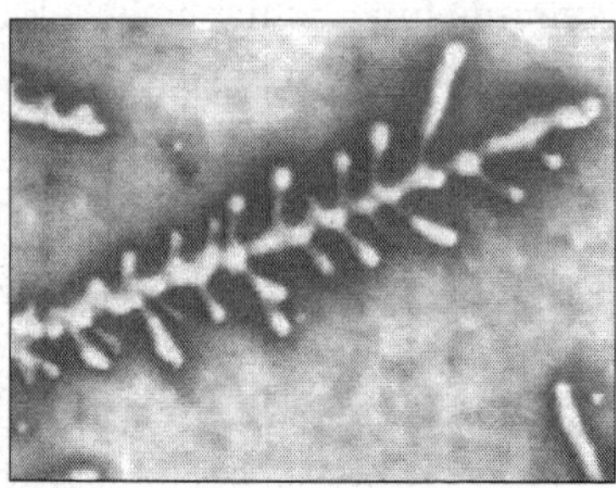

Figure 2. Mucor – mold fungus in psoriasis

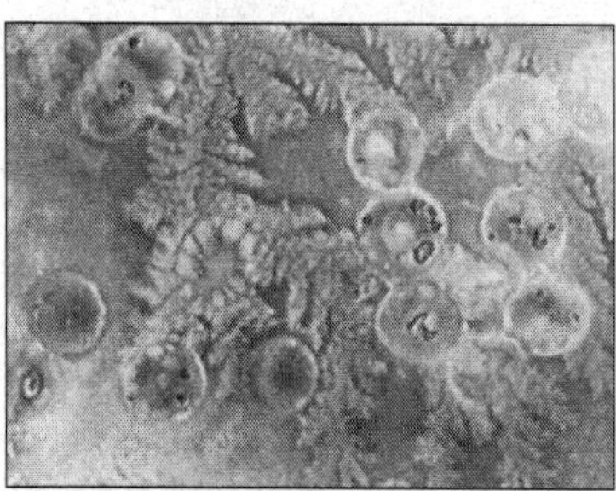

Figure 3. Aspergillus mold fungus in bronchiectasia

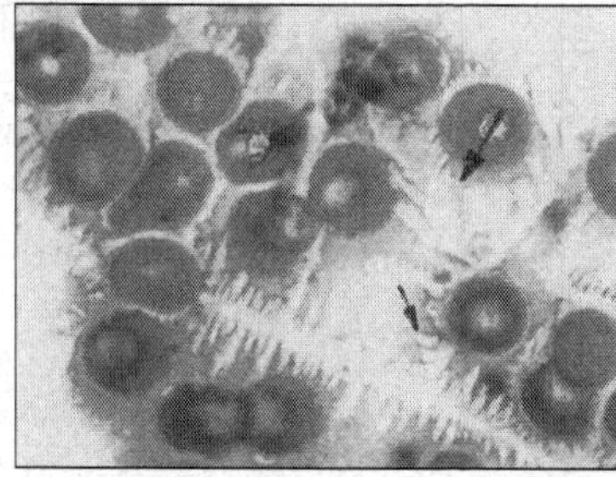

Figure 4. Aspergillus mold fungus in Gardner Syndrome. A tumor the size ofa fist had shrunk to 2.2 cm

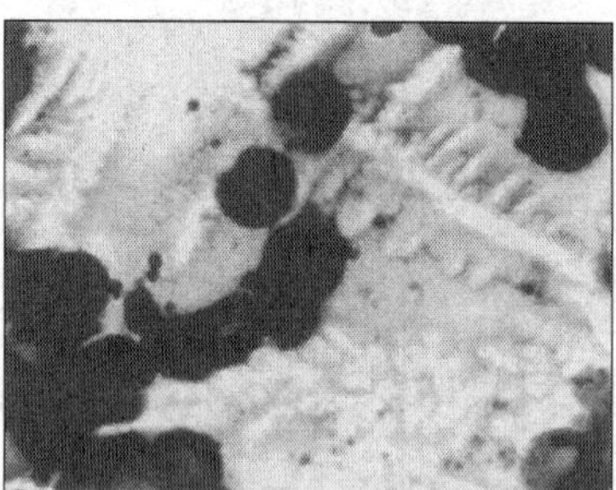

Figure 5. Mixed infection of Aspergillus mold fungus and Ascomycetes (sacfungi)

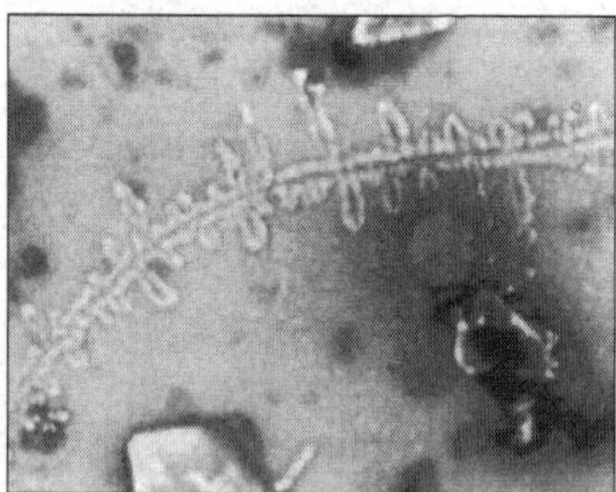

Figure 6. Ascomycetes in a stomach carcinoma

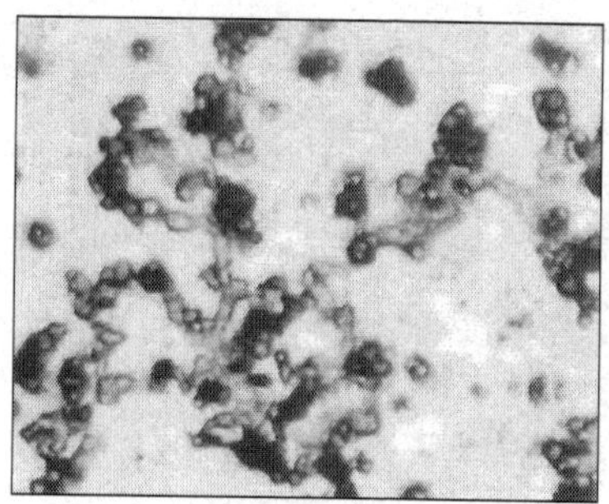

Figure 7. Exogenous Candida infection

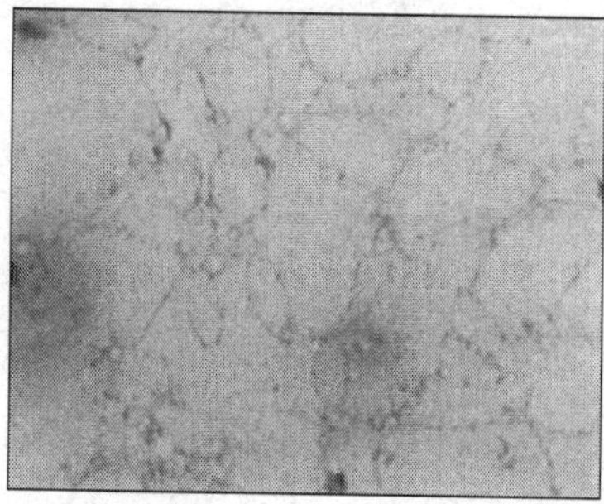

Figure 8. Endogenous Candida growth formation as it appears in the blood

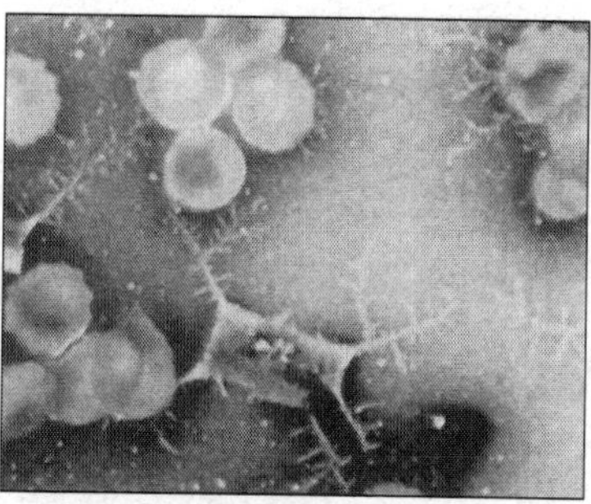

Figure 9. Stagnating drainage. Pseudo-crystals in the corner indicate the growthactivity of mycelia

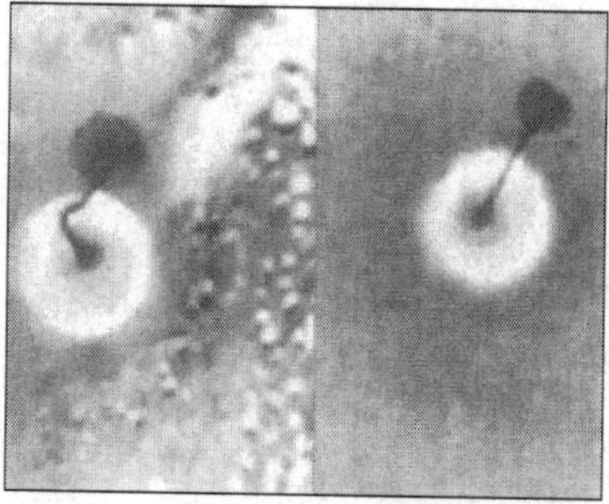

Figure 10. Basisdiomycet. Gilled mushrooms as they appeared in a two-year-oldboy's repeated infections

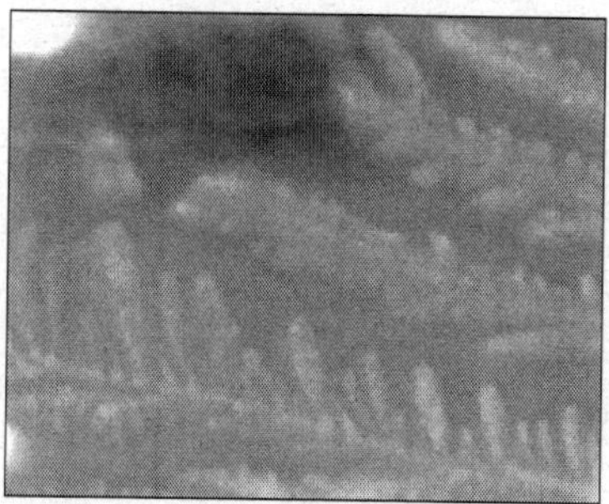

Figure 11. Ascomycetes in bush-like growths in a case of angina pectoris(bypass operation)

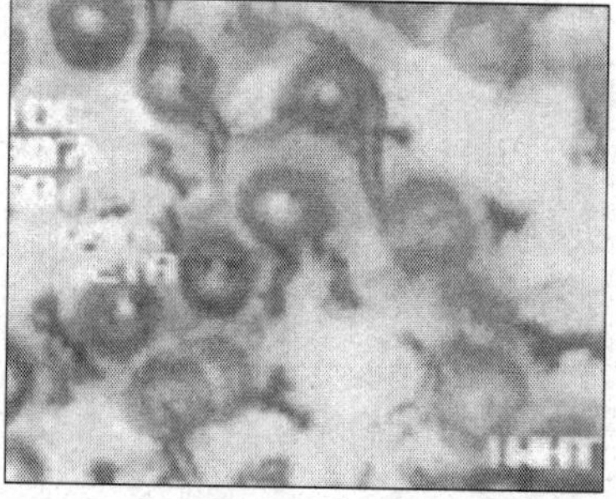

Figure 12. Spindle shapes seem particularly common in carcinomas and gravecases of immune deficiency

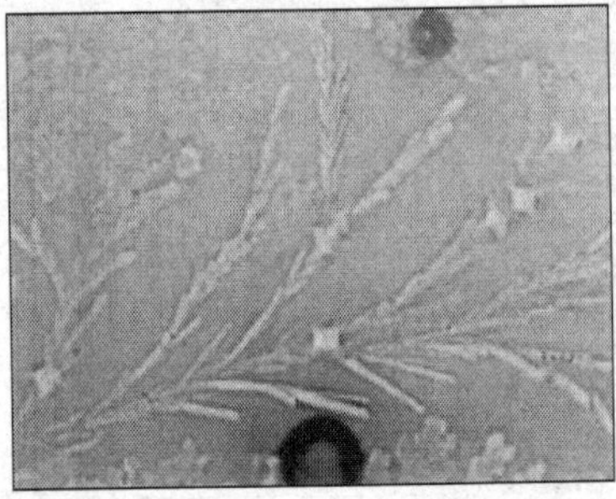

Figure 13. Penicillium mold fungus

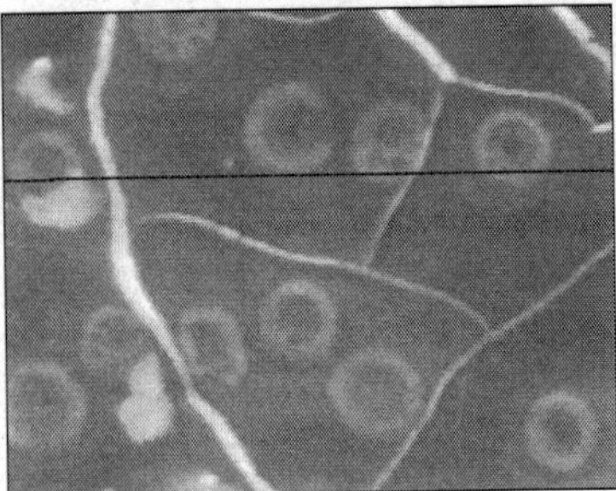

Figure 14. Hyphomycetes fungi

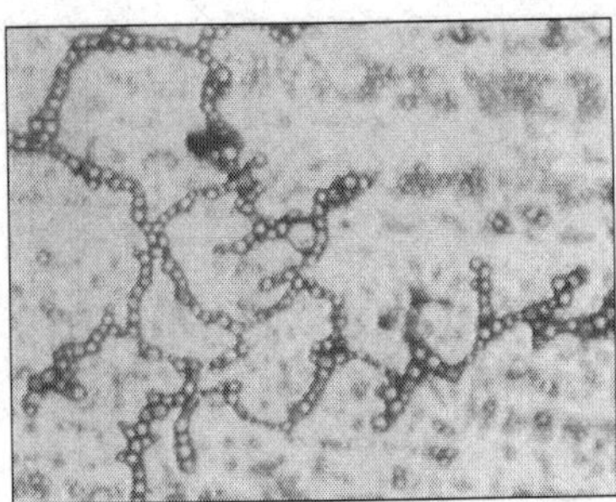

Figure 15. Streptomyces

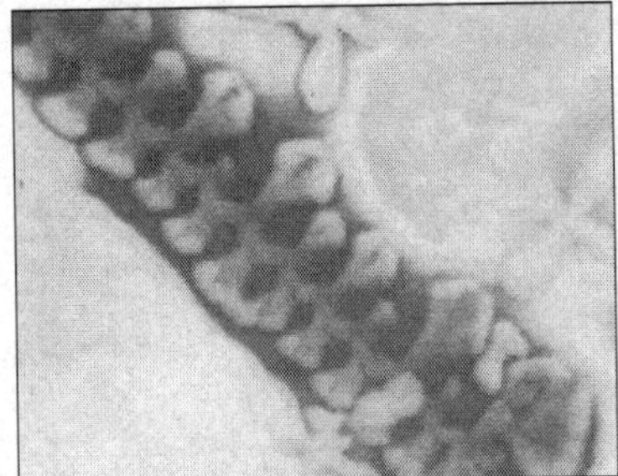

Figure 16. Ascomycetes with leaf-shaped sacs (asci)

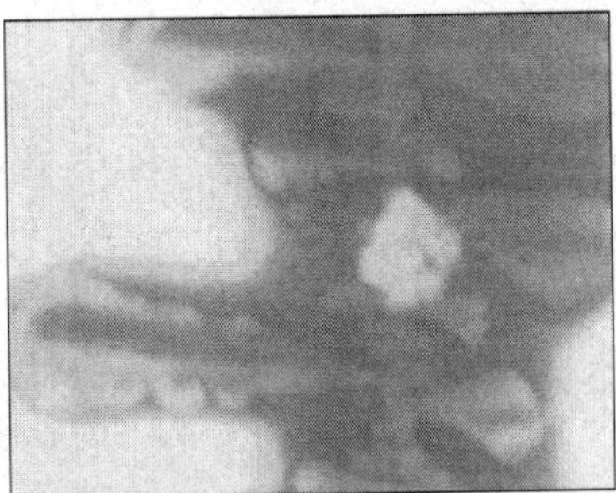

Figure 17. Ascomycetes (leaf-shaped sacs enlarged) in the case of a stomachcarcinoma metastasis

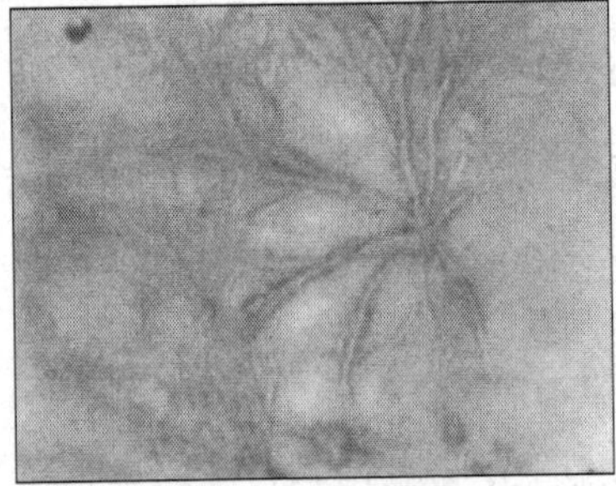

Figure 18. Ascomycetes, rare form, root-shaped mycelia

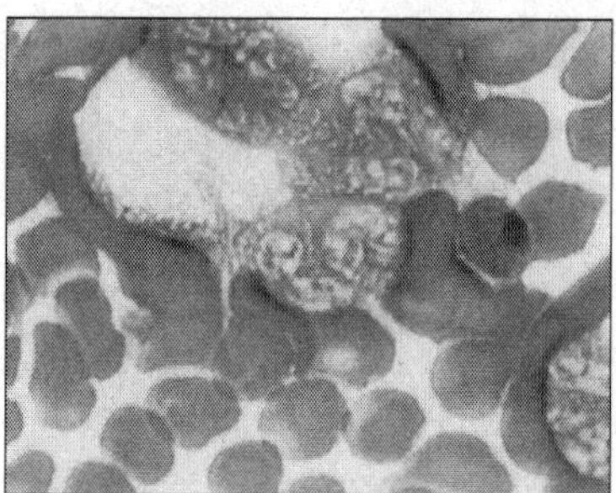

Figure 19. Proliferation of fungi in the protoplasm of leucocytes in the case ofthyroid tumor

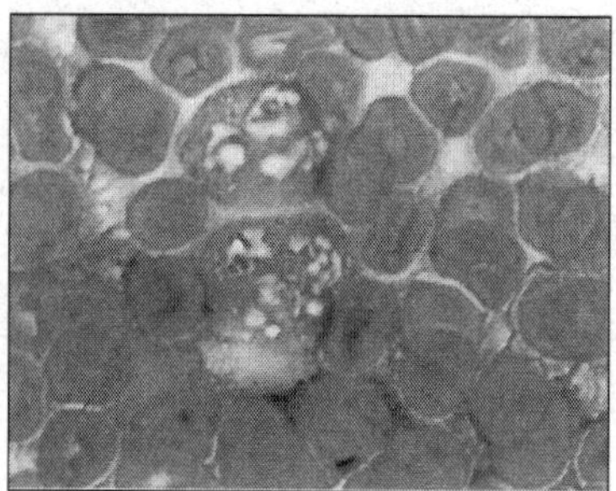

Figure 20. Fluorescent cluster of fungi in the protoplasm of leucocytes where the fungi have already attacked the nucleus

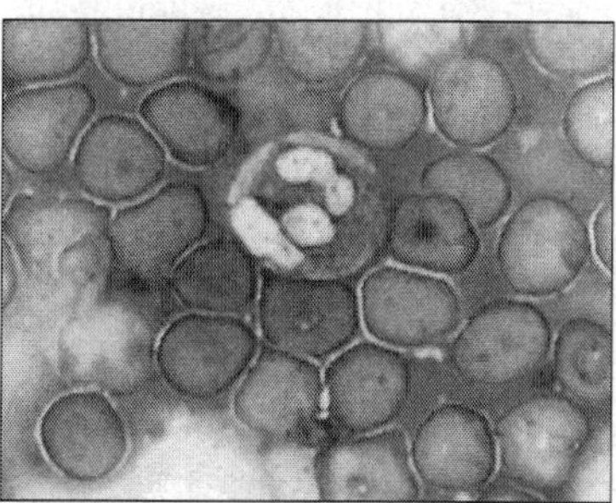

Figure 21. Pseudo-crystals; fluorescent mycotic substrate, resulting in thebloating of the nucleus

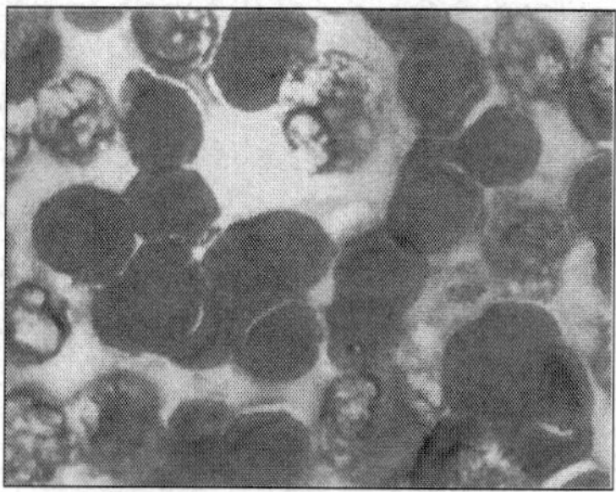

Figure 22. Large pseudo-crystalline pieces accumulating on top of the nucleus, which may pass into the serum

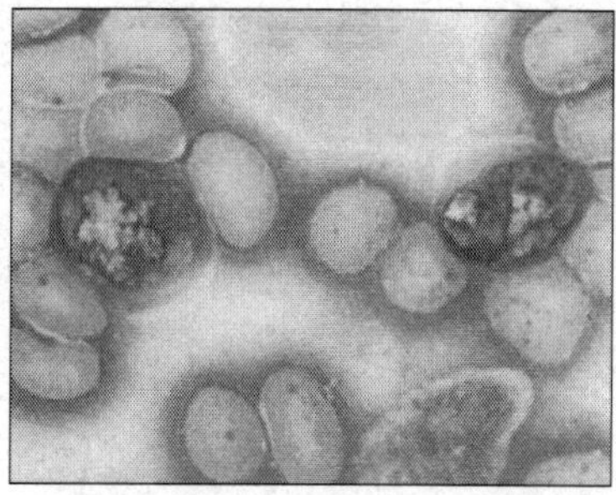

Figure 23. Cauliflower-like fungal structures on the nucleus. On the right-handside of the leucocyte on the nuclei it shows fluorescent bulges

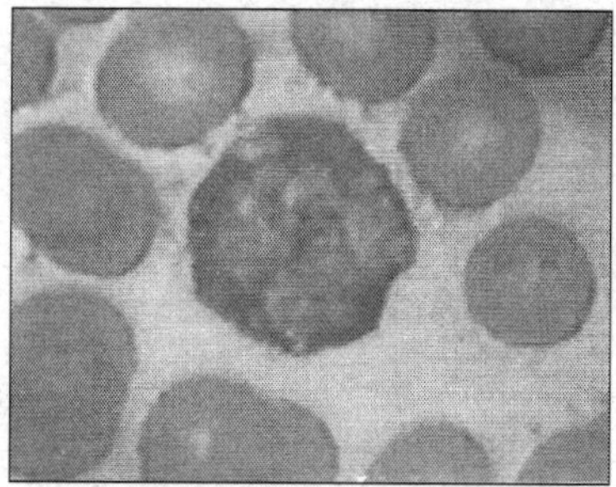

Figure 24. Tumor of the thyroid gland[4]

Notes

Foreword by Ervin Laszlo

1 Laszlo, E., *Science and the Akashic Field.* Inner Traditions, Rochester, Vermont, 2004.

2 Ho, M-W., *The Rainbow and the Worm: The Physics of Organisms.* World Scientific, Singapore, 1993.

3 The Nobel Prize in Physics in 2011 was given to Eric A. Cornell, Wolfgang Ketterle and Carl E. Wieman *for the achievement of Bose–Einstein condensation in dilute gases of alkali atoms, and for early fundamental studies of the properties of the condensates.*

4 Kwok, S., *Organic Matter in the Universe.* Wiley, 2011; Kwok, S. and Zhang, Y., 'Astronomers Discover Complex Organic Matter Exists throughout the Universe'. *Science Daily,* October 26, 2011.

5 Sagi, M., 'Healing Over Space and Time', in Laszlo, E., *The Akashic Experience: Science and the Cosmic Memory Field.* Inner Traditions, Rochester, Vermont, 2009.

Chapter 1

The New Way of Healing – the Transmission of Information

1 Laszlo, E., *The Creative Cosmos.* Floris Books, Edinburgh, 1993.

2 Laszlo, E., *Kozmikus kapcsolatok.* Magyar Könyvklub, Budapest, 1996; Bohm, D., *Wholeness and the Implicate Order.* Routledge and Kegan Paul, London, 1980.

3 Laszlo, E., *Science and the Akashic Field.* Inner Traditions, Rochester, Vermont, 2004.

4 Laszlo, E., *The Akashic Experience.* Inner Traditions, Rochester, Vermont, 2009.

5 Lipton, B., *The Biology of Belief.* Mountain of Love / Elite Books, Santa Rosa, California, 2005.

6 Cimbal, D., in Becker, G. and Massey, H., *The Living Matrix.* Innergy Collection, 2009.

7 Meissner, F., in Becker, G. and Massey, H., *The Living Matrix.* Innergy Collection, 2009.

8 Biava, P. M., *Il cancro e la ricerca del senso perduto.* Springer Verlag, Milan, 2008.

9 Fraser, P., Lipton, B., Cimbal, D., in Becker, G. and Massey, H., *The Living Matrix.* Innergy Collection, 2009.

10 Resch, G., Gutmann, V., *Wissenschaftliche Grundlagen der Homöopathie.* O-Verlag, Berg am Starnberger See, 1987.

11 Körbler, E., 'Die Universalrute VI. Zusammenfassung'. *Raum und Zeit Special 3,* pp. 23–28. 1990-93

Chapter 2

The Scientific Background of New Homeopathy

1 Hahnemann, S., *Organon der rationellen Heilkunde.* Dresden, in der Arnoldschen Buchhandlung, 1810.

2 Faraday, M., *Experimental Researches in Electricity, Vols. I and II.* 1839, 1844.

3 Maxwell, J. C., *'A dynamical theory of the electromagnetic field'.* Philosophical Transactions of the Royal Society of London, 1865.

4 Maxwell, J. C., *A Treatise on Electricity and Magnetism.* Oxford, at the Clarendon Press, 1873.

5 Laszlo, E., *The Connectivity Hypothesis.* State University of New York, 2003.

6 Prigogine, I., Order Out of Chaos: *Man's Dialogue with Nature.* Bantam, New York, 1984.

7 Katchalsky, A., Curran, P. F., *Nonequilibrium Thermodynamics in Biophysics.* Harvard University Press, 1965.

8 Laszlo, E., *The Connectivity Hypothesis.* State University of New York, 2003.

9 Cornell, E. A., Wieman, C. E., 'Bose–Einstein Condensates in a Dilute Gas; the First 70 Years and Some Recent Experiments'. Nobel Lecture, 1995.

10 Davis, K. B., Mewes, M. O., Andrews, M. R., van Druten, N. J., Durfee, D. S., Kurn, D. M., Ketterle, W., 'Bose–Einstein Condensation in a Gas of Sodium Atoms'. *Physical Review Letters* 75 (22): 3969–3973, 1995.

11 Engel, G. S., Calhoun, T. R., Read, E. L., Ahn, T. K., Mancal, T., Cheng, Y.-C., Blankenship, R. E., Fleming, G. R., 'Evidence for wavelike en-

ergy transfer through quantum coherence in photosynthetic complexes'. *Nature* 446, 782–786, 2007.

12 Behe, M. J., *Darwin's Black Box: The Biochemical Challenge to Evolution.* Touchstone Books, New York, 1998.

Chapter 3

The Conceptual Foundations of New Homeopathy

1 The physical constant of $h=6.64\times10^{-34}$ J which describes the proportionality constant between the energy *(E)* of a charged atomic oscillator and the frequency *(v)* of its associated electromagnetic wave is the quantum of action in quantum mechanics, also called the Planck constant.

2 Del Giudice, E., Pulselli, R. M., 'Structure of liquid water based on QFT'. *International Journal of Design, Nature and Ecodynamics.* Vol. 5 (1), 2010; Tedeschi, A., 'Is the living dynamics able to change the properties of water?' ibid.; Del Giudice, E., Tedeschi, A., 'Water and the autocatalysis in living organisms'. *Electromagnetic Biology and Medicine,* Vol. 16, 2009.

3 Telekolleg: Körbler, E., 'Die Neue Homöopathie VIII'. *Raum und Zeit Special 3,* pp. 71–73., 1990-93

4 Even the ancient Chinese had discovered that the first dorsal vertebra is the central information point in the spine; therefore they call this vertebra the *spider.*

5 Prigogine, I., Stengers, I., *Order Out of Chaos: Man's Dialogue with Nature.* Bantam Books, New York, 1984.

6 Systems in type 1 state are in thermodynamic equilibrium. Systems of a type 2 state have lost their thermodynamic equilibrium but can return to that state through physical processes. Systems in type 3 states, by contrast, are furthest removed from a state of thermodynamic balance but are able to sustain themselves in this new state.

Chapter 4

Körbler's Dowsing Rod

1 Aranyi, Lászlóné, *Az inga elmélete és gyakorlata* [The Theory and Practice of the Pendulum]. Private edition, 1991; Czeslaw Spychalski: *A varázsvessző tudománya* [The Science of the Dowsing Rod]. Háttér Lap- és Könyvkiadó, Budapest, 1990.

Chapter 6

Experiments for Transmitting Healing Information

1 Pichler, Ö. H. Mag., *Die Neue Homöopathie in Theorie und Praxis.* Ehlers Verlag, 2008.

2 Körbler, E., 'Die Neue Homöopathie VI. War "Ötzi" ein Heiliger?' *Raum und Zeit Special 3,* pp. 64–66. 1990-93.

3 Körbler, E., 'Die Neue Homöopathie II', pp. 50–54. 1990-93

4 Csiszár, R., Dr., 'Jelgyógyászat [Healing with Symbols] – Erich Körbler Neue Homöopathie – A kereszt mint gyógyító jel [The Cross as a Healing Symbol]'. *Természetgyógyász Magazin,* December 2010.

5 Körbler, E., 'Die Neue Homöopathie VI. War "Ötzi" ein Heiliger?' *Raum und Zeit Special 3,* pp. 64–66. 1990-93.

6 Körbler, E., 'Die Neue Homöopathie XIII. Das Tao der Psychologie'. *Raum und Zeit Special 3,* pp. 91–96. 1990-93.

7 Goethe, J. W., *Faust.* Szépirodalmi Könyvkiadó, Budapest, 1963.

Chapter 7

The Theory and Practice of Diagnosis and Therapy

1 Körbler, E., 'Universalrute III'. *Raum und Zeit Special 3,* p. 11. 1990-93.

Chapter 9

Körbler's Tree-Blossom Remedies

1 Körbler, E., 'Die Neue Homöopathie XV. Die Baumblüten-Information'. *Raum und Zeit Special 3,* p. 104. 1990-93.

2 Sági, M., Sági, I., 'Körbler-féle favirág-terápia. Új Homeopátia (7. rész)' [Körbler's Tree-Blossom Therapy. New Homeopathy (Part 7)]. *Természetgyógyász Magazin,* 1994/2, pp. 13–15.

3 By a 'living fossil' we mean plants (usually species or genus) which are also known from fossils and have survived through millennia, despite odds of extinction, in an almost unmodified form, or are members of a derivative line the relations of which have long died out. This is called the 'phenomenon of persistence'.

Chapter 10

Sound and Music as Healing Information

1 Sági, M., 'Hang és zene mint gyógyító információ' [Sound and Music as Healing Information]. *Természetgyógyász Magazin,* 2004/4, pp. 20–23.

2 Helmholtz, H., *Die Lehre von Tonempfindungen.* Vieweg, Braunschweig, 1863.

3 Stumpf, C., *Tonpsychologie.* 2 vols. Hirzel, Leipzig, 1883–90.

4 Révész, G., *Zur Grundlegung der Tonpsychologie.* Veit, Leipzig, 1913. Körbler, E., 'Die Neue Homöopathie IV'. *Raum und Zeit Special 3,* pp. 59–61. 1990-93

6 Platón, *Az állam* [Plato: The Republic], 2nd edn. Gondolat Könyvkiadó, Budapest, 1970.

7 Schopenhauer, A., *Die Welt als Wille und Vorstellung.* Leipzig, Brodhaus, 1818.

8 Halm, T., 'Hallástan' [The Study of Hearing]. *Physiologia acustica,* 1963.

9 Vitányi, I., *A zene pszichológiája* [The Psychology of Music]. Gondolat, Budapest, 1969.

10 Sági, M., *Esztétikum és személyiség* [Aesthetics and Personality]. Akadémiai Kiadó, Budapest, 1981.

11 Sági, M., 'Gyógyító információ' [Healing Information]. *Természetgyógyász Magazin,* 2001/10, pp. 26–31; Sagi, M., 'Informationsmedizin'. *Hagia Chora,* Sommer 2001, pp. 50–56. 2001.

Chapter 11

The Informational Aspect of Psychosomatic Problems

1 Körbler, E., 'Die Neue Homöopathie III'. *Raum und Zeit Special 3,* pp. 54–56. 1990-93.; Körbler, E., 'Die Neue Homöopathie XIII. Das Tao der Psychologie'. *Raum und Zeit Special 3,* pp. 91–96. 1990-93.; Körbler, E., 'Die Neue Homöopathie XVI. Psychosomatik und Placebo-Effekt'. *Raum und Zeit Special 3,* pp. 116–118. 1990-93.

2 Sperry, R. W., 'Mind–brain interaction: mentalism, yes; dualism, no'. *Neuroscience* 5 (2): 195–206, 1980.

3 Bánki, M. Cs., 'Atavizmus, csalás vagy a jövő nagy kérdése: a placebo hatás' [Atavism, Fraud or the Great Question of the Future. The Placebo Effect]. *Psychiatrica Hungarica,* 1994.9.3, pp. 271–273.

4 Shapiro, A. K. and Shapiro, E., *The Powerful Placebo: From Ancient Priest to Modern Physician.* Johns Hopkins University, Baltimore, 1997.

5 Spiro, H. M., *Doctors, Patients and Placebos.* Yale University Press, New Haven, 1986.

6 Roger C. Guillemin and Andrew V. Schally received a divided Nobel

Prize for Medicine or Physiology in 1977 for their discoveries concerning the peptide hormone production of the brain.

7 Cziboly, Á., Bárdos, Gy., 'A placebo fogalma, története, alkalmazása, valamint számos magyarázó elméletének áttekintése' [The Concept, History and Application of Placebo and a Review of a Number of Explanatory Theories]. *Magyar Pszichológiai Szemle,* 58: 381–416, 2003.

8 Köteles, F., Cziboly, Á., Fodor, D., Bárdos, Gy., 'A placebo terápiás felhasználásának etikai kérdései' [Ethical Questions Regarding the Use of Placebo in Therapy]. *Magyar Pszichológiai Szemle,* 62: 429–448, 2007. Impf.

9 Köteles, F., Bárdos, Gy., 'A placebo evolúciós szemmel' [Placebo from an Evolutionary Angle]. *Magyar Pszichológiai Szemle,* 62: 221–234, 2007. Impf.

10 Köteles, F., Bárdos, Gy., 'Nil nocere? A nocebo jelenség' [Nil Nocere? The Nocebo Effect]. *Magyar Pszichológiai Szemle,* 64: 697–727, 2009. Impf.

11 The publication closest to the present topic by this author is Kulcsár, Zs., 'Placebo hatás a pszichoszomatika nézőpontjából'. *Psychiatrica Hungarica,* 1994.9.3, pp. 279–282.

12 Bánki, M. Cs., 'Atavizmus, csalás vagy a jövő nagy kérdése: a placebohatás' [Atavism, Fraud or the Great Question of the Future. The Placebo Effect]. *Psychiatrica Hungarica,* 1994.9.3, pp. 271–273.

13 Cziboly, Á., Bárdos, Gy., 'A placebo fogalma, története, alkalmazása, valamint számos magyarázó elméletének áttekintése' [The Concept, History and Application of Placebo and a Review of a Number of Explanatory Theories]. *Magyar Pszichológiai Szemle,* 58: 381–416, 2003.

14 Bitter, I., 'Heveny szkizofrén és szkizoaffektív betegek negatív és pozitív szindrómájának vizsgálata placebo, haloperidol és benzotropil kezelés során' [Testing the Negative and Positive Syndrome of Acute Schizophrenic and Schizo-affective Patients after Treatment with Placebo, Haloperidol and Benzotropil]. PhD thesis, Pécs, 1994.

15 Fürst, Zs., *Gyógyszertan* [Pharmacology]. Medicina, Budapest, 1997.

16 Moseley, J. B. et al., 'A Controlled Trial of Arthroscopic Surgery for Osteoarthritis of the Knee'. *New England Journal of Medicine,* July 11, 2002, Vol. 347, No. 2.

17 Kirsch, I., Moore, T. J. et al., 'The emperor's new drugs: An analysis of antidepressant medication data submitted to the US Food and Drugs Administration Prevention and Treatment'. *American Psychological Association,* 2002, 5:23.

18 Cziboly, Á., Bárdos, Gy., 'A placebo fogalma, története, alkalmazása, valamint számos magyarázó elméletének áttekintése' [The Concept, History and Application of Placebo and a Review of a Number of Explanatory Theories]. *Magyar Pszichológiai Szemle*, 2003, 58: 381–416.

19 Coué, E., *Elméd gyógyító hatalma. Önszuggesztió és szuggesztió* [The Healing Power of the Mind. Self-suggestion and Suggestion]. Édition Hongroise, 1993.

20 The cell membrane absorbs the stimuli and then aligns the cell responses required for sustaining life. In fact it plays the part of the 'brain' of the cell. Integral membrane proteins (IMP) are 'push buttons' of perception which establish connections between impulses from the environment and the signaling pathways built from proteins and organizing the response.

21 Lipton, B. H. et al., 'Histamine-modulated transdifferentiation of dermal microvascular endothelial cells'. *Experimental Cell Research*, 1992, pp. 279–291.

22 Lipton, B. H. et al., 'Histamine-modulated transdifferentiation of dermal microvascular endothelial cells'. *Experimental Cell Research*, 1992, pp. 279–291.

Chapter 12

The Psychomeridian

1 Lipton, B., *The Biology of Belief.* Mountain of Love / Elite Books, Santa Rosa, California, 2005.

2 Körbler, E., 'Die Neue Homöopathie XIII. Das Tao der Psychologie'. *Raum und Zeit Special 3*, pp. 91–96. 1990-93.

3 Sági, M., Sági, I., 'A pszichoszomatika új megvilágításban. Új Homeopátia' [Psychosomatics in a New Light. The New Homeopathy]. *Természetgyógyász Magazin* 1993 / 12, pp. 10–11.

Chapter 14

The Diagnosis and Therapy of Mycosis

1 Beszedics, Gy., Szolnoki, L. Dr., 'A gombadiagnosztika az alapellátás szintjén' [Fungus Diagnostics in the Field of Basic Healthcare]. *Magyar Orvos*, May 2008, year XVI.

2 Dumrese, J. Dr. Med., Haefeli, B., *Pleomorphismus.* Haug Verlag, 1996; Haefeli, B., *Krebs muss nicht unser unabwendbares Schicksal sein!* Medinca-Verlag Zug, 1987; Haefeli, B., *Die Blut-Mykose Handbuch für Theorie und Praxis.* Medinca-Verlag Ch-Zug, 1985.

3 Scheller, S., Scheller, E., *Candidalismus?!* Günter Albert Ulmer Verlag, Tuningen, 2005.

4 *BHS Labor Bruno Haefeli für mikroanalytische Blut-Mykose-Forschung.* After Körbler's death, publishing house Ehlers signed a contract with B. Haefeli for publication of the mycosis images, so at first these were marketed in the form of mycosis cards for course participants. In 2005 they also published the mycosis cards in the form of a test package, complete with commentaries by B. Haefeli. The second edition of the test package was published in 2010.

Chapter 15

Diagnosis and Therapy of Allergies

1 Sági, M., Sági, I., 'Die Neue Homöopathie XIX. Wie man Allergien diagnostizieren und therapieren kann'. *Raum und Zeit,* 1994, No. 70, pp. 58–62. Also Sági, M., Sági, I., 'Allergiás megbetegedések szelíd gyógymódja. Új Homeopátia (6. rész)' [Gentle Cure of Allergic Diseases. Part 6]. *Természetgyógyász Magazin,* 1994/1, pp. 10–12.

2 Since 2004 the author has replaced 'psi-field' with the term 'Akashic field', because beyond the psi-phenomena this also includes and explains the Akasha dimension as represented in the original Sanskrit idea.

Chapter 16

Diagnosis and Therapy of Milk Allergy

1 Sági, M., Sági, I., 'Tejallergia az új homeopátia tükrében. Új Homeopátia' [Milk Allergy in the Mirror of New Homeopathy]. *Természetgyógyász Magazin,* 1996/2, pp. 41–44; also Sági, M., Sági, I., 'Die Neue Homöopathie XXI. Diagnose und Therapie von Milchallergien, Möglichkeiten bei Zivilizationskrankheiten'. *Raum und Zeit,* 1995, Nos. 11–12, pp. 88–93.

Chapter 17

The Impact and Measurement of Harmful Influences in the Everyday Environment

1 Chapter 17 is a revised version of the following articles published in 1996: Sági, M., Sági, I., 'Lakókörnyezetünk ártalmai az új homeopátia szemszögéből (1. rész). Új Homeopátia' [Hazards of Our Habitat from the Angle of New Homeopathy. Part 1]. *Természetgyógyász Magazin,* 1996/10, pp. 36–39; Sági, M., Sági, I., 'Lakókörnyezetünk ártalmai az

új homeopátia szemszögéből (2. rész). Új Homeopátia' [Hazards of Our Habitat from the Angle of New Homeopathy. Part 2]. *Természetgyógyász Magazin,* 1996/11, pp. 36–39; Sagi, M., 'Körperschprache'. *Hagia Chora,* Winter 1999/2000, pp. 15–17; Sagi, M., 'Die Kraft der Form'. *Hagia Chora,* Frühjahr 2000, pp. 44–47.

2 Spychalski, C., *A varázsvessző tudománya* [The Science of the Dowsing Rod]. Háttér Lap- és Könyvkiadó, Budapest, 1990.

3 Ho, M-W., Popp, F. A., Warnke, U., *Bioelectrodynamics and Biocommunication.* World Scientific, New York, 1994.

4 Warnke, U., 'Electromagnetic Sensitivity of Animals and Humans: Biological and Clinical Implications', in Ho, M-W., Popp, F. A., Warnke, U., *Bioelectrodynamics and Biocommunication.* World Scientific, New York, 1994.

5 It is capable of perceiving up to 3 billion Hz (3 GHz), which enables us to measure the strength of radio waves, the effect of CBs and mobile phones, as well as several types of radars.

6 Zehenter, Ch., 'Was taugen Glühbirne, Halogenlampe & Co.?' *Naturarzt,* 2009/3, p. 39; Borr, H., 'So telefonieren Sie strahlungsarm'. *Naturarzt,* 2010/12, p. 22; Maes, W., 'Energiesparlampen und ihre dunklen Seiten'. *Naturarzt,* 2010/12, p. 29; Wunsch, A., 'Gesundheitsfaktor Licht: stark unterschätzt!' *Naturarzt,* 2011/1, p. 17.

7 Radio frequency and microwave radiation, based on charts and tables published by the Swiss Agency for the Environment, Forests and Landscape, SAEFL.

8 Aschoff, D., *Elektromagnetische Eigenschaft des Blutes durch Reizzonen messbar verändert – Der Elektromagnetische-Bluttest.* Paffrath-Druck Remscheid, 1978, 3, mit Erfahrungen von Rothdach, München (2 Vorträge).

9 'Electromagnetic fields (300 Hz to 300 GHz)'. WHO, Geneva, 1993; König, Folkerts, *Elektrischer Strom als Umweltfaktor.* Pflaum Verlag, München, 1997.

Appendix I

An Interview with Erich Körbler by János Déri

1 Déri, J., 'Firkáld össze a lepedőt' [Why Not Draw All Over Your Sheet], in *Nulladik típusú találkozások* [Close Encounters of Type Zero], CO-NEXUS Print-teR Kft., Budapest, 1991, pp. 79–92.

Appendix II

Theses and Hypotheses Regarding Connections between Fungi and Cancer

by Bruno Haefeli Dedicated to the Present Volume

1 See Chapter 14. The method is based on research by Professor Günter Enderlein (1872–1968), a microbiologist who described the organic processes taking place in the living blood in his theory of paleomorphism in 1925. He pointed out that the various types of microbes living in our organism, bacteria, fungi and viruses, were constantly going through cyclic and never-ending transformation and in the healthy blood even those micro-organisms which become pathogenic break down and can revert to protein colloids. If, however, the blood becomes overly acidy, the organic processes taking place in a healthy blood milieu suffer and micro-organisms which had turned pathogenic can gain predominance, opening the way to the emergence of various diseases. This method renders latent bacteria, pathogenic fungi genuses and mycoparasites clearly visible.

Bibliography

Aranyi, L.-né. *Az inga elmélete és gyakorlata* [The Theory and Practice of the Pendulum]. Private edition, 1991.

Aschoff, D. *Elektromagnetische Eigenschaft des Blutes durch Reizzonen messbar verändert – Der Elektromagnetische-Bluttest.* Paffrath-Druck Remscheid, 1978, Aufl. 3, mit Erfahrungen von Rothdach, München (2 Vorträge).

Bánki, M. Cs. 'Atavizmus, csalás, vagy a jövő nagy kérdése: a placebohatás' [Atavism, Fraud or the Great Question of the Future. The Placebo Effect]. *Psychiatrica Hungarica,* 1994.9.3. pp. 271–273.

Barrow et al. *The Anthropic Cosmological Principle.* Oxford University Press, London and New York, 1986.

Becker, G., Massey, H. *The Living Matrix.* Innergy Collection, 2009.

Behe, M. J. *Darwin's Black Box: The Biochemical Challenge to Evolution.* Touchstone Books, New York, 1998.

Beszedics, Gy., Szolnoki, L. Dr.'A gombadiagnosztika az alapellátás szintjén' [Fungus Diagnostics on the Level of Basic Health Care]. *Magyar Orvos,* 2008. May, year XVI.

Biava, P. M. *Il cancro e la ricerca del senso perduto.* Spriger, Milano, 2008.

Bitter, I. 'Heveny szkizofrén és szkizoaffektív betegek negatív és pozitív szindrómájának vizsgálata placebo, haloperidol és benzotropil kezelés során' [Testing the Negative and Positive Syndrome of Acute Schizophrenic and Schizo-affective Patients after Treatment with Placebo, Haloperidol and Benzotropil]. PhD thesis, Pécs, 1994.

Bohm, D. *Wholeness and the Implicate Order.* Routledge and Kegan Paul, London, 1980.

Borr, H. 'So telefonieren Sie strahlungsarm'. *Naturarzt,* 2010/12, p. 22.

Cornell, E. A.,Wieman, C. E. 'Bose–Einstein Condensates in a Dilute Gas; the First 70 Years and Some Recent Experiments'. Nobel Lecture, 1995.

Coué, E. *Elméd gyógyító hatalma. Önszuggesztió és szuggesztió* [The Healing Power of Your Mind. Self-suggestion and Suggestion]. Édition Hongroise, 1993.

Cziboly, Á., Bárdos, Gy. 'A placebo fogalma, története, alkalmazása, valamint számos magyarázó elméletének áttekintése' [Testing the Negative and Positive Syndrome of Acute Schizophrenic and Schizoaffective Patients after Treatment with Placebo, Haloperidol and Benzotropil]. *Magyar Pszichológiai Szemle,* 58: 381–416, 2003.

Csiszár, R. Dr. 'Jelgyógyászat [Healing with Signs]. Erich Körbler Neue Homöopathie. A kereszt, mint gyógyító jel [The Cross as a Healing Sign]'. *Természetgyógyász Magazin,* Budapest, December 2010.

Davis, K. B., Mewes, M. O., Andrews, M. R., van Druten, N. J., Durfee, D. S., Kurn, D. M., Ketterle, W. 'Bose–Einstein Condensation in a Gas of Sodium Atoms'. *Physical Review Letters 75,* 1995 (22): 3969–3973.

Del Giudice, E., Pulselli, R. M. 'Structure of liquid water based on QFT'. *International Journal of Design, Nature and Ecodynamics.* Vol. 5 (1), 2010; A. Tedeschi, 'Is the living dynamics able to change the properties of water?' ibid; Del Giudice, E., Tedeschi, A. 'Water and the autocatalysis in living organisms'. *Electromagnetic Biology and Medicine,* Vol. 16, 2009.

Déri, J. 'Firkáld össze a lepedőt' [Why Not Draw All Over Your Sheet]. In *Nulladik típusú találkozások* [Close Encounters of Type Zero], CO-NEXUS Print-teR Kft., Budapest, 1991, pp. 79–92.

Dumrese, J. Dr., Haefeli, B. *Pleomorphismus.* Haug Verlag, 1996.

Engel, G. S., Calhoun, T. R., Read, E. L., Ahn, T. K., Mancal, T., Cheng, Y.-C., Blankenship, R. E., Fleming, G. R. 'Evidence for wavelike energy transfer through quantum coherence in photosynthetic complexes'. *Nature* 446, 782–786, 2007.

Faraday, M. *Experimental Researches in Electricity.* Vols. I and II. 1839, 1844.

Fürst, Zs. *Gyógyszertan* [Pharmacology]. Medicina, Budapest, 1997.

Goethe, J. W. *Faust.* Szépirodalmi Könyvkiadó, Budapest, 1963.

Haefeli, B. *Die Blut-Mykose Handbuch für Theorie und Praxis.* Medinca. Verlag Ch-Zug, 1985.

Haefeli, B. *Krebs muss nicht unser unabwendbares Schicksal sein!* Medinca. Verlag Zug, 1987.

Haefeli, B. *Mykosekarten Testset.* ISBN 978-3-934-196-85-8 Ehlers Verlag GmbH, Wolfratshausen, BHS Labor für mykroanalytische Blut-Mykose-Forschung, CH-6030 Ebikon, 2007.

Hahnemann, S. *Organon der rationellen Heilkunde.* In der Arnoldschen Buchhandlung, Dresden, 1810.

Halm, T. 'Hallástan'. *Physiologia acustica,* 1963.

Helmholtz, H. *Die Lehre von Tonempfindungen.* Vieweg, Braunschweig, 1863.

Ho, M-W. *The Rainbow and the Worm: The Physics of Organisms.* World Scientific, Singapore, 1993.

Ho, M-W., Popp, F. A., Warnke, U. *Bioelectrodynamics and Biocommunication.* World Scientific, New York, 1994.

Katchalsky, A., Curran, P. F. *Nonequilibrium Thermodynamics in Biophysics.* Harvard University Press, 1965.

Kirsch, I., Moore, T. J. et al. 'The emperor's new drugs: An analysis of antidepressant medication data submitted to the US Food and Drugs Administration Prevention and Treatment'. *American Psychological Association,* 5:23, 2002.

König, Folkerts. *Elektrischer Strom als Umweltfaktor.* Pflaum Verlag, München, 1997.

Körbler, E. 'Die Neue Homöopathie II'. *Raum und Zeit Special 3,* pp. 50–54.

Körbler, E. 'Die Neue Homöopathie III'. *Raum und Zeit Special 3,* pp. 54–56.

Körbler, E. 'Die Neue Homöopathie VI. War "Ötzi" ein Heiliger?' *Raum und Zeit Special 3,* pp. 64–66.

Körbler, E. 'Die Neue Homöopathie VIII'. *Raum und Zeit Special 3,* pp. 71–73.

Körbler, E. 'Die Neue Homöopathie XIII. Das Tao der Psychologie'. *Raum und Zeit Special 3,* pp. 91–96.

Körbler, E. 'Die Neue Homöopathie XV. Die Baumblüten-Information'. *Raum und Zeit Special 3,* p. 104.

Körbler, E. 'Die Neue Homöopathie XVI. Psychosomatik und Placebo-Effekt'. *Raum und Zeit Special 3,* pp. 116–118.

Körbler, E. 'Die Universalrute III'. *Raum und Zeit Special 3,* p. 11.

Körbler, E. 'Die Universalrute VI. Zusammenfassung'. *Raum und Zeit Special 3,* pp. 23–28.

Köteles, F., Bárdos, Gy. 'A placebo evolúciós szemmel' [Placebo from an Evolutionary Angle]. *Magyar Pszichológiai Szemle,* 62: 221–234, 2007. Impf.

Köteles, F., Bárdos, Gy. 'Nil nocere? A nocebo jelenség' [Nil Nocere? The Placebo Phenomenon]. *Magyar Pszichológiai Szemle,* 2009. Impf.

Köteles, F., Cziboly, Á., Fodor, D., Bárdos, Gy. 'A placebo terápiás felhasználásának etikai kérdései' [Ethical Questions of the Use of Placebo in Therapy]. *Magyar Pszichológiai Szemle,* 62: 429–448, 2007. Impf.

Kulcsár, Zs. 'Placebo hatás a pszichoszomatika nézőpontjából' [The Placebo Effect from the Perspective of Psychosomatics]. *Psychiatrica Hungarica,* 1994.9.3, pp. 279–282.

Kwok, S. *Organic Matter in the Universe.* Wiley, 2011.

Kwok, S., Zhang, Y. 'Astronomers Discover Complex Organic Matter Exists throughout the Universe'. *Science Daily,* October 26, 2011.

Laszlo, E. *The Creative Cosmos.* Floris Books, Edinburgh, 1993.

Laszlo, E. *The Whispering Pond: A Personal Guide to the Emerging Vision of Science.* Element Books, Dorset, UK and Rockport, 1996, p. 182.

Laszlo, E. *The Connectivity Hypothesis.* State University of New York, 2003.

Laszlo, E. *Science and the Akashic Field.* Inner Traditions, Rochester, Vermont, 2004.

Laszlo, E. *The Akashic Experience.* Inner Traditions, Rochester, Vermont, 2009.

Laszlo, E. *New Science for a New World,* 2013. (MS)

László, M. Dr. *Candidiasis. Divat vagy a XXI. század betegsége?* White Golden Book Kft., 2002.

Lipton, B. *The Biology of Belief.* Mountain of Love / Elite Books, Santa Rosa, California, 2005.

Lipton, B. H. et al. 'Histamine-modulated transdifferentiation of dermal microvascular endothelial cells'. *Experimental Cell Research,* 1992, 179–291.

Maes, W. 'Energiesparlampen und ihre dunklen Seiten'. *Naturarzt,* 2010 / 12, p. 29.

Maxwell, J. C. 'A dynamical theory of the electromagnetic field'. *Philosophical Transactions of the Royal Society of London,* 1865.

Maxwell, J. C. *A Treatise on Electricity and Magnetism.* Oxford, at the Clarendon Press, 1873.

Moseley, J. B. et al. 'A Controlled Trial of Arthroscopic Surgery for Osteoarthritis of the Knee'. *New England Journal of Medicine,* July 11, 2002, Vol. 347, No. 2.

Pichler, Ö. H. Mag. *Die Neue Homöopathie in Theorie und Praxis*. Ehlers Verlag, 2008.

Platón. *Az állam* [The Republic]. 2nd edition. Gondolat Kiadó, Budapest, 1970.

Prigogine, I. *Order Out of Chaos: Man's Dialogue with Nature*. Bantam, New York, 1984.

Resch, G., Gutmann, V. *Wissenschaftliche Grundlagen der Homöopathie*. O-Verlag, Berg am Starnberger See, 1987.

Révész, G. *Zur Grundlegung der Tonpsychologie*. Veit, Leipzig, 1913.

Sági, M. *Esztétikum és személyiség* [Aesthetics and Personality]. Akadémiai Kiadó, Budapest, 1981.

Sági, M. 'Körperschprache'. *Hagia Chora*, Winter 1999/2000, pp. 15–17.

Sági, M. 'Die Kraft der Form'. *Hagia Chora*, Frühjahr 2000, pp. 44–47.

Sági, M. 'Informationsmedizin'. *Hagia Chora*, Sommer 2001, pp. 50–56.

Sági, M. 'Gyógyító információ'. *Természetgyógyász Magazin*, 2001/10, pp. 26–31.

Sági, M. 'Hang és zene mint gyógyító információ' [Sound and Music as Healing Information]. *Természetgyógyász Magazin*, 2004/4, pp. 20–23.

Sági, M. 'Healing Over Space and Time'. In Laszlo, E. *The Akashic Experience: Science and the Cosmic Memory Field*. Inner Traditions, Rochester, Vermont, 2009.

Sági, M., Sági, I. 'Új Homeopátia. A pszichoszomatika új megvilágításban' [The New Homeopathy. Psychosomatics in a New Light]. *Természetgyógyász Magazin*, 1993/12, pp. 10–11.

Sági, M., Sági, I. 'Wie man Allergien diagnostizieren und therapieren kann. Die Neue Homöopathie XIX'. *Raum und Zeit*, 1994. No. 70, pp. 58–62.

Sági, M., Sági, I. 'Allergiás megbetegedések szelíd gyógymódja. Új Homeopátia (6. rész)' [Gentle Cure of Allergic Diseases. The New Homeopathy. Part 6]. *Természetgyógyász Magazin*, 1994/1, pp. 10–12.

Sági, M., Sági, I. 'Körbler-féle favirág-terápia. Új Homeopátia 7. rész' [Körbler's Tree-Blossom Therapy. The New Homeopathy. Part 7]. *Természetgyógyász Magazin*, 1994/2, pp. 13–15.

Sági, M., Sági, I. 'Diagnose und Therapie von Milchallergien, Möglichkeiten bei Zivilizationskrankheiten. Die Neue Homöopathie XXI'. *Raum und Zeit*, 1995, Nos. 11–12, pp. 88–93.

Sági, M., Sági, I. 'Tejallergia az új homeopátia tükrében. Új Homeopátia' [Milk Allergy in the Mirror of New Homeopathy]. *Természetgyógyász Magazin*, 1996/2, pp. 41–44.

Sági, M., Sági, I. 'Lakókörnyezetünk ártalmai az új homeopátia szemszögéből (1. rész). Új Homeopátia' [Hazards of Our Habitat from the Angle of New Homeopathy. (Part 1). The New Homeopathy]. *Természetgyógyász Magazin*, 1996/10, pp. 36–39.

Sági, M., Sági, I. 'Lakókörnyezetünk ártalmai az új homeopátia szemszögéből (2. rész). Új Homeopátia' [Hazards of Our Habitat from the Angle of New Homeopathy. (Part 2). The New Homeopathy]. *Természetgyógyász Magazin*, 1996/11, pp. 36–39.

Scheller, S., Scheller, E. *Candidalismus?!* Günter Albert Ulmer Verlag, Tuningen, 2005.

Schopenhauer, A. *Die Welt als Wille und Vorstellung*. Brodhaus, Leipzig, 1818.

Shapiro, A. K., Shapiro, E. *The Powerful Placebo: From Ancient Priest to Modern Physician*. Johns Hopkins University, Baltimore, 1997.

Sperry, R. W. 'Mind–brain interaction: mentalism, yes; dualism, no'. *Neuroscience* 5 (2): 195–206, 1980.

Spiro, H. M. *Doctors, Patients and Placebos*. Yale University Press, New Haven, 1986.

Spychalski, C. *A varázsvessző tudománya* [The Science of the Dowsing Rod]. Háttér Lap- és Könyvkiadó, Budapest, 1990.

Stumpf, C. *Tonpsychologie*, 2 vols. Hirzel, Leipzig, 1883–90.

Vitányi, I. *A zene pszichológiája* [The Psychology of Music]. Gondolat, Budapest, 1969.

Warnke, U. 'Electromagnetic Sensitivity of Animals and Humans, Biological and Clinical Implications'. In Ho, M.-W., Popp, F. A., Warnke, U. *Bioelectrodynamics and Biocommunication*. World Scientific, New York, 1994.

Wunsch, A. 'Gesundheitsfaktor Licht: stark unterschätzt!' *Naturarzt*, 2011/1, p. 17.

Zehenter, Ch. 'Was taugen Glühbirne, Halogenlampe & Co.?' *Naturarzt*, 2009/3, p. 39.

O is a symbol of the world, of oneness and unity; this eye represents knowledge and insight. We publish titles on general spirituality and living a spiritual life. We aim to inform and help you on your own journey in this life.

Visit our website: http://www.o-books.com

Find us on Facebook:
https://www.facebook.com/OBooks

Follow us on Twitter: @obooks